All
Blood
Counts

A manual for blood conservation and patient blood management

Edited by

Dafydd Thomas

John Thompson

Biddy Ridler

tfm Publishing Limited, Castle Hill Barns, Harley, Nr Shrewsbury, SY5 6LX, UK. Tel: +44 (0)1952 510061; Fax: +44 (0)1952 510192 E-mail: nikki@tfmpublishing.com; Web site: www.tfmpublishing.com

Editing & design:	Nikki Bramhill BSc Hons Dip Law
First Edition:	© 2016
Paperback	ISBN: 978-1-903378-95-3
E-book editions:	© 2016
ePub	ISBN: 978-1-910079-49-2
Mobi	ISBN: 978-1-910079-50-8
Web pdf	ISBN: 978-1-910079-51-5

Printed by Gutenberg Press Ltd., Gudja Road, Tarxien, PLA 19, Malta Tel: +356 21897037; Fax: +356 21800069

Contents

Contributors

Olugbenga Akinkugbe LLB MA MRCPCH Specialty Registrar in Paediatrics, Imperial College Healthcare NHS Trust, London, UK

John Barbara MA MSc PhD FRSB FRCPath Emeritus Microbiology Consultant to the National Blood Service, National Health Service Blood and Transplant, London, UK; Visiting Professor, University of Plymouth and University of the West of England, Bristol, UK

M. Ann Benton MA FRCP FRCPath Consultant Haematologist ABMU Health Board, Wales and National Clinical Lead for Transfusion, Welsh Blood Service, UK

Paula Bolton-Maggs DM FRCP FRCPath Medical Director SHOT, Manchester Blood Centre, Manchester, UK

Karim Brohi BSc FRCA FRCS Professor of Trauma Sciences, Centre for Trauma Sciences, Queen Mary University of London, UK

Bruce Campbell MS FRCP FRCS Past Chair of the Interventional Procedures and Medical Technologies Advisory Committees, National Institute for Health and Care Excellence (NICE), London, UK

Fernando Canilllas del Rey MD PhD Department of Orthopaedic Surgery, Hospital "Cruz Roja", Madrid, Spain

Abhishek Chauhan MRCP Specialty Trainee Gastroenterology, Queen Elizabeth Hospital, Birmingham, UK

Ben Clevenger MBBS BSc MRCP FRCA Clinical Research Associate, Division of Surgery and Interventional Science, University College London, London, UK

Tony Davies BSc (Hons) MSc CSci FIBMS Patient Blood Management Practitioner, NHS Blood & Transplant and Serious Hazards of Transfusion scheme, Manchester, UK

Heidi Doughty MBA FRCP FRCPath Consultant Adviser in Transfusion Medicine, Centre of Defence Pathology, Royal Centre of Defence Medicine, Queen Elizabeth Hospital Birmingham, UK and NHS Blood and Transplant, Birmingham, UK

Lewis Gall BMSc (Hons) MRCS Trauma Clinical Research Fellow, Centre for Trauma Sciences, Queen Mary University of London, UK

Jane Graham MBChB MRCP FRCPath PGCMedEd Haematology Specialty Trainee Doctor (ST7), NHS Blood and Transplant/Central Manchester University Hospitals NHS Foundation Trust, Manchester, UK

Hannah Grainger BSc (Hons) MSc PGCE (PCET) Cell Salvage Co-ordinator, Welsh Blood Service, Cardiff, UK

John Grant-Casey BSc RN Programme Manager, National Comparative Audit of Blood Transfusion, NHS Blood and Transplant, Oxford, UK

Andrea Harris RGN BSc MSc Regional Lead, Patient Blood Management, NHS Blood and Transplant, Birmingham, UK

Catherine Howell RGN Chief Nurse, Diagnostic & Therapeutic Services, NHS Blood and Transplant, Bristol, UK

David Howell BSc PhD Formerly Head of Surveillance, National Transfusion Microbiology Laboratories, National Health Service Blood and Transplant, London, UK

Beverley J. Hunt FRCP FRCPath MD Professor of Thrombosis & Haemostasis, King's College University; Consultant, Guy's & St Thomas' NHS Foundation Trust, London, UK

David Inwald FRCPCH FFICM PhD Consultant and Honorary Senior Lecturer in Paediatric Intensive Care, Imperial College Healthcare NHS Trust, London, UK

Tariq Iqbal MD FRCP Consultant Gastroenterologist, Queen Elizabeth Hospital, Birmingham, UK

Phil Learoyd Honorary Historian, British Blood Transfusion Society; Past — Scientific and Technical Training Manager, NHS Blood and Transplant (NHSBT), (retired 2009), Leeds, UK

Barbara Macafee BSc MBChB FRCA Consultant Anaesthetist, Belfast Health and Social Care Trust, Belfast, UK

Stuart McKechnie MBChB BSc (Hons) FRCA FFICM DICM PhD Consultant in Anaesthesia & Intensive Care, Nuffield Division of Anaesthetics, John Radcliffe Hospital, Oxford, UK

Manuel Muñoz MD PhD Professor, Peri-operative Transfusion Medicine, School of Medicine, University of Málaga, Málaga, Spain

Michael F. Murphy MD FRCP FRCPath Professor of Blood Transfusion Medicine, University of Oxford; Consultant Haematologist, NHS Blood & Transplant and Oxford University Hospitals NHS Foundation Trust, Oxford, UK

Helen New PhD FRCP FRCPath Consultant in Paediatric Haematology and Transfusion Medicine, Imperial College Healthcare NHS Trust/NHS Blood and Transplant, London, UK

Alistair F. Nimmo MB ChB FRCA Consultant Anaesthetist, Royal Infirmary of Edinburgh, Edinburgh, UK

Bernard Norman MB BS FRCA Consultant Anaesthetist, Chelsea and Westminster NHS Foundation Trust, London, UK

Kate Pendry MBChB FRCP FRCPath Consultant Haematologist, NHS Blood and Transplant/Central Manchester University Hospitals NHS Foundation Trust, Manchester, UK

Toby Richards BSc FRCS MD Professor of Surgery, Division of Surgery and Interventional Science, University College London, London, UK

Biddy Ridler MB ChB Blood Conservation Specialty Doctor, Royal Devon and Exeter Hospital, Exeter, UK

Megan Rowley MB BS FRCP FRCPath Consultant Haematologist, NHS Blood and Transplant/Imperial College Healthcare NHS Trust and Honorary Senior Lecturer, Imperial College, London, UK

Akshay Shah BMedSci (Hons) BM BS MSc MRCP NIHR Academic Clinical Fellow and Specialty Registrar, Anaesthesia & Intensive Care, Nuffield Division of Anaesthetics, John Radcliffe Hospital, Oxford, UK

Karen Shreeve RN RM MA Manager, Better Blood Transfusion, Welsh Blood Service, Cardiff, UK

Arunesh Sil MS (ENT) MRCS DOHNS Medical Advisor, Baxter Healthcare, Newbury, UK

Simon Stanworth MD DPhil Consultant Haematologist and Senior Lecturer, NIHR Oxford Biomedical Research Centre, Oxford University Hospitals NHS Foundation Trust and The University of Oxford, UK

Julie Staves BSc (Hons) FIBMS Transfusion Laboratory Manager, Oxford University Hospitals NHS Foundation Trust, Oxford, UK

Paul M. Stevenson Hospital Liaison Committee, Exeter, UK

Richard Telford BSc (Hons) MBBS FRCA Consultant Anaesthetist, Royal Devon and Exeter Hospital/Peninsula Medical School, Exeter, UK

Dafydd Thomas MB ChB FRCA Director of Cardiac Intensive Care, Morriston Hospital, Swansea, UK

John Thompson MS FRCSEd FRCS Consultant Surgeon, Royal Devon and Exeter Hospitals, University of Exeter Medical School, Exeter, UK

Claire Todd BSc MBChB (Hons) MRCP FRCA ST7 Anaesthetics, Royal Devon and Exeter Hospital/Peninsula Medical School, Exeter, UK

Jonathan Wallis BA MB BS FRCP FRCPath Consultant Haematologist, Freeman Hospital, Newcastle-upon-Tyne, UK

Foreword

In June 2012 I had the pleasure of chairing a conference held at the Royal College of Pathologists entitled "Patient Blood Management: The Future of Blood Transfusion", under the joint auspices of the Department of Health, the National Blood Transfusion Committee and NHS Blood and Transplant. The aim of the day was to build on our previous NHS "Better Blood Transfusion" initiatives, to promote best practice in the appropriate use of blood transfusion. Resource implications, data collection, the different methods available and key performance indicators were debated.

Since then a lot has happened. It has become clear that patient blood management (PBM) is not only a paradigm for the conservation of a precious resource. Elements such as the correction of pre-operative anaemia can improve clinical outcomes and reduce morbidity and mortality. Physical and psychological "prehabilitation" can reduce cancelled operations and improve our patients' experiences. Simple interventions, care packages and education can be highly effective and reduce expenditure.

The NHSBT/Royal College of Physicians National Comparative Audit team have recently completed an audit of PBM. The results show a very wide variation in the uptake of the different components of PBM and similar data have emerged worldwide, especially from the United States of America and Australia.

The editors of this book, a sequel to the best selling "Manual for Blood Conservation", have drawn on a wide range of experts to provide examples of best practice in all the components of a comprehensive PBM programme. I do hope that clinicians, nursing and ancillary staff involved in perioperative care will enjoy reading it, so that they may work with their managers to implement this important initiative.

Professor Sir Bruce Keogh KBE, FRCS, FRCP
Medical Director, National Health Service

Chapter 1

Historical perspective

Phil Learoyd
Honorary Historian, British Blood Transfusion Society; Past — Scientific and Technical Training Manager, NHS Blood and Transplant (NHSBT), (retired 2009), Leeds, UK

- "The discovery of ABO groups was not directly related to improving the safety of transfusion."

- "Delays were commonly encountered regarding the implementation of new techniques."

- "Blood provision — many changes have been implemented related to the needs of war."

- "Blood safety has always been an issue."

The provision of blood for transfusion

Introduction

Whilst the pioneering work of Jean-Baptiste Denys in France and Richard Lower in England dates from 1667, it was not until the beginning of the 19th Century that James Blundell began using blood transfusion primarily as a method for the treatment of postpartum haemorrhage. It was, however, to be the introduction of sterile methodologies, the development of practical anticoagulation and the discovery of the ABO blood group system at the beginning of the 20th Century that paved the way for more modern practical blood transfusion procedures.

However, it would be a mistake to assume that the resolution of these problems immediately led to improved technologies, increases in transfusion events and a reduction in the adverse effects of transfusion. This delay may be exemplified by the opening comment of the Ministry of Information film *Blood Transfusion* that was produced by Paul Rotha in 1941, 40 years after the discovery of the ABO blood groups: "Today, doctors and research workers are at last able to place blood transfusion therapy in its right perspective with other kinds of therapeutic medicine".

Prior to the end of the First World War

Whilst the discovery of the ABO blood groups by Karl Landsteiner in 1901 is often quoted as the seminal moment in the development of safer blood transfusions, the original work was not conducted with this as its objective and blood transfusion did not in fact become the focus of Landsteiner's work until after 1921 when he was working in America. In addition, it would be more than half a century later that the nature, origins and significance of ABO antibodies would be appreciated and the structure of the A and B antigens understood [1].

Effective anticoagulation of blood by citrate was identified independently by Hustin (1914), Agote (1915) and Lewisohn (1915). However, again, there were delays in its general acceptance and a move away from direct donor to recipient transfusion methods. It is probable that this was at least partly due to the fact that the use of citrated blood was associated with an increased frequency of febrile transfusion reactions, subsequently shown to be due to the bacterial contamination of the distilled water used to make the citrate anticoagulant as well as inadequately cleaned transfusion equipment, rather than to the citrate itself [2].

The American surgeon Oswald Robertson (1886-1966) set up a 'blood depot' and used citrate-dextrose blood stored in ice boxes at casualty clearing stations during the First World War [3]. One of his English surgical colleagues during the war, Mr Geoffrey Keynes, became convinced that blood transfusion not only saved the lives of soldiers who were in shock from blood loss but that it could also help in the provision of possible life-saving surgery. After the war when working at St Bartholomew's Hospital in London, Keynes was surprised to find that his medical colleagues placed little importance on the value of blood transfusion [4].

The nature of the trench warfare that was such a feature of the First World War meant that some medical units could be placed near to the front line enabling direct donor to patient transfusion to be used for wounded soldiers as required. However, the subsequent changes in the methods of waging war led to the need for greatly increased mobility. The use of citrate anticoagulant enabled blood to be donated, stored and transported to a wounded soldier at a distant location — which characterised transfusion in the Second World War.

After the First World War

Percy Lane Oliver (1878-1944) who was a co-founder of the Camberwell Division of the British Red Cross began to organise a voluntary (unpaid) blood donor panel in 1921 following a request by King's College Hospital for volunteer blood donors. The Red Cross Blood Transfusion Service expanded rapidly under his leadership and was given official recognition by the British Red Cross in 1926. The blood of potential donors was grouped at any one of the hospitals that wanted to make use of the service. The volunteer donors also received a brief medical examination that basically ensured that they had no history of transmissible

3

disease and that they had accessible veins. A 'donor records' index was created by Oliver, which included the donor's name, address, blood group, and details of when and where the donor had been called to donate in the past. Donors were called wherever possible in 'rotation' though the decision to use a particular donor was based not only on their blood group but also on how far they had to travel to donate their blood. Oliver used a 'transfusion feedback' form that was completed by the surgeon who made the request for blood and he also issued a certificate to the donor for each donation given (Figure 1). In 1934, this scheme was extended to providing the donor with a medal together with a bar for every ten donations given (Figure 2). In addition, Percy Oliver with the help of Mr. Geoffrey Keynes also drew up rules for the treatment of donors and the method of blood extraction, which formed the basis of an article published in the *Lancet* in 1926 [5]. It would, however, be incorrect to assume that all blood donors

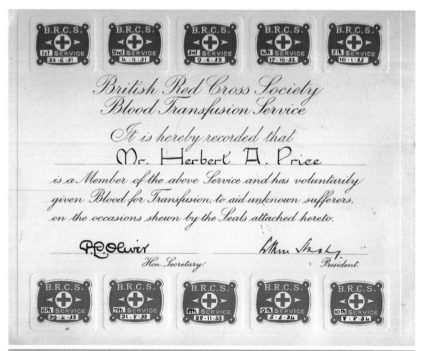

Figure 1. British Red Cross blood donation certificate (BBTS Archive).

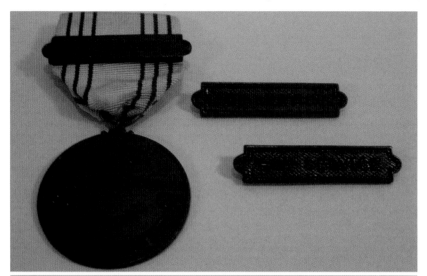

Figure 2. British Red Cross blood donor medal (BBTS Archive).

used in the UK during the 1920s and 1930 were volunteers, as many hospitals paid so-called 'professional blood donors'; the fees for individual donations varied around the country [6].

Percy Oliver delivered lectures on the Society's activities and also advised a large number of provincial hospitals in England on how to set up their own panel of voluntary non-remunerated blood donors during the 1920s and 1930s but was disappointed by the rather slow growth of these services outside London, which he attributed to a lack of facilities and to a shortage of surgeons with experience of taking and giving blood. At the first Congress of the International Society of Blood Transfusion (ISBT) in 1935, Dr. Arne paid tribute to the British Red Cross Service set up by Percy Oliver with the following statement: "It is the British Red Cross in London that the honour is due to having been the first in 1921 to solve the problem of the blood donor by organising a blood transfusion service available at all hours and able to send to any place a donor of guaranteed health and whose blood group has been duly verified. This service whose encouraging experiences were watched by Red Cross Societies of other nations served both as a model and inspiration for the organisation of similar services in seven other countries" [7].

The April 1937 edition of the British Red Cross Society *Blood Transfusion Service Quarterly Circular* bulletin includes a report by Dr. F. Duran Jorda that identifies his experiences and problems in setting up a blood banking system in Barcelona to support the army and civilians during the Spanish Civil War (1936-1939). The report includes a discussion of the logistics of transporting refrigerated stored blood to wounded soldiers. Whilst there appears to have been some resistance during the 1920s-1930s in the UK to the use of stored donor blood, a number of other countries including America, Russia and Spain were routinely using stored blood. Possibly related to the changing events in Europe, the 1937 Congress of the ISBT held in Paris emphasised the need to have stocks of stored blood available in the event of war.

The outbreak of World War II changed the views and methods of blood provision using stored blood in England. A leading figure in facilitating this change was Dr. (later Dame) Janet Vaughan, who was convinced by Dr. Jorda's argument that it was essential to store blood in emergencies. Using blood taken into sodium citrate solution, Dr. Vaughan and colleagues in 1939 showed that blood stored for several days was no more likely to cause reactions than blood taken into the same anticoagulant and used immediately [8]. Dr. Vaughan and her colleagues also produced comprehensive plans for the creation of four blood storage depots to serve London in the event of war. These plans were formally adopted by the government in April 1939. The directors in charge of these depots would later emphasise the importance of carefully cleaning all transfusion equipment, of using double-distilled water for the manufacture of citrate anticoagulant, and of employing an aseptic technique for taking donor blood.

In 1938, the War Office decided to set up an Army Blood Supply Depot to provide blood and plasma for its troops 'anywhere in the world'. This was a fundamental development as far as World War II was concerned especially since Germany had decided on a system of bleeding donors 'as required' that resulted in blood shortages. The Army Blood Transfusion Service under the command of Dr. (later Sir) Lionel Whitby opened its own blood depot in Southmead Hospital, Bristol, on the 3rd September 1939;

the date of the outbreak of World War II. This system was also to be used later during the war by the Americans, who set up a blood depot in the UK that was not only used to facilitate the bleeding of their own troops stationed in the UK but also subsequently acted as a distribution centre for blood delivered from the US.

In 1939, the Directors of the London depots in conjunction with the Medical Research Council (MRC) decided to standardise transfusion equipment, resulting in the production of the MRC standard blood bottle. This was essentially a modified milk bottle, slightly narrower in the middle, with an aluminium screw cap lined with a rubber diaphragm. A metal band that secured a hanging loop was attached to the bottom of the bottle that had marks at 180ml and 540ml for measuring the volumes of anticoagulant and collected blood, respectively (Figure 3).

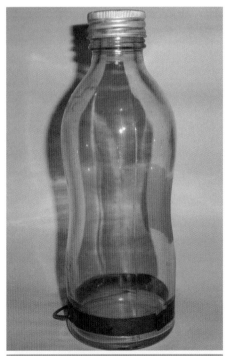

Figure 3. Medical Research Council blood bottle (BBTS Archive).

Blood donating sets and transfusion giving sets at the time were made from rubber tubing fitted with metal needles; a filter of knitted cotton was incorporated into giving sets (Figure 4). These sets were re-used, i.e. the needles were resharpened after each use, the tubing washed through and the whole assembly heat sterilised (autoclaved). This system was in use until the introduction of disposable plastic blood packs.

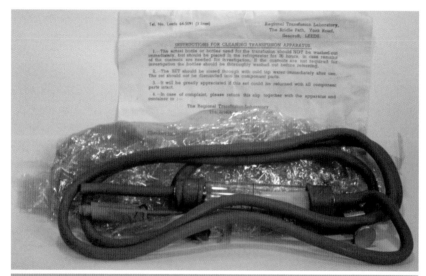

Figure 4. Rubber tubing blood donation giving set (BBTS Archive).

Initial work performed in America in 1916 [9] led to glucose being used as a red cell preservative — however, caramelisation of the glucose was an initial problem when a glucose-citrate mixture was autoclaved. Even though this anticoagulant was shown to be successful in other countries, the UK continued to use a simple citrate-saline solution. By 1940, a final concentration of 0.3% glucose in a glucose-citrate mixture was the accepted standard blood preservative, which although shown in the US to be effective for storing blood for 3 weeks, was initially used in the UK to store blood for only 2 weeks [6].

In 1942, work by Ms. (later Professor) Maureen Young at the South London Blood Depot initially identified that glucose heated in an acid solution did not caramelise. Further work using citric acid and disodium citrate resulted in the development of an acid-citrate dextrose (ACD) anticoagulant by Loutit and Mollison in 1943. This remained the standard worldwide anticoagulant until the introduction of citrate-phosphate dextrose (CPD) in 1957, which extended the storage time of blood from 21 days to 28 days. The licensing and subsequent introduction of citrate-phosphate dextrose adenine (CPD-A) in the early 1980s extended the maximum shelf-life of blood to 35 days when stored at 4°C ± 2°C.

Although research by the Imperial Chemical Industries resulted in the manufacture of polythene in 1941, it was not until the early 1950s that Professor Carl Walter in the US designed a disposable 'blood bag'. This development provided the major advantage of being a closed system, thereby reducing the risk of bacterial contamination whilst at the same time providing an easy method of separating plasma (and subsequently platelets) from red cells after centrifugation by squeezing the bag. This initial work led to the founding of the Fenwal Company and by the early 1960s most large hospitals in America and Canada were using plastic blood bags. However, due primarily to post-war cost constraints, there was a more gradual change-over to this technology in the UK and it was not until 1975 that plastic packs were introduced throughout the UK [6].

It was not possible for the UK to revert to a hospital-based blood donor service due to the fundamental changes that had already taken place during the Second World War. The rational solution was to supply hospitals with blood from 12 regional centres (i.e. on a similar basis to how the London Depots had done during the war) that were controlled nationally by the Ministry of Health (MoH). This change took place on the 26th September 1946 when the MoH created the National Blood Transfusion Service. This was not the case however for many other countries.

Blood grouping

Early blood grouping problems can be identified to be due, at least in part, to the variability in strength of locally sourced reagents and their subsequent deterioration in avidity during storage. The introduction and use of commercial grouping reagents resulted in improved reliability with respect to specificity, strength and storage capability. The subsequent development of monoclonal antibodies produced using hybridoma technology improved the consistency of grouping reagents even further. This change was of course mirrored by the introduction of increasingly sensitive blood grouping technologies, from direct agglutination methods initially on glass opaque tiles and small ('precipitin') tubes, to the development of microplate and modern column ('card') technologies.

Some of the initial blood grouping problems were not helped by the use of conflicting ABO blood group nomenclatures (group O was originally called C by Landsteiner) that were developed independently by different workers, i.e. Jansky (Prague): I (O), II (A), III (B), IV (AB); and Moss (USA): I (AB), II (A), III (B), IV (O). This confusing situation was at least one of the reasons for the preferential use of group O blood as the 'universal donor'. Initially, therefore, this inevitably resulted in a great variation in the frequency with which donors gave blood, i.e. being more based on the donor being group O rather than on the donor's health related to the frequency with which they donated. What is now recognised as the international designation of ABO blood group nomenclature (i.e. O, A, B and AB) was originally suggested at the 1937 Congress of the ISBT but was not adopted by the British Red Cross until 1939.

Pre-transfusion matching

The changes in the sensitivity and reproducibility of blood grouping techniques have been mirrored by the ability of laboratory techniques to detect clinically significant antibodies in the patient. The discovery of the anti-human globulin (AHG) test by Coombs, Mourant and Race in 1945 [10] was pivotal in providing a means of detecting immunoglobulin G (IgG) immune antibodies present in the patient. Although the test was originally performed in tubes, manual methods were replaced by semi-automated microplate and automated column technology systems. Changes to this technology also involved the increasing use of automated computerised laboratory equipment, which when linked to electronic patient identification systems resulted in changes to how blood was provided for patients, e.g. from specifically cross-matched and labelled donations to the introduction of 'type and screen' and 'electronic matching' methodologies.

Blood donation safety

The introduction of product liability in 1988 and the subsequent creation of the Medicines Control Agency (which became the Medicines and Healthcare Products Regulatory Agency in 2003) had major repercussions on the UK Blood Services. One aspect of this change has been the introduction of increasingly complex and regulated collection and processing methodologies for donated blood and components, together with the increasingly sophisticated and sensitive (automated) serological and microbiological testing of every donation. These changes have been mirrored in many countries.

Pivotal to the implementation of these changes has been a drive to actively reduce the occurrence of errors relating to the provision of blood and blood products for patients. Haemovigilance (which in the UK has involved the introduction of the Serious Hazards of Transfusion [SHOT] scheme in 1996 and later the Serious Adverse Blood Reactions and Events [SABRE] data collection system), together with the quality objective of continuous improvement, has been instrumental in focusing effort, changing attitudes and implementing quality improvements in many countries.

Historically, one of the biggest changes to blood donation safety has been that related to transfusion transmitted infections (TTI), which has involved changes to blood donor eligibility (i.e. Donor Selection Guidelines) and the introduction of increasingly sophisticated mandatory and discretionary microbiology testing technologies for an ever increasing number of TTI types, together with increasingly complex mechanisms of statistical process monitoring.

From the time of Percy Oliver, who collected data on the incidence of syphilis of donors within his panel when they were re-examined after every 10 donations (no case of syphilis was ever discovered), the safety of donated blood has always been an issue. The effects of various factors such as the use of paid vs. unpaid donors, donor selection criteria, blood donation methodology and the sensitivity of TTI test systems, have been and continue to be debated in discussions regarding patient safety and their clinical management.

Conclusions

The history of allogeneic blood transfusion is one that has involved innovation, vision and research in a large number of diverse and to some degree separate disciplines, that frequently questioned establish beliefs. Whilst individual topic areas and specific periods of higher activity can be highlighted as important, there is no single 'eureka' moment that defines the development and implementation of blood transfusion into the procedures that we see today. Advances continue to be made, especially in the use of alternative treatment options and new products, which ensure that the history of transfusion remains incomplete. The implementation of automation and computerisation, together with changes to the testing and donor selection processes, have improved the safety of the procedure, but there continues to be a need to use this resource sensibly and wisely to ensure that supply and demand as well as patient safety requirements are achieved.

Checklist summary

✓ Practical therapeutic blood transfusion has only been developed over the last 75 years.

✓ Percy Lane Oliver developed the concept of the 'voluntary blood donor' in the UK in the 1920s-1930s.

✓ World War I and World War II can be seen as 'tipping points' in changing methods of blood provision and transfusion practice.

✓ The first standard anticoagulant (ACD) was introduced in the early 1940s.

✓ Plastic blood bags were used in the USA from the 1960s.

✓ Historically, changes in blood safety can be identified to be associated with the introduction of increasingly sophisticated/sensitive methodologies, computerised systems and the quality objective of continuous improvement.

References

1. Boulton FE. Blood transfusion; additional historical aspects. Part 1. The birth of transfusion immunology. *Transfus Med* 2013; 23(6): 375-81.
2. Lewisohn R, Rosenthal N. Prevention of chills following the transfusion of citrated blood. *JAMA* 1933; 100(7): 466-9.
3. Robertson OH. Transfusion with preserved red cells. *BMJ* 1918; 1(2999): 691-5.
4. Keynes G. *The Gates of Memory*. Oxford, UK: Clarendon Press, 1981.
5. Gibson PC. The technique of blood transfusion. *Lancet* 1926; 208(5373): 375-6.
6. Gunson HH, Dodsworth H. Fifty years of blood transfusion. *Transfus Med* 1996; 6(1): 28.
7. Hanley F. *The Honour is Due*. Surrey, UK: JRP, 1998.
8. Elliot GA, Macfarlane RG, Vaughan JM. The use of stored blood for transfusion. *Lancet* 1939; 233(6025): 384-7.
9. Rous P, Turner JR. The preservation of living red blood cells *in vitro*. 1. Methods of preservation. *J Exp Med* 1916; 23: 219-37.
10. Coombs RRA, Mourant AE, Race RR. A new test for the detection of weak and 'incomplete' Rh agglutinins. *Br J Exp Pathol* 1945; 26: 255-66.

Chapter 2

Transfusion transmitted infections

David Howell BSc PhD
Formerly Head of Surveillance, National Transfusion Microbiology Laboratories, National Health Service Blood and Transplant, London, UK
John Barbara MA MSc PhD FRSB FRCPath
Emeritus Microbiology Consultant to the National Blood Service, National Health Service Blood and Transplant, London, UK; Visiting Professor, University of Plymouth and University of the West of England, Bristol, UK

- "Before any transfusion the balance of risk versus benefit should be assessed."

- "New infectious agents are continually emerging and some of these are likely to pose a threat to transfusion safety."

- "Climate change and rapid global travel have enhanced the threat from emerging agents."

- "Surveillance and reporting of post-transfusion infections will lead to interventions to reduce risks even further."

Background

The potential risks to recipients of blood transfusion are similar to and often less than risks from other activities that are acceptable to the public, such as playing football or travelling by car (Figure 1); successive interventions have reduced the risks from transfusion even more. Nevertheless, it is still necessary to appraise the recipients of blood and its components of the risks, alternatives and any potential hazards from such alternatives. When discussing the risks with the patient it is necessary to consider the particular circumstances of the recipient. Different advice might be given depending on the severity of their illness and potential life span, i.e. the balance between risks and benefits.

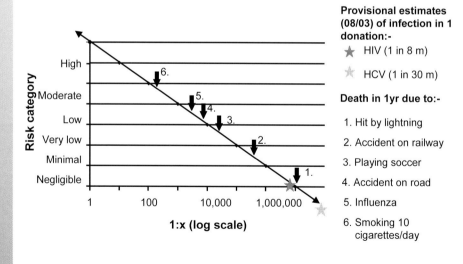

Figure 1. Risk from transfusion related to other risks (personal communication from K. Soldan and J. Barbara).
Subsequent to the date of this analysis, residual infectious risk from transfusion will have reduced even further due to enhanced testing technology.

Safe donated blood is an expensive resource and there has been much work on development of effective alternatives. These include cell salvage, pre-operative autologous donation and subsequent transfusion, and 'artificial' blood components, which are all discussed elsewhere. It is not part of the remit of this chapter to discuss infectious risks to staff arising from using these techniques. Hospital staff should be aware that blood donors are a highly selected and tested population and their donated blood is much less likely to be infectious for human immunodeficiency virus (HIV), hepatitis B virus (HBV) or hepatitis C virus (HCV) than the general hospital population. There will be a much greater risk from a needle-stick accident involving the patient than there would be from a needle-stick accident involving donated blood.

What makes a microbial agent important to blood safety?

Any risk will depend on which blood component is involved, as some agents are associated with particular components; for example, human T-cell leukaemia virus (HTLV) and cytomegalovirus (CMV) are associated with white cells. The main factors predisposing an agent to transfusion transmission are:

- Presence in blood.
- Persistence. Some organisms, such as hepatitis A virus (HAV), have a viraemic phase but it is relatively short, and thus any risk of transmission is small, often sub-clinical. The donor is effectively symptomless (potential donors who feel unwell tend not to donate).
- Significant morbidity/mortality. If an agent is not pathogenic (e.g. CMV in immunocompetent recipients), testing is unnecessary.
- Prevalence and incidence in the recipient population. If the majority of the population is already infected then there would be an argument for screening recipients and offering vaccination, if available.

There are also practical considerations:

- Assays must be available that can be afforded within the context of the overall health budget.

- The performance of the assay must be compatible with the requirements of mass, rapid microbial testing.
- The total assay time must be considerably less than the shelf life of the blood product.

Which agents are relevant to transfusion?

The significance of these agents will vary geographically. Each country should assess its own priorities and ascertain the relevant significance of the agents of concern in their own particular context.

Viruses

- HBV might be automatically included as a significant risk for all countries. However, in future, this might not be the case in a country with a policy of universal post-natal HBV screening and vaccination, or with a high prevalence of hepatitis B infection such that most of the population will have been infected by the time they are adults. Specific policies would then be needed for younger recipients.

Other viruses for which most countries test are:

- HCV.
- HIV 1 and 2 (with various subtypes of HIV 1).

Other viruses that may be included in testing programs are:

- HTLV. Japan was one of the first countries to introduce screening because of a high incidence in the population.
- CMV is a risk to immunocompromised patients, e.g. low birth weight neonates, bone marrow transplant patients. It is usual for these patients to receive blood screened and found to be negative for CMV antibody. However, although not proven by prospective studies, leucodepletion is likely to provide levels of safety equivalent to screening.

- West Nile Virus (WNV) is transmitted by mosquitoes. The United Kingdom (UK) Blood Services dealt with this potential threat to safety by excluding prospective donors who had visited the USA during the mosquito season. To reduce unnecessary loss of donations, nucleic acid testing (NAT) for WNV is performed when a donor has reported a visit to the USA (or other areas where the infection is common) during the relevant season.
- Hepatitis E virus (HEV) has been found to be transmitted by transfusion [1]. Blood screened negative may be appropriate for immunocompromised patients.

Other viruses are known to be transmitted by transfusion, but only infrequently for most recipients, e.g. HAV, parvovirus B19, dengue. The problem of risk of very occasional transmission by transfusion of non-persistent agents with a short period of viraemia is exemplified by a report of probable transmission by transfusion of the Ross River virus in Australia [2]. Zika is another arthropod-borne virus, recognised for many years, but which has recently reached epidemic levels of infection in South America, especially in Brazil. It is spreading into North America and may also become a problem in other warm countries where the mosquito vector exists. Although symptoms are usually mild it appears to cause microcephaly in babies born to mothers infected early in pregnancy. As a precaution, the UK Blood Services have implemented a 28-day donation ban for travellers returning from Zika-affected countries. Other blood services are also likely to do so.

Bacteria

The only bacterium for which specific screening is implemented is *Treponema pallidum* (syphilis). Syphilis was the first routine transfusion microbiology screen to be introduced. There has been discussion about its cost/benefit but the screening is unlikely to be withdrawn because of the perception that it is a "life-style marker".

Interventions to reduce bacterial risk have been implemented in developed countries.

Bacterial contamination of a blood donation can be either endogenous or exogenous as outlined below:

- Syphilis would be an example of endogenous infection. Other endogenous bacterial infections are not generally a problem for the transfusion service because the potential donor will feel unwell and will not donate. However, some transmissions of *Yersinia enterocolitica* from red cells (often nearing the end of their shelf life) have been reported.
- The pattern of exogenous contamination is changing. There have been improvements in manufacturing and processing (e.g. the withdrawal of water baths to warm/thaw blood) leading to fewer 'pinhole' type failures and associated contamination with organisms such as pseudomonads. More common was the identification of skin contaminants arising from inadequate arm cleansing prior to venepuncture to obtain the blood donation. This has led many Blood Services to instigate enhanced routine donor arm cleansing and also to introduce diversion of the first 20ml of the donation so that the skin bacteria contaminating the venepuncture needle are flushed away into a pouch separate from the blood collection bag. Bacterial screening of platelets has also been introduced in many countries. Pathogen reduction (PR) processes have been introduced in some countries while others are reviewing its possible implementation.

Parasites

The importance of parasites with regard to transfusion safety depends on location but risks are changing with greatly increased global travel. Several parasitic diseases are potentially transmissible by transfusion, e.g. malaria, toxoplasmosis, babesiosis, leishmaniasis). Prevention, in a non-endemic area, of transmission of parasitic disease by transfusion is achieved by exclusion from donation for a suitable period.

The main problem is malaria; in the UK, donor exclusion would lead to the loss of a large number of donations. Current policy is to use an exclusion period together with an assay for release of blood donated by individuals who may have been exposed to malarial infection.

Prions

These 'proteinacious infectious agents' generated considerable concerns in respect of transfusion safety. Although tragic for the individuals concerned, fortunately only a very small number of transfusion recipients have so far been identified as having been infected:

- Variant Creutzfeldt-Jakob disease (vCJD) presumed to have been caused by transfusion has been reported in four recipients of blood components [3]. In the first case [4] in 1996, before the introduction of leucodepletion, a patient in the UK aged 62 was transfused with five units of red cells at the time of surgery. One of the units had been donated by a 24-year-old individual who developed symptoms of vCJD 3 years and 4 months later. Six and a half years after the transfusion the recipient started to show symptoms of vCJD and died 13 months later. It is important to note that it appears that the donor would therefore have been infectious 3 years before symptoms developed with an incubation period for transfusion transmitted disease of 6 years. The chance of the disease in the recipient being due to diet is 1:15,000 to 1:30,0000 [4]. From the 5th April 2004, the UK Blood Services have excluded the recipients of transfusion from blood donation while also sourcing plasma from non-endemic countries.

- All four cases were prior to leucodepletion; the experimental work of Gregori *et al* [5] showing a 42% reduction of prion infectivity in the scrapie-infected hamster model suggests that leucodepletion does have a beneficial effect. This hypothesis is strengthened by the findings from transmissible spongiform encephalopathy (TSE) transmissions in sheep that the level of infectivity of prion in blood is low.

- In 2008, a haemophilia patient had evidence of vCJD in his spleen at post-mortem. Although he had no signs or symptoms of vCJD or other neurological disease when alive, he had received factor VIII linked to a donor who later developed clinical vCJD [6]. A risk assessment indicated that factor VIII was the likeliest source of infection.

- The first reported case of bovine spongiform encephalopathy (BSE) in a cow in the USA (that had been imported from Canada) with the possibility of material from this animal entering the human food chain. This single case will not affect the UK's decision to source plasma from the USA.

Surveillance data [7] show that in the UK there has been just one case of vCJD between 2012 and the end of 2015 (with no cases in the last 2 years). The number of cases of bovine spongiform encephalopathy (BSE) in the UK shows similar trends [8]. The disease has not been completely eliminated from cattle but superior food hygiene will greatly reduce the spread to humans.

Other 'emerging' infections

WNV, severe acute respiratory syndrome (SARS), human *Herpes* virus 8 (HHV8), TT virus (TTV), SEN virus (SEN-V) and the so-called hepatitis G virus (HGV/GB virus-C) have all been suggested as a threat to the safety of the blood supply. Consensus opinion is that some of these agents are not a significant risk. However, it is without doubt that "dozens of new infectious diseases are likely to emerge" [9] and that some of these emerging infections will pose a threat to transfusion safety. It is for this reason that efforts to improve transfusion safety may well be directed towards approaches such as pathogen reduction and donor selection rather than additional donation testing.

Any additional testing introduced to improve the safety of the blood supply will have an associated cost, not just in purchasing and performing the assay but also in handling the inevitable false-positive reactions. False-positive donations involve a direct, associated cost (reference testing, contacting the donor, etc), but more importantly, will exclude blood from hospital shelves. In most instances in the UK's low-risk populations, only a small proportion of 'reactive' donor samples prove to be positive.

Residual risk

The risk to the recipients of blood donation will depend on several factors and will be different in different countries. For a given agent the factors are:

- Numbers of infected individuals in the general population.
- Efficiency of donor selection, i.e. numbers of infected individuals in the donor population.

- The rate of new infections.
- Immunity in recipients.
- Problems associated with donation testing:
  - testing errors — much reduced because of enhanced process control;
  - assay failures — in 1996, it was reported that an HIV assay from a reputable manufacturer had failed to detect seven samples that were positive;
  - falsification of results — in 1997, it was reported that the staff of a major blood centre in the USA were falsifying test results to enhance their remuneration.

    Surveillance and quality control have improved and none of the above issues have been reported recently.
- Supplementary tests added to improve detection such as polymerase chain reaction (PCR); usually for HCV, HIV and HBV. Other tests, e.g. HIV p24 antigen, anti-HBc, and alanine aminotransferase (ALT) are also available.
- Bacterial screening for release of product. Pathogen reduction with commercial systems is becoming increasingly available.

The following do not provide any direct input to blood safety but should be linked into a feedback mechanism designed to improve the efficiency of the testing:

- Haemovigilance schemes. In the UK, the Serious Hazards of Transfusion (SHOT) scheme directly assesses the residual risk of acute, symptomatic complications.
- Statistical control for the testing process and active/efficient quality control schemes.

Blood safety in the UK is further complicated because, following HCV litigation, blood is now regulated by the Consumer Protection Act 1987. It is important that blood safety must have adequate financial resources available.

It is obviously unethical to carry out formal transmission experiments studying the infectivity of a given agent in human patients. However, much information has been obtained from retrospective studies on human recipients of HCV-infected blood. Similar work is undertaken following the introduction of any new screening test. The introduction of HTLV screening in the UK in 2002 led to a review exercise [10] which, although involving small numbers, provided information on the efficiency of leucodepletion for increasing transfusion safety.

The current safety of the blood supply is such that prospective studies are no longer feasible because of the large numbers of transfused units that need to be followed to produce meaningful results. One of the last studies in the UK was reported by Regan *et al* [11], who followed the recipients of 20,000 units of red cells between 1990 and 1995. No transfusion infection was identified. It is now necessary to use complex statistical methods to measure blood safety. Such estimates are depicted in Table 1. These methods will rely on assumptions with wide margins of error. In the UK, Soldan [12] reported an estimated frequency of infectious units entering the blood supply in England to be 1:260,000 for HBV, 1:8 million for HIV and 1: 30 million for HCV. The highest and lowest estimates for HBV differed by a factor of 13. The risks will continue to decrease [13].

Table 1. Calculated residual risks of transmission of infections by transfusion.

		England 1993-2001 [12]	USA window period [14]	Italy 1996-2000 [15]	Spain 1997-99 [16]
HBV	1:	260,000	63,000	-	74,000
HCV	1:	30 million	103,000	127,000	149,000
HIV	1:	8 million	493,000	435,000	513,000

Conclusions

Blood transfusion in the developed world is safe but never completely without risk. Risks are greater in developing countries but the costs of improvements in safety need to be considered in relation to the availability of resources within the overall budget. It is likely that the risk from bacterial contamination and from new/emerging agents will mean that a greater importance is given to pathogen inactivation.

It is without doubt that in the developed world the current risk of infectious complications following transfusion is minimal compared with the risks associated with the overall transfusion process.

Checklist summary

✔ There will always be a risk associated with blood transfusion.

✔ The biggest risk will be due to clerical/identification errors.

✔ The risk associated with transfusion transmitted infections is usually only a small part of the overall risk.

✔ The magnitude of this risk will depend on local circumstances.

✔ It is important to monitor new/emerging pathogens.

✔ Alternative interventions to testing (such as pathogen reduction) merit serious consideration.

References

1.   Hewitt PE, Ijaz S, Brailsford SR, et al. Hepatitis E virus in blood components: a prevalence and transmission study in southeast England. Lancet 2014; 384: 1766-73.

2.   Hoad VC, Speers DJ, Keller AJ, et al. First reported case of transfusion-transmitted Ross River virus infection. Med J Aust 2015; 202(5): 267-70.

3.   Hewitt PE, Llewelyn CA, Mackenzie J, Will RG. Creutzfeldt-Jakob disease and blood transfusion: results of the UK Transfusion Medicine Epidemiological Review study. Vox Sang 2006; 91(3): 221-30.

4.   Llewelyn CA, Hewitt PE, Knight RSG, et al. Possible transmission of variant Creutzfeldt-Jakob disease by blood transfusion. Lancet 2004; 363: 417-21.

5.   Gregori L, McCombie N, Palmer D, et al. Effectiveness of leucoreduction for removal of infectivity of transmissible spongiform encephalopathies from blood. Lancet 2004; 364: 529-31.

6.   Health Protection Report, 20th Feb 2009; 3: 7.

7.   http://www.cjd.ed.ac.uk/documents/figs.pdf.

8.   http://www.oie.int/animal-health-in-the-world/bse-specific-data/number-of-cases-in-the-united-kingdom/.

9.   News Round Up. New infectious diseases will continue to emerge. *Br Med J* 2004; 328: 186.

10.   Hewitt PE, Davison K, Howell DR, Taylor GP. Human T-lymphotropic virus lookback in NHS Blood and Transplant (England) reveals the efficacy of leucoreduction.*Transfusion* 2013; 53: 2168-75.

11.   Regan FAM, Hewitt PE, Barbara JAJ, Contreras M. Prospective investigation of transfusion transmitted infection in recipients of over 20,000 units of blood. *Br Med J* 1999; 320: 403-6.

12.   Soldan K, Barbara JAJ, Ramsey ME, Hall AJ. Estimation of the risk of hepatitis B virus, hepatitis C virus and human immunodeficiency virus infectious donations entering the blood supply in England 1993-2001. *Vox Sang* 2003; 84: 274-86.

13.   Dodd RY. Current risk for transfusion transmitted infections. *Curr Opin Hematol* 2007; 14(6): 671-6.

14.   Schreiber GB, Busch MP, Kleinman SH, Korelitz JJ. The risk of transfusion transmitted infections. *N Engl J Med* 1996; 334: 1685-90.

15.   Velati C, Romano L, Baruffi L, *et al*. Residual risk of transfusion-transmitted HCV and HIV infections by antibody screened blood in Italy. *Transfusion* 2002; 42: 989-93.

16.   Alvarez M, Oyonarte S, Rodriguez PM, Hernandez JM. Estimated risk of transfusion-transmitted viral infections in Spain. *Transfusion* 2002; 42: 994-8.

Further reading

1.   Caspari G, Gerlich WH, Gurtler L. Pathogen inactivation of cellular blood products - more security for the patient or less? *Transfusion Medicine and Haemotherapy* 2003; 30: 261-3.

2.   Dzik WH. Transfusion safety in the hospital. *Transfusion* 2003; 43: 1190-9.

3.   Glyn SA, Kleinman SH, Wright DJ, Busch MP. International application of the incidence rate/window period model. *Transfusion* 2002; 42: 966-72.

4.   Wagner SJ. Transfusion-transmitted bacterial infection: risks, sources and interventions. *Vox Sang* 2004; 86: 157-63.

5.   Yomtovian R. Bacterial contamination of blood: lessons from the past and road map for the future. *Transfusion* 2004; 44: 450-60.

6.   Kitchen AD, Chiodini PL. Malaria and blood transfusion *Vox Sang* 2006; 90(2): 77-84.

7.   Joint United Kingdom (UK) Blood Transfusion and Tissue Transplantation Services Guidelines for the Blood Transfusion Services in the UK. www.transfusionguidelines.org/.

8.   Bennett P, Daraktchiev M. vCJD and transfusion of blood components: an updated risk assessment. London, UK: Health Protection Analytical Team, Department of Health.

9.   Zia M, Besa EC. Transfusion-transmitted diseases. http://emedicine.medscape.com /article/1389957-overview.

10.   WHO Screening blood for transfusion transmissible infections. http://www.who.int/ bloodsafety/ScreeningDonatedBloodforTransfusion.pdf.

11.   Barbara JAJ, Regan FAM, Contreras MC, Eds. *Transfusion Microbiology*. Cambridge, UK: Cambridge University Press, 2008.

Chapter 3

Changing demographics — projected impact on blood supplies/Blood Stock Management Scheme (BSMS)

Megan Rowley MB BS FRCP FRCPath
Consultant Haematologist, NHS Blood and Transplant/Imperial College Healthcare NHS Trust and Honorary Senior Lecturer, Imperial College, London, UK

- "Demand for blood fluctuates as we change and improve clinical practice."

- "Measuring and monitoring the demand for blood helps us manage blood stocks more effectively."

- "Audits give us a snapshot of where blood is being transfused; demand for blood in medical patients is increasing at the same time as surgical blood usage is going down."

- "Clinical benchmarking has the potential to demonstrate that blood is being used safely and wisely."

- "Predicting future demand for blood is an evolving but as yet imprecise process."

Background

The demand for blood to support elective and emergency healthcare in developed countries is high. In developed countries it is unusual to get a shortage of blood that impacts on clinical practice. Collection, processing, testing and distribution of blood components is streamlined and efficient. Modern hospital transfusion laboratories are well versed at getting the '*right* blood to the *right* patient at the *right* time'. However, the hospital clinician, and the patient who needs a transfusion, see little of the efforts behind the scenes that go into ensuring that the supply of blood components matches clinical demand. A better understanding of how much blood is available and where it is needed requires close cooperation and sharing of information.

Blood services have a good understanding of the usual patterns of the demand for blood and blood components, and the factors that affect the availability and suitability of blood donors. This information is used to plan service delivery, including donor recruitment and blood service inventory management. Blood services monitor trends but also need to be proactive in working with hospitals to increase their knowledge of where and why blood is transfused. Minimising wastage of blood is an equally important part of our stewardship of the blood supply. Predicting future demand for blood components, based on the implications of changing clinical practice as well as the changing demographics of our populations, is an evolving but as yet imprecise process.

This chapter is about understanding how the demand for blood can be measured and monitored, and how we can use information on blood usage and wastage to manage blood stocks effectively.

Evidence

A blood service has the responsibility of collecting enough blood for the population it serves. A hospital has a responsibility for obtaining enough blood for the patients in its care and clinicians have a responsibility for good patient blood management on behalf of their patients.

The use of computer databases and electronic blood management systems provides an opportunity to collect real-time data that informs the blood service, the hospital and the patients of trends in blood usage and how they match good practice.

How much blood is there?

Blood services issue data

Statistics on the number of blood donations collected and blood components issued per year are monitored by blood services. In 2013, the four UK blood services issued approximately 2.7 million blood components, of which 76% were red cells, 11% platelets and 12% frozen components. The population served by the UK blood services is approximately 63 million.

Figures 1 and 2 show the red cells and platelets issued to hospitals in England and North Wales by the NHS Blood and Transplant (NHSBT)

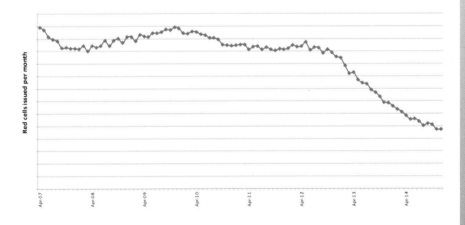

Figure 1. Red cells issued from NHSBT from 2007 to 2014 during which time demand for this component decreased by approximately 10%.

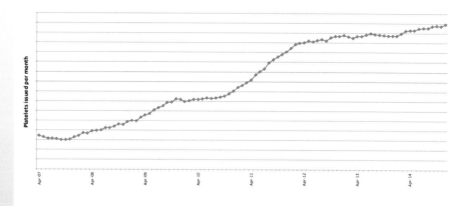

Figure 2. Platelets issued from NHSBT from 2007 to 2014 during which time demand for this component increased by approximately 25%.

over a 7-year period. These large changes in clinical use are a big challenge when planning future blood supplies. To predict whether trends in blood component usage will continue requires an understanding of changes in clinical demand, a change in population demographics or perhaps change driven by financial constraints on hospitals. It might be claimed that the reduction in red cell issues represents the improvement in patient blood management, but demand data alone are insufficient to make that assumption!

Blood supply levels

For red cell stock levels, blood services provide a graphical or pictorial representation on their public website showing how many units of blood are currently held in stock demonstrating the expected fall in stock reflecting donor availability during holiday periods. The Welsh Blood Service (https://www.welsh-blood.org.uk) shows how many days' supply there is for each of the eight blood groups, based on average demand. A 7-day supply or more is coded 'green' for adequate but fewer than 7 days is coded 'amber'.

By constantly monitoring blood supply levels, the blood services move to prevent critical stock levels by notifying hospital transfusion departments of impending shortage and suggesting enhanced local blood conservation measures (without the need to cancel any procedures), at the same time mobilising blood donors using direct contact and public campaigns. With this cooperation and coordination, the stock levels rapidly improve.

Blood Stock Management Scheme (BSMS)

The Blood Stock Management Scheme (http://www.bloodstocks.co.uk) was established 15 years ago to "improve blood inventory management across the blood supply chain, by enabling both hospitals and blood services to benchmark their services against their peers". Over this time it has set out to "improve standards of hospital stock management practice through education on blood stock management, recommendations on best practice to reduce wastage and to monitor the entire supply chain from donor to patient".

Data on the daily unreserved stock levels of blood components and reason for wastage are submitted by hospital transfusion departments using the web-based Vanesa software. In 2015, the scheme was expanded to include frozen components as well as adult red cells and platelets.

The scheme's annual report can be used to review national trends in usage and wastage in the blood services as well as in hospitals. The "issuable stock index" represents the number of days' stock held at the participating hospital. In the BSMS 2012-14 [1] report, this was around 6-8 days. Holding a lower stock correlates with lower wastage (quoted as "wastage as a percentage of issue" or WAPI). In the recent BSMS report, WAPI for red cells is around 2% on average with variation between UK countries and different hospitals. The commonest reason for wastage of red cells is time-expiry; approximately two-thirds to three-quarters of wastage is because the 35-day shelf life of red cells has been exceeded. For platelets, where the WAPI is around 4% on average, there is much more variation both in wastage rates and reasons for wastage. Lower stockholding, however, is not always desirable or feasible, as it may not allow the hospital transfusion laboratory to meet clinical demand for blood in a timely manner.

How much blood do we need?

Blood donation and issue rates per 1000 population

In 2008, a WHO initiative entitled "Universal Access to Safe Blood Transfusion" [2] noted that there was considerable global inequality in the timely access to safe blood. It states that "Of the estimated 80 million units of blood donated annually worldwide, less than 45% is collected in developing countries, home to 80% of the world's population" and that the "average number of blood donations per 1000 population is 10 times higher in high-income countries than low-income countries". The report further stated that "the equivalent of 1-3% of the population should donate blood to meet a country's needs". In the UK, it is estimated that 4% of the population are blood donors.

A similar index relating the number of blood units issued per 1000 population provides another method of defining transfusion demand. In 2011, data published by the European Blood Alliance [3] showed a surprisingly wide variation between similar European countries ranging from 32.2 red cells per 1000 population for the Netherlands and 57.2 for Germany. In this year, the UK issued 34.2 red cells per 1000 population.

There is considerable interest in the factors that might influence blood usage in developed countries and discussion about what the correct level should be. A high index might be taken to suggest inappropriate transfusion and/or excessive wastage, whereas a low index might represent restriction because an inadequate blood supply does not meet clinical demand.

Blood group profile of the patient population

The blood supply has to match the blood group profile of the population being transfused. There is additional demand for group O RhD negative blood because it can be transfused in an emergency to patients whose blood group is unknown. The distribution of blood groups within a population is known to vary with ethnic diversity, for example, 35% of UK blood donors are group A and 37% are group O, with approximately 15% being group RhD negative. But in Asian populations, group B is much more common than group A and RhD negative is very rare.

Table 1. Blood group distribution from the Blood Stocks Management Scheme survey of 101 hospitals and 1,339,911 patient blood groups over 12 months in 2007-2008 [4]. The London region is highlighted to show the variation in distribution compared to the national profile. This can be taken into account when planning regional blood supply and hospital blood inventory.

Region	Blood group distribution (%)							
	O+	O-	A+	A-	B+	B-	AB+	AB-
England (all)	38	8	33	7	9	2	3	<1
East Midlands	35	9	35	8	8	2	3	<1
East of England	36	9	34	9	8	2	3	<1
London	39	6	31	5	14	2	4	<1
North East	39	9	31	7	8	2	2	<1
North West	39	8	32	6	10	2	3	<1
South Central	37	7	33	7	9	2	3	<1
South East Coast	37	8	35	7	8	2	3	<1
South West	37	8	35	8	8	1	3	<1
West Midlands	37	8	33	7	9	2	3	<1
Yorkshire and The Humber	37	8	33	7	9	2	3	<1

To help understand whether national statistics for blood donors could be used to predict demand in the patient population, the BSMS undertook a survey of hospital transfusion departments [4] and the profile of blood groups in the hospital population was broken down into regional subgroups. Table 1 shows a higher proportion of group B and lower proportion of group O RhD negative patients are represented in the London region. This is assumed to be due to the ethnic diversity in London, and probably other urban areas. It is another factor that can be used to match supply with demand.

Where does blood go?

Surveys of blood usage

Until recently our knowledge of the patient groups who received the most blood components was patchy and often anecdotal.

A group from Northern Ireland categorised the adult recipients of blood transfusion using case note review and identified the key characteristics of patients who were transfused [5]. Two-thirds of the recipients were aged 60 years or over. The conditions most commonly represented amongst the transfused patients were gastrointestinal 29%, haematological 15%, and musculoskeletal 13%. Overall, 71% of red cells were given to medical patients and 29% to surgical patients.

In a series of three simple surveys designed to map blood usage in the North of England [6], the age, gender and reason for transfusion for each red cell unit were recorded on pre-printed paper forms over two 2-week periods in 1999/2000, 2004 and 2009. In 2009, the mean age of transfused patients (similar to the previous surveys) was 63.2 years (95% CI 62.5-63.9 years) with a small peak in the first year of life due to neonatal transfusions and another small peak of women transfused during the childbearing years. The same age distribution was noted in a similar national survey undertaken over two 1-week periods in 2014 (see Figure 3).

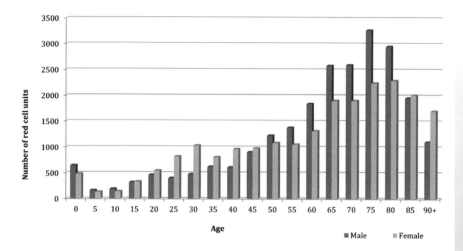

Figure 3. National survey of red cell use in English hospitals 2014 [7], with age and gender distribution of transfused patients.

In these "Where does blood go?" surveys, the number of red cells transfused to surgical patients progressively decreased, specifically in 50-80-year-old patients, whilst blood use in the medical and obstetric & gynaecology categories remained stable. The proportion of patients with a medical diagnosis increased from 52% in 1999/2000 to 62% in 2004 and 64.2% in 2009. The overall transfusion rate at the time of the first survey was 45.5 per 1000 population and decreased to 36 per 1000 population in 2009. The authors document the change in surgical practice during that time with increasing blood conservation measures and reflect on the increasing age of the population that is likely to account for the increasing proportion of blood use in medical patients.

The 2014 national "Where does blood go?" survey [7] shows a reduced red cell transfusion rate of 31.5 units per 1000 population and a higher median age of transfused patients at 69 years (IQR 51-80). The specialty and diagnosis was obtained for the majority of 46,111 units of red cells (representing 73-75% of all of the red cells issued by NHSBT in the weeks where the survey was carried out) and 67% of red cells were transfused to medical patients. 27.1% was transfused to patients with a haematological diagnosis and within that 4.5% of the blood was given to patients with thalassaemia and sickle cell disease. 27.4% was transfused to patients with non-haematological anaemia including renal, critical care, chronic disorders and anaemias that could be treated with alternatives to transfusion such as those with iron deficiency (2.7%). Within the surgical categories, 6% went to patients having cardiothoracic surgery, 4.8% trauma (including fractured femur 2.8%), 3.9% orthopaedics (including 3% for joint replacement surgery) and, finally, 3.8% to GI surgery.

All of this data helps to plan future blood collection strategies as well as providing target areas for blood conservation. Patterns of blood use will inevitably change however and continuous data collection with this level of detail is desirable in the future.

Audits of blood use

Clinical audit has been used to provide a snapshot of transfusion practice. Over the last 10 years the National Comparative Audit of Blood Transfusion has undertaken a number of 'appropriate use' audits including the use of platelets in haematology patients, red cells in total hip replacement, the general use of fresh frozen plasma (FFP), red cells in children and neonates, the use of O RhD negative red cells and transfusion in medical patients. These large multicentre audits provide an overview of transfusion practice in the UK and allow local and regional comparison of performance against national standards. Demographic information on blood transfusion is collected as part of every audit and recommendations are made to improve practice.

Each audit shows considerable variability in transfusion practice between hospitals and the level of 'inappropriate use'. A summary of these audits is shown in Table 2 (http://hospital.blood.co.uk/audits/national-comparative-audit/).

Table 2. National Comparative Audit of Blood Transfusion data on inappropriate use of blood components when compared against standards taken from national guidelines.

Audit	Year	Hospitals (participation rate)	Cases	Inappropriate use	Standards
Red cells in hip surgery	2007	139/167 (83%)	7465	48% of transfusions	BOA (2005)
Upper gastrointestinal bleeding	2007	217/257 (84%)	6750	15% of red cell transfusions 42% of platelets and 27% of fresh frozen plasma	BSG (2002)
Fresh frozen plasma	2009	186/248 (75%)	5023	43% of transfusions to adults, 48% to children and 62% to infants	BCSH (2004)
Platelets in haematology patients	2011	139/153 (91%)	3296	27% of transfusions	BCSH (2003)
Red cells in adult medical patients	2012	135/156 (86.5%)	9126	20% transfused for potentially reversible anaemia	BCSH (2001)

BOA = British Orthopaedic Association

BSG = British Society for Gastroenterology

BCSH = British Committee for Standards in Haematology

How can we influence blood usage and wastage?

Continuous high-level issue data with national and regional indices of blood usage and wastage allow us to follow trends in blood and blood component usage, but it is benchmarking data and information about 'why' and 'where' blood is being used and wasted that can be used to drive change.

Inventory management by blood services

Demand planning

Blood services set annual contracts with hospitals and require to be informed if significant change in blood component usage is anticipated. In practice this does not happen because demand planning for blood in hospitals is not that well developed, so blood services set collection targets based on trends in blood component issues in-year and respond reactively through demand planning groups to change in demand.

The BSMS has enabled demand planning to be more robust since its introduction in 1999 and it has proved vital to sufficiency in the blood supply.

Vendor managed inventory

An NHSBT initiative of vendor managed inventory (VMI) system is being piloted, whereby electronic links to a hospital transfusion department's laboratory information management system (LIMS) and electronic fridge management systems enable the blood service to monitor and automatically replenish blood components when stock levels fall below agreed safe levels. Unexpected emergency demand or specialist components for named patients continue to be ordered through an electronic blood ordering system. This has benefits for the blood service and the hospital transfusion department.

Inventory management by hospitals

Benchmarking

There are two successful models of regional benchmarking that can be used to guide good clinical practice and improve stockholding of blood components.

In Scotland, there is an automated system that extracts data from Scottish blood banks and combines this with other available epidemiological information in a data warehouse. This is the Scottish "Account for Blood" which is used to produce regular and ad hoc reports to the hospital, the blood service and the national transfusion committee. Information is used to prioritise quality improvements and target areas of potential reduction in demand.

The Blood Stocks Management Scheme has been previously described. Hospitals can use the software to benchmark their stock management performance against others in a similar usage category or geographical area.

Lessons can be learned from the information gathered by the BSMS in relation to the blood supply. The most recent BSMS annual report covering 2012-2014 [1] recommends a more agile approach to changes in demand for blood components. For example, where demand is temporarily reduced when wards are closed or surgery is cancelled, or supply is reduced due to the availability of donors, blood services and hospitals should be changing the blood stock inventory in a timely and responsive manner.

O RhD negative red cells

One example of using benchmarking and auditing to improve practice is the management of O RhD negative blood. Only 8% of the population is O RhD negative and by preferentially recruiting O RhD negative blood donors and asking them to donate regularly, the blood services are able to collect between 10-12% of their blood as O RhD negative. The BSMS

41

monitors the O RhD negative issues to hospitals as a proportion of total red cells. Ideally this should be less than 10.5% and it is suggested that hospitals achieve this by limiting its use to patients with 'acceptable' indications based on national guidelines.

In two national audits of the use of O RhD negative red cells in 2008 and 2010 [8], O RhD negative blood was transfused to patients in whom there was at least one acceptable indication in 79.3%. The commonest reason for transfusing O RhD negative red cells to non-O RhD negative patients who did not meet any of the above criteria was to prevent time-expiry of over-ordered units. The BSMS ran a series of workshops for biomedical scientists working in transfusion laboratories in 2013 and developed stockholding management advice for emergency O RhD negative blood with the aim of reducing demand for this scarce component [9].

Clinicians can help by establishing the blood group of emergency and unknown patients as soon as possible and by considering developing a policy to give O RhD positive blood to unknown adult males.

Wastage targets

Blood components may be wasted in the laboratory because components expire or there is some failure in cold chain management, which requires them to be discarded. BSMS wastage categories that apply to clinical areas include "Out Of Temperature Control", "Medically Ordered, Not Used" and "Surgically Ordered, Not Used". Transfusion teams can compare their local wastage rates with national rates and rates of similar hospitals and act to improve/reduce wastage if it seems excessive.

In London, the Regional Transfusion Committee (RTC) set up a working group to look at platelet usage and wastage, which was higher than in other English regions. The approach taken by the London Platelet Action Group (LoPAG) was to ask hospitals with low platelet wastage how it had been achieved, to share that practice across all of the regional hospitals by developing "Ten Top Tips" [10] and disseminating these via local platelet champions.

Biomedical scientist (BMS) empowerment

Northern Ireland has undertaken comprehensive audit of blood usage in all its hospitals and has introduced a standardised blood request form that has reduced inappropriate requests for blood by empowering biomedical scientists to challenge requests that do not meet pre-agreed criteria.

The English National Blood Transfusion Committee (NBTC) has suggested blood component requests are mapped to indication codes for red cells, platelets, plasma and FFP either manually, again using BMSs in the transfusion laboratory to challenge requests, or via electronic requesting algorithms.

Electronic blood management

IT systems to improve patient safety and control the cold chain can also be used to track blood usage within a hospital and to guide blood usage. Electronic ordering (ordercomms) systems can be used to challenge requests for blood if the latest blood count does not meet the local policy for transfusion triggers and give the prescriber an opportunity to review the decision. This has been shown to reduce inappropriate blood use as well as record the decision to override the recommendations [11].

In 2011, an NBTC survey of IT systems [12] used to support blood transfusion was completed by 118/160 (74%) of hospitals. Only 21% were using electronic ordering (ordercomms) of blood components and the "diagnosis" or "procedure" data field was often free text and not mandatory to complete. Further, 22% of respondents had included the indication codes in their blood transfusion laboratory information management system (BT-LIMS) or ordercomms systems and these were mandatory fields in a much smaller proportion. So although the IT systems are available to monitor and influence blood usage, they are not always configured to provide this functionality.

Clinical benchmarking

Blood transfusion laboratory information management systems (BT-LIMS) can be used to identify which patient has received a blood component, and this information is frequently used to provide financial information for cross-charging blood usage (and wastage) to departments within the hospital who are caring for that patient. Trends in usage, particularly if provided at a specialty or individual consultant level, form the basis of discussion for changes in service delivery as well as blood conservation measures. These clinical accounts for blood can be further developed to include indication codes, diagnostic codes and procedure codes from the patient administration system (PAS) or the BT-LIMS and it may be possible to give transfusion rates per clinical team or per surgical procedure. Some have successfully configured IT systems to link blood count data with transfusion so the pre- and post-transfusion haemoglobin can be compared to pre-agreed triggers and targets. This could be done for platelet counts and coagulation screens as well.

Clinical accounts for blood have been used by many hospital transfusion teams to engage clinicians who prescribe blood, consultants and junior medical staff, with policy review and feedback about poor practice. The ability to review trends in practice is helpful with managers as well, particularly in these times of austerity!

Key performance indicators (KPIs) for blood transfusion

Hospitals transfusion committees should consider the most useful indicators for their clinical practice as well as choosing those where it is possible to collect information automatically — without too much time-consuming manual data manipulation.

The following have proved useful and should be considered:

- % of patients transfused for the top 5-10 surgical procedures.
- % of patients transfused above the Hb threshold.
- % of patients transfused to a Hb >100g/L.
- % of single-unit transfusions.

Conclusions

Donors and patients have every expectation that blood is used safely and appropriately. Every healthcare professional involved with the transfusion of a blood component to a patient should have an understanding of the limitations of the blood supply and how to make best use of a precious resource by using it wisely and not wasting it. The ready availability of accurate and easily understandable data on blood usage and wastage helps blood services and hospitals share good practice and plan ahead. In the future it is hoped that IT systems and databases will be improved so that information already collected can be used in a clinically directed way to improve patient care.

Checklist summary

✓ Understand your own practice:
- who is getting transfused in your hospital?
- how does your transfusion practice compare with standards?
- how does your blood usage and wastage compare with others?

✓ Understand the limitations of the blood supply:
- how could you reduce blood usage if there were to be a shortage?
- what measures are in place to manage blood stocks effectively?
- use benchmarking data to compare usage and wastage;
- share good practice.

✓ Is demand for transfusion likely to change in the future?
- service developments;
- change in the patient population;
- inform the blood service.

✓ Develop local systems for monitoring and guiding transfusion practice:
- participate in the Blood Stocks Management Scheme;
- implement clinical accounts for blood;
- decide on some key performance indicators.

References

1.   MacRate EB, Ed, Taylor C, on behalf of the Blood Stocks Management Scheme (BSMS) Steering Group. The 2012-2014 BSMS Report, 2014. http://www.blood stocks.co.uk/reports/annualreports/index.asp.

2.   Universal Access to Safe Blood Transfusion. World Health Organization, 2008 http://www.who.int/bloodsafety/universalbts/en/.

3.   van Hoeven LR, Jansse MP, Rautmann G. The collection, testing and use of blood and blood components in Europe 2011. Directorate for the Quality of Medicines and HealthCare of the Council of Europe (EDQM), 2011. https://www.edqm.eu/en/blood-transfusion-reports-70.html.

4.   Blood Group Distribution Survey, 2008. Blood Stocks Management Scheme. http://www.bloodstocks.co.uk/usefulresources/bloodgroupdistribution/index.asp.

5.   Barr PJ, Donnelly M, Morris K, *et al*. The epidemiology of red cell transfusion. *Vox Sang* 2010; 99: 239-50.

6.   Tinegate H, Wallis JP, on behalf of the Northern Regional Transfusion Committee. Ten-year pattern of red blood cell use in the North of England. *Transfusion* 2013; 53: 483-9.

7.   National Red Cell Survey 2014. http://hospital.blood.co.uk/audits/national-comparative-audit/national-comparative-audit-reports/.

8.   Foukaneli D, Grant-Casey J. Re-audit of the use of Group O RhD negative red cells, 2010. http://hospital.blood.co.uk/media/26868/nca-re-audit_of_the_use_of_group_o_rhd_negative_red_cells_doc_2010.pdf.

9.   MacRate E, on behalf of the Blood Stocks Management Scheme. Red cells for emergency use. Best practice from BSMS regional roadshows. http://www.bloodstocks.co.uk/pdf/red_cells_for_emergency_use.pdf.

10. Moss R, for the London Platelet Action Group. Top tips to reduce platelet usage and wastage, 2012. http://hospital.blood.co.uk/media/2289/3b812bb0-0c86-48a1-b216-25b100aa3443.pdf.

11. Haspel RL, Uhl L. How do I audit hospital blood product utilization? *Transfusion* 2012; 52: 227-30.

12. Murphy M, Taylor C, Hyare J, on behalf of the National Blood Transfusion Committee. Survey of IT systems in Hospital Transfusion Laboratories, September 2011 http://www.transfusionguidelines.org.uk/uk-transfusion-committees/national-blood-transfusion-committee/better-blood-transfusion.

Chapter 4

What patients and the public need to know about blood conservation — and why they need an advocate

Biddy Ridler MB ChB
Blood Conservation Specialty Doctor, Royal Devon and Exeter Hospital, Exeter, UK

- "Patients now have access to more information, but still need an interpreter." [1]

- "People need to know."
  Myrtle, aged 76, 1.11.13

- "There will be a tipping point."
  Julia, age not stated, 6.11.13

- "Those of us who have the knowledge and expertise in blood conservation must ensure that people are appropriately informed."

- "There have been no large studies regarding/concerning what people know, or want to know, about blood conservation."

- "If possible, involve people in discussions about blood conservation before they become patients."

Background

There is an increasingly negative imbalance between the supply and demand for blood transfusion, together with much debate about its inherent risks and benefits. Very little information is currently available about whether the patient, and indeed the general population, is aware of this extremely concerning and complex problem and how it can be addressed.

According to the World Health Organisation (WHO) June 2013 factsheet, the blood donation rate in high-income countries is 39.2 donations per 1000 population; 12.6 donations in middle-income and 4.0 donations in low-income countries [2]. Worldwide, in 71 countries over 90% of these donations come from voluntary unpaid donors. In the UK, this figure is 100%, as neither payment nor family/directed donation is permitted by the National Blood Transfusion Committee (NBTC). There are, however, a further 73 countries where over 50% of the blood supply is from paid or family donors.

In the UK, only 4% of the population are blood donors, but up to 30% will need a blood transfusion at some stage in their lives [3]. This need is particularly required for the older population; as medical treatments improve so people in this upper age group live longer. This figure reflects the WHO data for high-income countries worldwide. Unfortunately, the upper age limit for which it is safe clinically to donate is 65 (for first-time healthy donors in the UK, but similar elsewhere), so there is an inevitable and growing deficit of blood donors (Figure 1). This threat to what is usually perceived by many as a stable and secure supply of blood can therefore only become more critical in the future as demographics play an increasingly major role.

Whilst it would be unwise to alarm either patients or the general public at large, it is incumbent on those involved in healthcare to provide information (as for any other medical treatment [4]) on the risks and benefits of blood transfusion together with those alternatives which are available to conserve precious blood stocks. This information should form the basis for informed consent, so that the patient is always very much at the centre of any subsequent decision-making about their clinical management.

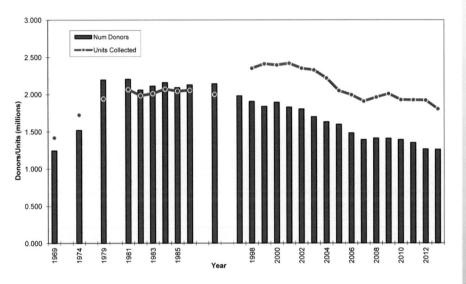

Figure 1. Long-term trend in the number of active blood donors in the UK. *Reproduced with kind permission from Crispin Wickenden, Head of Donor Insight, NHS Blood & Transplant.*

Evidence

The process of blood conservation aims to keep the precious stocks of donor blood for those patients who really need it and for whom there is no safe alternative. Whilst there is no argument that donor blood can save lives and improve health, there is now increasing evidence that transfusion carries with it many risks [5] and may not in fact be the optimum treatment of choice.

Although information about receiving a blood transfusion is available for patients [6], there have been no large studies on what people know, or want to know, about blood conservation. Only one small pilot study has ever been performed, looking at patients' perceived hazards of transfusion [7].

As for any other clinical intervention, it is important to discuss with the patient the risks and benefits regarding blood transfusion. There has been much debate on informed consent for patient blood management. Interestingly, only 6% of the respondents to the UK Advisory Committee on the Safety of Blood, Tissues and Organs (SaBTO) 2011 report were from those "with an interest in patient safety", i.e. patients, patient associations, hospital governors and risk managers [8].

Following the UK Department of Health document "Better Blood Transfusion 3" [9], the National Blood Transfusion Committee set up a Patient Involvement Working Group (PWIG) to address patient involvement in blood transfusion, but this currently does not address specifically whether the general public is aware of all the challenges facing the availability of blood and how it is managed.

There is an analogy here with the global supply of oil and other global energy sources: there is only a finite supply, it is costly and dependent on market forces, it must be used wisely, there are both risks and benefits, and so alternatives must be sought.

How to do it

Involve people before they become patients

Once anyone commences on the 'patient pathway' for any clinical treatment they will inevitably (and of course appropriately) be provided with a large quantity of information. This will be about their condition, risks and benefits, management options, hospital stay arrangements, social/ discharge care and many other details. Each patient can then use this information to help to guide their own decision for their own care, and also to have the opportunity to ask further questions if unsure. In addition, they may well have carried out their own research via the internet and printed media. Furthermore, they may have sought and/or received information from their general practitioner, family, friends and colleagues. In the light of all this acquired information, it may therefore not necessarily be the most optimal time to provide them with details about blood conservation, although this subject may well arise anyway at some point in the whole process. It should be noted, however, that an increasing number of patients are concerned enough (and not always necessarily on religious grounds) to challenge whether or not they need transfusion. These patients may question their possible treatment with donor blood, and ask for details about alternatives.

Need to know basis

Many clinical areas, including patient blood management, are moving towards patient-centred and individualised treatment as much as medical, logistical and financial aspects allow. This approach is dependent on each individual patient — what they already know, how much of that information they believe, what worries them and what they want to know.

Although there is high-standard, peer-reviewed national and/or local information on blood transfusion available from varied sources, patients (and the public) may well need some guidance as to what is relevant to them personally.

What we don't know, however, is what people, even when they are not actual patients, know about the current blood conservation strategies. Would they want to know more and if so would it affect their attitude towards having a blood transfusion if they or their family needed one?

Patient advocacy

Health professionals should try to involve their patients as much as possible in the decision process for treatment. There is, however, a plethora of information on all topics, including blood-related ones, out there in the public domain both from the internet and sources such as newspapers and journals, television and social media.

This is where the role of the patient advocate is so important. Whoever is caring for the patient (and it is increasingly a team approach) should take on the responsibility for studying the existing evidence, evaluating that which is robust and relevant, and then informing the patient accordingly. If there is a gap in the evidence — such as whether the public generally know, or even care, about blood and its associated issues — then research should be undertaken accordingly.

Research

Our patients and the public at large have a wealth of information about health-related topics freely available should they wish to pursue them.

Those of us working in the blood conservation/blood management arena are acutely aware that, despite current efforts, the supply of blood is fragile and may well be an escalating cause for concern in the future. Anecdotal evidence from the public and patient domain, and also more worryingly from health professionals, has shown a sometimes frightening lack of basic knowledge about blood. This includes the assumption that "blood will always be there when I need it" and that a blood transfusion is always the default option. Very few people are aware of how and why we must conserve our precious blood supply and seek alternatives such as cell salvage to save the blood for those who have no other option.

One might compare blood conservation awareness with Road Safety — we should all be aware of the basic rules and regulations which affect us all. These measures exist to provide clear, sensible and pertinent information, and the guidance for everyone who uses the roads whether as pedestrian, cyclist, driver or any other user. We ignore at our peril.

Although there has been much clinical progress and product development around blood conservation over recent years, these vary both nationally and worldwide. As quoted at the start of this chapter — "people need to know". Obviously we would not want to scare them, nor blind them with science, but rather allow them to ask questions of us to provide answers. Simply raising their awareness of the practicalities of blood management could help guide their attitude. For example, what if there are adverse weather conditions such as high snowfall or floods, or the nation falls victim to a flu epidemic? In those situations how can the blood donors and donor teams access the venues? How can any blood reach hospitals? These 'pinch-points' are only a few examples of the many potential problems which could affect the supply of blood for our patients. None of us can assume now, or more importantly in the future, that donor blood will automatically be available as and when we need it. It is therefore incumbent on those of us who have the knowledge and expertise in blood conservation to ensure that people be informed <u>before</u> they become patients and thus potential users of blood.

In the 1980s, there was high-profile worldwide publicity about the acquired immune deficiency syndrome (AIDS), one of the most devastating pandemics ever recorded. This highly successful campaign led to a major increase in the awareness of AIDS, the formation of powerful pressure groups, education of the public in ways they could avoid contracting the disease and the development of therapies to treat and perhaps eventually eradicate this life-threatening condition. Could not a similar approach be used to raise public awareness about the potential threat to the supply of blood and its current problems?

If we ask what people know, or would like to know, about blood conservation, then we might be able to use this information to enhance their perception (and ours) of this potentially major problem. In addition, we may well have enough answers to encourage debate and also provide educational resources for everyone involved both now and in the future.

We might then be able to develop these resources into an educational package which could be available in many different formats. These would depend on how people prefer their information to be presented to them. It could be as an online resource linked to an approved national forum such as the NHS Blood and Transplant (NHSBT) Patient Involvement Working Group, or added to an official public blood website. Some may prefer a printed patient information leaflet (PIL), or would like a blood conservation professional to deliver a presentation at a local meeting or focus group. The latter method would have the advantage of a 'face to face' approach with the opportunity to ask questions and receive answers. Perhaps inspired employers, business groups, local organisations and educational establishments (schools, colleges, and universities) could provide an initial forum for discussion. It would be useful if any of these methods raised the level of interest to inspire more patient representation on blood management groups and committees. A good starting point for any or all of these actions could be at the primary care level. In addition, patients and the public in general could be approached via hospital coordinators and managers who organise such interest groups at secondary care level. Inviting the general public (whether or not they are actually patients at the time) to state what they know, or would like to know, about blood conservation might help to provide a framework for their present knowledge and education. Most importantly though, in the spirit of patient involvement in their treatment, there will be a process for continued and improving patient empowerment in the whole process of blood management for the future.

Conclusions

Our patients, and the public in general, have a right to know about the implications surrounding blood conservation. Awareness of how increasingly fragile blood stocks are currently managed, together with information about alternatives to blood transfusion, will help empower them to make decisions for their own, individual, blood management.

It is therefore incumbent on all professionals working in this specialty to not only enhance their own knowledge so that they can act as advocates for their patients, but also help to disseminate such knowledge into the wider public arena.

Further research will assist us to find out what people know about blood conservation, what they would like to know and how they would prefer to receive this information.

Checklist summary

✓ Ensure our own knowledge of blood conservation is sound and relevant.

✓ Interpret the facts appropriately for each individual patient.

✓ Involve the patient in that discussion, thereby providing informed consent.

✓ Think about finding out what people outside the clinical arena know about blood conservation.

✓ Consider developing educational packages in differing formats.

References

1. Doctors in society - medical Professionalism in a Changing World. Technical supplement to a report of a Working Party of the Royal College of Physicians of London, December 2005. http://www.rcplondon.ac.uk/sites/default/files/documents/docs_in_socs_tech_navigable.pdf.

2. Blood Safety and Availability. Fact sheet N° 279. Updated June 2013. World Health Organisation (WHO). http://www.who.int/mediacentre/factsheets/fs279/en/.

3. Give blood. http://www.blood.co.uk/index.aspx.

4. "No decision about me without me". Liberating the NHS, 2012. https://www.gov.uk/government/uploads/system/uploads/attachment_data/file/213823/dh_117794.pdf.

5. Serious Hazards of Transfusion (SHOT). http://www.shotuk.org/.

6. "Will I need a blood transfusion?" National Health Service Blood and Transplant (NHSBT), 2013. http://hospital.blood.co.uk/library/pdf/Will_I_need_blood_tx_13_06_26.pdf.

7. Khan MM, Watson HG, Dombrowski SU. Perceived hazards of transfusion: can a clinician tool help patients' understanding? *Transfus Med* 2012; 22(4): 294-7.

8. Patient Consent for Blood Transfusion - Advisory Committee on the Safety of Blood Tissues and Organs (SaBTO) October 2011. London, UK: Department of Health, 2011. http://www.dh.gov.uk/en/Publicationsandstatistics/Publications/Publications PolicyAndGuidance/DH_130716.

9. Better Blood Transfusion 3. Health Service Circular. London, UK: Department of Health, 2007; 001: summary #4. http://www.dh.gov.uk/prod_consum_dh/groups/dh_digitalassets/documents/digitalasset/dh_080803.pdf.

Chapter 5

Haemovigilance in 2020?

Dafydd Thomas MB ChB FRCA
Director of Cardiac Intensive Care, Morriston Hospital, Swansea, UK
Paula Bolton-Maggs DM FRCP FRCPath
Medical Director SHOT, Manchester Blood Centre, Manchester, UK

- "Identify yourself, identify the correct patient and record your intervention."

- "Treat blood components for transfusion with the same respect as any other pharmaceutical product."

- "Give the right dose at the right time and only when clinically indicated."

- "Observe the effect in the patient whether positive or negative."

- "If unsure about the process or procedure — just ask!"

Background

The observation that transfusion of blood can be problematic as well as life-saving was appreciated by Blundell and other workers in the field — even prior to the development of a sophisticated blood service — because a significant proportion of treated individuals died. It is true to say that it is unclear whether Blundell's patients died of hypovolaemic shock or as a consequence of transfusion-associated complications. It took more than one and a half centuries before a more focused approach was adopted to monitor blood transfusion safety.

Haemovigilance is a term that has been used, initially by the French blood service, to encapsulate a system of monitoring adverse effects of transfusion of blood and blood components. It was developed as a result of the emergence of transfusion-transmitted viral infections in the 1970s and 80s (hepatitis and AIDS) and incorporates surveillance from donor to recipient.

It is surprising that even in the modern age of easier communication between countries and the almost instantaneous ability to keep in contact with each other by email, that countries have developed haemovigilance schemes that differ slightly in their ways of reporting categories of incidents, that essentially are a human species-specific reaction to blood transfusion and blood transfusion-associated problems.

Communication difficulties also occur at a grass roots level because the transfusion process has nine individual steps and requires participation by several individuals from different professional groups. Different professionals may not understand each other's scientific language. In addition, shift systems and patient transfers between wards as a result of more subspecialisation increase the number of times that transfer of care occurs, thus increasing the opportunity for communication failure.

When reports are submitted to haemovigilance schemes, regardless of the country in which the reporting scheme was devised, it can be seen how similar the reported problems are. It is also very obvious that there are generic issues that apply to the problems that arise. They fall into a small number of categories involving issues that seem to recur time and time again despite adequate training and competency assessments. These basic issues require an attention to detail, but even then there will always be unanticipated events related to allergic, acute and delayed transfusion reactions. It is the mark of a good haemovigilance reporting system that trends and signals are noted so that these occurrences can be investigated and hopefully change clinical processes for the benefit of safer blood transfusion practices.

In a recently published book on haemovigilance, René de Vries succinctly outlined the basic tenets of haemovigilance which has been reproduced below in diagrammatic form (Figure 1) [1].

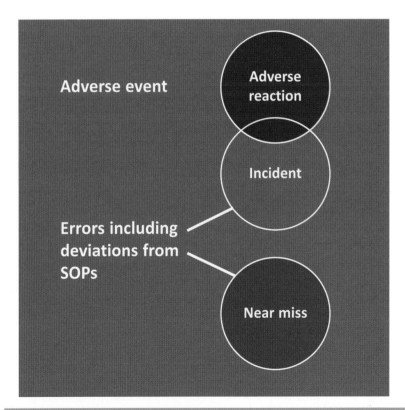

Figure 1. The basic tenets of haemovigilance.
SOPs = standard operating procedures.

As an explanation to this diagram it is important to grasp the four basic definitions shown. These definitions have mostly been taken directly from the introductory chapter of the book, *Hemovigilance*, to keep them consistent, as considerable debate was initiated to reach their current form [1]. (The definition of an adverse event, however, has been modified slightly to reflect the definition used by SHOT.)

An **adverse event** is any untoward occurrence associated with the collection, testing, processing, storage and distribution of blood or blood components that might lead to death or life-threatening, disabling or incapacitating conditions for patients or which results in, or prolongs, hospitalization or morbidity. It may or may not be the result of an error or an incident and may or may not result in an adverse reaction in a donor or a recipient.

An **incident** is a case in which the patient is transfused with a blood component that did not meet all the requirements for a suitable transfusion for that patient, or that was intended for another patient. Incidents thus comprise transfusion errors and deviations from standard operating procedures (SOPs) or hospital policies that have led to mistransfusions. It may or may not lead to an adverse reaction.

An **adverse reaction** is an undesirable response or effect in a patient or donor temporally associated with the collection or administration of blood or blood component. It may, but need not, be the result of an incident.

A **near miss** is an error or deviation from standard procedures or policies that is discovered before the start of the transfusion and that could have led to a wrongful transfusion or to a reaction in a recipient.

In 2004, the National Patient Safety Agency advocated seven steps to patient safety. These steps are as follows:

- Build a safety culture.
- Lead and support your staff.
- Integrate your risk management activity.

- Promote reporting.
- Involve and communicate with patients and the public.
- Learn and share safety lessons.
- Implement solutions to prevent harm.

Observations from the UK haemovigilance system (Serious Hazards of Transfusion — SHOT)

Over the last 19 years SHOT has promoted six of these steps [2]. Implementing solutions to prevent harm has to occur at the hospital or treatment centre, as it is only the practitioners and scientists at this level that can ensure their safety processes are followed.

Implementing translational change of the observed and reported negative occurrences during the preparation and administration of blood components into safer practice is fraught with difficulty. Human factors inevitably play a part in the errors that occur as well-trained, motivated and apparently competent staff continue to make mistakes. SHOT has highlighted improvements in the preparation and screening of blood components which is commendable, yet it has also highlighted that despite training and competency assessment, human errors still occur during the transfusion process. Perhaps we can encourage adoption of ideas from industry to enlighten us about how a change in design and process can lead to improved safety. Recent presentations outlining the safety culture in the airline industry have led to improved passenger safety, yet it cannot ever be 100% assured. Anaesthetists are aware of some significant developments that have led to improved safety. These days most anaesthetic machines have electronic self-checks and connections of piped gases do not allow oxygen pipes to be incorrectly sited in a nitrous oxide outlet (non-interchangeable screw threads [NIST]). Unfortunately, these changes in design were prompted by incidents involving patient harm as a result of incorrectly connected oxygen supplies [3].

Joint UK haemovigilance

Recently, discussions between the UK's Medicines and Healthcare products Regulatory Agency before (MHRA) and SHOT have led to a more unified approach to reporting, in an attempt to eliminate the duplication of reporting the same incident several times to different bodies. Those reporting on transfusion incidents will already have noticed a more streamlined approach to incident reporting which is only the first phase of developing a comprehensive but more streamlined system for UK haemovigilance. The simplification and streamlining of the transfusion process needs to be standardized in the way in which reports are completed. Until recently, reporting was divided with a requirement to report adverse events to the MHRA under their Serious Adverse Blood Reactions and Events reporting (SABRE). The MHRA has the role as the competent authority in the UK reporting on serious adverse events (SAEs) to the European Parliament following the introduction of the Blood Safety and Quality Regulations (2005) [4].

Patient safety

A recent safety campaign launched in England aims to halve avoidable harm in the next 3 years. There are five safety pledges:

- **To put patient safety first**. Commit to reduce avoidable harm in the NHS by half and make public the goals and plans locally.
- **Continually learn**. Make their organisations more resilient to risks, by acting on the feedback from patients and try constantly measuring and monitoring how safe their services are.
- **Honesty**. Be transparent with people about their progress to tackle patient safety issues and support staff to be candid with patients and their families if something goes wrong.
- **Collaborate**. Take a leading role in supporting local collaborative learning so that improvements are made across all of the local services that patients use.

- **Support**. Help people understand why things go wrong and how to put them right. Give staff time and support to improve and celebrate the progress.

To achieve further improvement in the quality of transfusion it is essential that all clinical and laboratory staff understand their responsibility to report adverse incidents. Overall, the reports received by a haemovigilance system can be broadly categorized into a number of categories as highlighted in repeated haemovigilance reports. The illustration below is taken from the SHOT report for incidents reported in 2014 (but does not show data for near miss, handling and storage errors or those where the patient received the correct components despite errors)(Figure 2) [2].

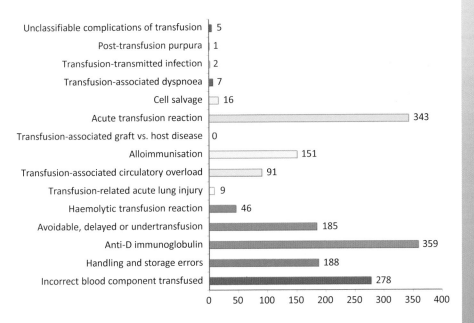

Figure 2. SHOT report for incidents reported in 2014 [2]. Cases reviewed in 2014, n = 1681.

The pattern of incidents has remained fairly constant over the years with correct patient identification being an ongoing issue leading to many of the other errors. If, however, it were necessary to pick six obvious failings in blood component use identified from year on year reporting to SHOT, that would improve patient safety it would be:

- Identifying the patient correctly.
- The correct labelling of blood samples for group and antibody screen and correct labelling and identification of the component to be transfused.
- Treatment of acute transfusion reactions combined with appropriate resuscitation.
- A strict and well-adhered to protocol for communication between clinicians and blood laboratories.
- Increasing awareness of circulatory overload.
- A comprehensive understanding of the use of anti-D immunoglobulin (anti-D Ig) treatment for RhD negative women of childbearing potential.

All of these well-defined processes have been clarified in guidelines with procedural steps which, if followed, can prevent avoidable incidents that often result in patient harm [5].

The triangle of care and correct patient ID

As a model of best practice when initiating clinical care in medicine, it is a good principle to "task and finish" patient episodes. If one deconstructs this to its simplest form, if a carer is doing anything to a patient there are three elements that need to be undertaken. It is essential that the carer is qualified and authorised to undertake the procedure, and positively identifies that the patient is the right patient and that the drug and dose or intervention or procedure is identified and delivered correctly. This may be described as the triangle of care. If one adds behaviour to this in that the carer completes the task before moving on to the next one, there is an inherent safety in avoiding multitasking.

Applying this principle to the clinical situation, when venesecting a patient to obtain a sample for cross-matching for a suitable blood component:

- The carer has to be competent and authorized to be taking the blood.
- The patient needs to be identified correctly by a process of open questioning, asking them to state their last name and their first, and their date of birth. If previously registered, their NHS number will be available from the hospital Patient Administration System (PAS), and the patient must be informed about why blood is being taken.
- The blood sample needs to be labelled completely and correctly before moving away from that patient.
- The culture within the clinical environment needs to ensure that practitioners comply with this complete process before being expected to undertake another task.

The various haemovigilance systems throughout the world repeatedly demonstrate a failure to identify the patient correctly at times of blood sampling and later at the time of component administration. These are the two key points where patients must be correctly identified. If all practitioners completed their tasks as trained, there would be fewer problems. Failures occur due to the pressure of work, when practitioners within the laboratory environment and in clinical interactions are multitasking using work arounds and short cuts. These human factors will always remain a problem until the culture within the organisation changes, to offer carers and laboratory staff a suitable environment to complete the task they have started before being asked to complete another.

Clinical overload is the most commonly offered reason for major incidents involving patient harm. We hear frequently about emergency departments being overstretched with an overwhelming number of patients presenting with relatively minor injuries. It may not be the answer to provide larger and better-staffed emergency departments but to examine why so many patients present directly to a secondary care establishment.

The National Institute for Health and Care Excellence (NICE) is developing guidelines for safe staffing and the recommendation is for a ratio of one nurse to four patients in minor injuries, with one to one in triage/major injuries and one to two in resuscitation areas.

The more recent interest in human factors has shown that humans cannot be made more perfect — at least not in the short term and that attention needs to be diverted towards improving the working environment and looking at the ergonomics involved in common and crucial tasks to minimize risks [6, 7].

Looking to the future it will be possible to record data over an adequate wireless environment and thus electronically capture the event with minimum effort, and it would be recorded to the second, minute, hour and day on which the event occurred. This would be an incredible audit of care. It is likely that the various machines used to perform basic observations such as pulse, PaO_2 and blood pressure will be similarly enabled and so there will be no need to record these events by writing them down.

Current processes are susceptible to human factors leading to errors of sample labelling and checking. The use of electronic devices to help improve the process are already established in some hospitals and trusts. There is a need for resilient and widely available WiFi within hospitals to fully appreciate the advantages of such a system.

Electronic devices need to be widely available so that all transfusion events can be recorded easily. Observations could be recorded in a similar way onto tablets or phones allowing complete retrieval of key information. Such a system would provide denominator data as well as the numerator data on adverse incidents. In addition, the performance of each practitioner could be assessed and audited, thus providing useful supporting information for appraisal. Of course, the same electronic devices can be used for many other similar functions within similar clinical situations where busy healthcare workers need to record the administration of treatments in addition to sample labelling, and to ensure that they correctly label and identify.

The schematic diagram overleaf outlines this simple triangle of care discussed above (Figure 3).

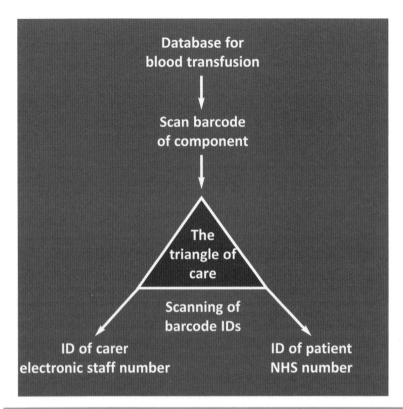

Figure 3. The simple triangle of care.

All IDs can be scanned if the information is barcoded — which it currently is, as patients have printed wristbands with barcoded numbers, staff have barcoded badges and blood components have a number of barcodes on the bag. As we look forward, then the steps in the transfusion chain have to be followed in a precise order and the data need to be collected electronically preferably over the WiFi or when the scanning device is next placed in its docking station it can be recharged and the data uploaded to the relevant database. As mentioned earlier, some hospitals already have such systems and it would make data collection and recording more streamlined and less dependent on paper records [8].

The advantage of such systems is that audit becomes easy to perform and individual data on carer and patient easier to retrieve.

Recent SHOT reports have shown that some of the current systems also have their shortcomings, but on balance provide a considerable improvement in the documentation of each process.

Acute transfusion reactions

Acute reactions

When an acute reaction occurs it may be allergic or haemolytic and the following steps need to be undertaken:

- Immediately discontinue the transfusion but maintain venous access.
- Observe for hypotension, renal failure, and disseminated intravascular coagulation (DIC).
- Ensure a forced diuresis, administer hydration with crystalloid solutions (3000ml/m^2/24h), and osmotic diuresis with 20% mannitol (100ml/m^2/bolus, followed by 30ml/m^2/h for 12h).
- If a coagulopathy develops with bleeding it will require treatment, using fresh frozen plasma (FFP), correction of low fibrinogen with cryoprecipitates or fibrinogen concentrate if available, and/or platelet infusion.

Acute haemolytic reactions which are non-antibody-mediated may display less severe symptoms, but nevertheless the ensuing haemoglobinuria will still require treatment with ongoing diuresis to avoid acute renal damage.

Allergic reactions

In allergic reactions, pruritis associated with hives or a rash is commonly treated with diphenhydramine and is usually effective. The route (oral or intravenous) and the dose (25-100mg) depend on the severity of the reaction and the weight of the patient.

In anaphylactic reactions resulting in severe hypotension or bronchospasm, a subcutaneous injection of epinephrine (0.3-0.5ml of a 1:1000 aqueous solution) is standard treatment. If the patient is sufficiently hypotensive to raise the question of the efficacy of the subcutaneous route, epinephrine (0.5ml of a 1:10,000 aqueous solution) may be administered intravenously.

Although no documented evidence exists that intravenous corticosteroids are beneficial for the management of acute anaphylactic transfusion reactions, theoretical considerations cause most clinicians to include an infusion of hydrocortisone or prednisolone in an attempt to depress the immune response.

Anti-D immunoglobulin (anti-D Ig) incidents

The errors reported to SHOT related to anti-D Ig show both a lack of understanding by various practitioners and a lack of compliance with recommended guidance [9, 10].

A 17-year analysis of adverse events related to anti-D Ig administration showed that 61% of cases related to late administration or omission of anti-D Ig and 31% of cases where there was inappropriate use of anti-D Ig [10]. In 73% of the cases, midwives and nurses were identified as making the primary error. Additionally, 23.5% of the reports involved errors originating in the laboratory, whilst 3.5% involved medical staff often at a senior level.

Health care workers need to be allowed to speak up and ask when they are unsure about what to do.

The openness that results from this can lead to more discussion and the educational opportunity to learn what should be done according to recommended guidance. The production of a flow chart for anti-D issues has provided a clear and useable guide that needs to be available in all clinical areas, especially obstetric and gynaecology wards, antenatal clinics and emergency departments (Figure 4).

Anti-D Administration Flowchart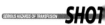

Always confirm
• the woman's identity
• that the woman is RhD Negative using the latest available laboratory report
• that the woman does not have immune anti-D using the latest available laboratory report
• that a blood sample has been taken to confirm group & antibody screen, (but do not wait for results before administration of anti-D Ig)
• that informed consent for administration of anti-D Ig is recorded in notes

Potentially Sensitising Events (PSEs) during pregnancy

Gestation less than 12 weeks	**Gestation LESS than 12 weeks**
• Therapeutic termination of pregnancy • ERPC / Instrumentation of uterus • Ectopic / Molar Pregnancy • Miscarriage / vaginal bleeding associated with severe pain	Administer at least **250iu** anti-D Ig within 72 hours of event. Confirm product / dose / expiry and patient ID pre administration No need for a Kleihauer / FMH Test at <12 weeks
Regardless of Gestation All the above, plus;	**Gestation 12 to 20 weeks**
• Amniocentesis, chorionic villus biopsy /cordocentesis • Antepartum haemorrhage / PV bleeding • External cephalic version • Fall or abdominal trauma (sharp / blunt, open or closed) • At diagnosis of Intrauterine death • In-utero therapeutic interventions (transfusion, surgery, insertion of shunts, laser)	Administer at least **250iu** anti-D Ig within 72 hours of event. Confirm product / dose / expiry and patient ID pre administration No need for a Kleihauer / FMH Test at <20 weeks
Administer anti-D Ig for a PSE irrespective of whether RAADP has already been given	**Gestation 20 weeks to term** Request a Kleihauer / FMH Test and immediately administer at least **500iu** anti-D Ig within 72 hours of event. Confirm product / dose / expiry and patient ID pre administration
Does the Kleihauer / FMH Test indicate that further anti-D Ig is required ?	Administer more anti-D Ig following discussion with laboratory
For continuous vaginal bleeding at least **500iu** anti-D Ig should be administered at a minimum of 6-weekly intervals, irrespective of the presence of detectable anti-D, and a Kleihauer requested every two weeks in case more anti-D is needed	

Routine Antenatal Anti-D Prophylaxis (RAADP)

For Routine Antenatal Anti-D Prophylaxis (**Irrespective** of whether anti-D Ig already given for PSE)	Take a blood sample to confirm group & check antibody screen – do not wait for results before administering anti-D Ig
	Administer **1500iu** anti-D Ig at 28 – 30 weeks **OR** At least **500iu** at 28 weeks **and** at least **500iu** at 34 weeks
	Confirm product / dose / expiry and patient ID pre administration

At Delivery   (or at diagnosis of Intra Uterine Death >20 weeks AND at delivery)

Is the baby's group confirmed as RhD positive ? OR Are cord samples not available ?	Request a Kleihauer / FMH Test
	Administer at least **500iu** anti-D Ig within 72 hours of delivery Confirm product / dose / expiry and patient ID pre administration
Transfusion Laboratory staff will advise if further anti-D Ig is required	Administer more anti-D following discussion with laboratory

Figure 4. A flow chart for the management of anti-D Ig incidents. *Reproduced with permission from SHOT.*

Conclusions

Haemovigilance has shown that adverse events continue to occur throughout the transfusion process. Merely monitoring the occurrence of such events does not improve patient safety.

Many of the areas where events occur are related to human factors where well-trained workers deviate from the recommended processes, either due to inattention, distraction or downright violation of the pathway in an attempt to complete a task more quickly.

Constant vigilance of the adverse events that occur within an organisation will hopefully give useful information on how these events may be decreased or eliminated altogether, by changing the working environment at a local level to make it easier to "do the right thing".

Checklist summary

✓ Always ensure you know who the patient is and the reason for the transfusion.

✓ Inform the patient of the reason for the transfusion.

✓ Record the event in the notes whether paper or electronic.

✓ Do not get distracted when labelling or checking the identification (ID) of the patient or the blood component.

✓ Ensure (where possible) you know the patient's transfusion history.

✓ Record all observations fully and ensure the fate of the blood component is documented.

✓ Keep up-to-date, especially with the treatment of acute transfusion reactions.

✓ If you are unsure ask for help!

References

1. De Vries RP, Faber JC, Eds. *Hemovigilance. An Effective Tool for Improving Transfusion Safety.* Oxford, UK: Wiley-Blackwell, 2012.

2. PHB Bolton-Maggs, Ed. Poles D, *et al.* on behalf of the Serious Hazards of Transfusion (SHOT) Steering Group. The 2014 Annual SHOT Report, 2015.

3. Subrahmanyam M, Mohan S. Safety features in anaesthesia machine. *Indian J Anaesth* 2013; 57(5): 472-80.

4. The Blood Safety and Quality Regulations, 2005. ISBN 0110990412. http://www.legislation.gov.uk/uksi/2005/50/made.

5. British Committee for Standards in Haematology (BCSH); Harris AM, Atterbury CLJ, Chaffe B, *et al.* BCSH guideline on the administration of blood components, 2009. http://www.bcshguidelines.com/documents/Admin_blood_components_bcsh_05012010.pdf.

6. England N. Human factors in healthcare - a concordat from the National Quality Board, 2013. http://www.england.nhs.uk/wp-content/uploads/2013/11/nqb-hum-fact-concord.pdf/1-22.

7. Clinical Human Factors Group (CHFG). First do no harm: closing the gap in patient safety, 2014: 1-66. http://chfg.org/news/a-roadmap-for-further-embedding-human-factors-in-the-nhs.

8. Davies A, Staves J, Kay J, *et al.* End-to-end electronic control of the hospital transfusion process to increase the safety of blood transfusion: strengths and weaknesses. *Transfusion* 2006; 46(3): 352-64.

9. British Committee for Standards in Haematology (BCSH); Quereshi H, Masset E, Kirwan D, *et al.* Guideline for the use of anti-D immunoglobulin for the prevention of haemolytic disease of the fetus and newborn. *Transfus Med* 2014; 24: 8-20.

10. Davies T, Bolton-Maggs P, Poles D, Keidan J. Seventeen years' analysis of adverse events associated with anti-D immunoglobulin (Ig). http://www.shotuk.org/wp-content/uploads/ISBT-2015-TD-Seventeen-years-analysis-of-adverse-events-associated-with-anti-D-immunoglobulin.pdf.

Chapter 6

Patient safety

Michael F. Murphy MD FRCP FRCPath
Professor of Blood Transfusion Medicine, University of Oxford; Consultant Haematologist, NHS Blood & Transplant and Oxford University Hospitals NHS Foundation Trust, Oxford, UK

Julie Staves BSc (Hons) FIBMS
Transfusion Laboratory Manager, Oxford University Hospitals NHS Foundation Trust, Oxford, UK

- "Developing robust methods for the avoidance of error is the best way to improve transfusion safety".

- "The standard manual bedside transfusion process is overly complex and is completed correctly for less than 50% of transfusions."

- "Bedside processes such as patient identification, sample labelling and the pre-transfusion bedside checks are only safe if performed <u>at the bedside</u>."

- "Making use of information technology makes the right thing to do the easy thing to do."

- "Excellence in transfusion safety requires rigorous training and active monitoring of practice and these are facilitated by the use of information technology."

- "Clinical decision support has major potential to minimise inappropriate blood use."

Background

The main challenges for the hospital transfusion service are ensuring:

- Patient safety including the avoidance of errors such as 'wrong blood transfusions', and the effective use of blood.
- Robust methods for documentation and monitoring practice.
- Good blood stock management and low wastage.
- Adequate staff training.
- Rapid availability of blood for those patients who need it urgently.

Patient safety is paramount. However, haemovigilance schemes worldwide continue to demonstrate that errors in the transfusion process result in patient morbidity and mortality. Once a decision to transfuse a patient has been made, it is essential to have complete accuracy during all the stages of the transfusion process, which is complex and involves many different staff (Figure 1). Errors made at any stage, including blood sample collection, laboratory testing and handling of samples, blood retrieval from blood transfusion refrigerators and during the pre-transfusion bedside check can result in transfusion of blood to the wrong patient.

The risk of ABO incompatible red cell transfusion, which is an avoidable event, is many times greater than the risk of human immunodeficiency virus (HIV) or hepatitis C virus (HCV) transmission by blood [1]. It has been one of the leading causes of death from transfusion reported to the Food and Drug Administration (FDA) in the United States [2], and to the Serious Hazards of Transfusion (SHOT) scheme [3] in the United Kingdom since national reporting of transfusion fatalities and serious incidents began in 1996/97. There has been little change in the number of ABO incompatible red cell transfusions reported to SHOT in the last 10 years (Figure 2). However, the true incidence of wrong transfusion is undoubtedly even higher than reported to haemovigilance schemes due to failure to recognise many errors. Baele *et al* uncovered numerous instances of wrong transfusion that went unrecognised [4]. With active tracking, they estimated that the true frequency of some form of error in bedside blood administration was 30-fold higher than those reported using passive reporting systems.

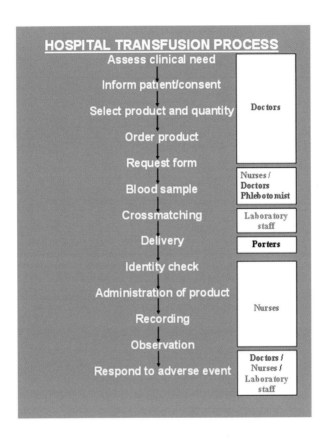

Figure 1. Steps in the hospital transfusion process, and the staff predominantly responsible for each step.

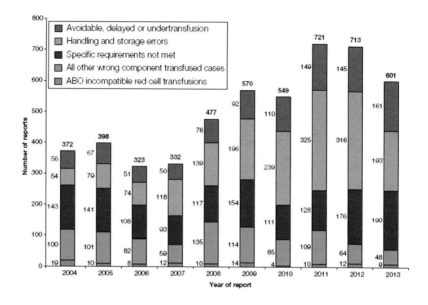

Figure 2. Cumulative data for blood component error-related reports to SHOT 2004 to 2013, subdivided according to the type of error. *Reproduced with permission from the 2013 SHOT Annual Report, 2014. Bolton-Maggs PHB, Ed, Poles D, Watt A, Thomas D, on behalf of the Serious Hazards of Transfusion Steering Group.*

The College of American Pathologists published results of two large observational audits — one conducted in 1994 and one in 2000 [5]. These audits assessed the frequency with which basic elements of the bedside check were correctly performed including positive patient identification, and matching wristband identification to the blood compatibility label. The frequency that checks failed to be performed was a major concern; the audit of over 4000 transfusions in 2000 found that all components of patient identification were correctly performed in only 25% of transfusions. Essentially the same results were found in a large international multicentre trial [6].

The most important factor in wrong blood transfused incidents is misidentification of the patient, blood sample or blood unit at the time of blood sample collection, compatibility testing in the laboratory or in the collection and administration of blood (Figure 3) [7]. Such errors include:

- The conscious patient is not asked to state his/her name and date of birth, and these are not checked against the same details on the wristband and other written documentation, such as the request form and the medical notes.
- The patient is not wearing an identification wristband.
- The patient's details on the wristband are illegible.
- Staff do not check the details on the wristband.
- Staff rely on self-identification of the patient.
- A surrogate identifier such as bed number is used to identify the patient.
- Labelling sample tubes away from the bedside.

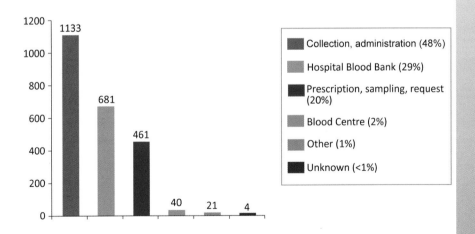

Figure 3. Distribution of errors in incorrect blood component transfused (IBCT) incidents reported to the Serious Hazards of Transfusion (SHOT) scheme between 1996 and 2003 (number of cases = 1393, number of errors = 2340).

- Failure to take patient identification to the blood fridge when collecting blood or to complete correct collection process.
- Carrying out procedures for two patients at the same time, e.g. labelling samples, laboratory testing or collecting or administering blood.
- Interruptions and/or distractions when undertaking any of these procedures.

Retrieval of the wrong blood from the blood refrigerator is a major cause of wrong blood transfusion. This primary error in the identification of the correct blood unit for collection and transport to the ward or operating theatre is not detected at the bedside due to inadequate checking that the unit is intended for the patient. Laboratory errors include using the wrong patient sample for testing and technical errors in blood grouping. Another important error is a failure to ensure that 'special requirements' for transfusion are met; for example, irradiated blood for patients with Hodgkin's disease or those receiving purine analogue drugs such as fludarabine. Most of these errors are due to poor communication from the clinical team to the laboratory.

How to do it

The British Committee for Standards in Haematology (BCSH) *Guideline on the Administration of Blood Components*[8] describes the key steps for safe transfusion (summarised in the *Handbook of Transfusion Medicine*[9] and in Table 1). Figure 4 illustrates the pre-transfusion identity check between the patient and blood component.

The key principles of safe transfusion practice are:

- **Positive patient identification**. A patient identification band such as a wristband must be worn by all patients undergoing transfusion. It should contain the patient's first name, last name, date of birth and unique patient identification number. In emergencies or where the patient cannot be identified, the patient's gender and unique patient identification number should be used. Discrepancies in patient identification at any stage of the process must be investigated and

Table 1. Safe blood administration. *Reproduced with permission from the Handbook of Transfusion Medicine [9], adapted from the BCSH guideline on the administration of blood components [8].*

Positive patient identification	Positive patient identification at all stages of the transfusion process is essential. Minimum patient identifiers are: • Last name, first name, date of birth, unique identification number. • Whenever possible ask patients to state their full name and date of birth. For patients who are unable to identify themselves (paediatric, unconscious, confused or language barrier) seek verification of identity from a parent or carer **at the bedside**. This must exactly match the information on the identity band (or equivalent). • All paperwork relating to the patient must include, and be identical in every detail, to the minimum patient identifiers on the identity band.
Patient information and consent for transfusion	Where possible, patients (and for children, those with parental responsibility) should have the risks, benefits and alternatives to transfusion explained to them in a timely and understandable manner. Standardised patient information, such as national patient information leaflets, should be used wherever possible.
Pre-transfusion documentation	Minimum dataset in patient's clinical record: • Reason for transfusion (clinical and laboratory data). • Summary of information provided to patient (benefits, risks, alternatives) and patient consent.
Prescription (authorisation)	The transfusion 'prescription' must contain the minimum patient identifiers and specify: • Components to be transfused. • Date of transfusion. • Volume/number of units to be transfused and the rate or duration of transfusion. • Special requirements (e.g. irradiated, CMV negative).
Requests for transfusion	Must include: • Minimum patient identifiers and gender. • Diagnosis, any significant comorbidities and reason for transfusion. • Component required, volume/number of units and special requirements. • Time and location of transfusion. • Name and contact number of requester.
Blood samples for pre-transfusion testing	**All patients being sampled must be positively identified.** • Collection of the blood sample from the patient into the sample tubes and sample labelling must be a continuous, uninterrupted event involving one patient and one trained and competency assessed healthcare worker. • Sample tubes must not be pre-labelled. • The request form should be signed by the person collecting the sample.

Continued

Table 1 *continued.* **Safe blood administration.** *Reproduced with permission from the Handbook of Transfusion Medicine* [9], *adapted from the BCSH guideline on the administration of blood components* [8].

Collection and delivery of blood component to clinical area	• Before collection, ensure the patient (and staff) is ready to start transfusion and there is good venous access. • Only trained and competent staff should collect blood from the transfusion laboratory or satellite refrigerator. • Authorised documentation with minimum patient identifiers must be checked against the label on the blood component. • Minimum patient identifiers, date and time of collection and staff member ID must be recorded. • Delivery to clinical area without delay.
Administration to patient	• The final check must be conducted next to the patient by a trained and competent healthcare professional **who also administers the component**. • All patients being transfused must be positively identified. • Minimum patient identifiers on the patient's identity band must exactly match those on the blood component label. • All components must be given through a blood administration set (170-200µm integral mesh filter). • Transfusion should be completed within 4 hours of leaving controlled temperature storage.
Monitoring the patient	Patients should be under regular visual observation and, for every unit transfused, **minimum** monitoring should include: • Pre-transfusion pulse (P), blood pressure (BP), temperature (T) and respiratory rate (RR). • P, BP and T 15 minutes after start of transfusion — if significant change, check RR as well. • If there are any symptoms or signs of a possible reaction — monitor and record P, BP, T and RR and take appropriate action. • Post-transfusion P, BP and T — not more than 60 minutes after transfusion completed. • Inpatients observed over next 24 hours and oupatients advised to report late symptoms (24-hour access to clinical advice).
Completion of transfusion episode	• If further units are prescribed, **repeat the administration/identity check with each unit**. • If no further units are prescribed, remove the blood administration set and ensure all transfusion documentation is completed.

Check the laboratory-generated label against the patient's identity band

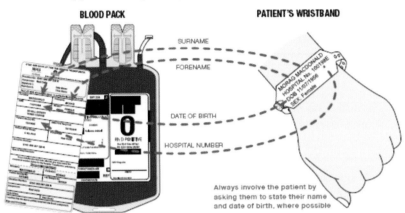

BLOOD PACK **PATIENT'S WRISTBAND**

SURNAME

FORENAME

DATE OF BIRTH

HOSPITAL NUMBER

Always involve the patient by asking them to state their name and date of birth, where possible

Figure 4. How to perform an identity check between the patient and blood component. *Reproduced with permission* [9].

resolved before moving to the next stage. The patient wristband should be printed from the hospital patient administration system, and the details checked with a patient or carer before being attached to the patient. Ideally, the wristband should have a barcode containing the patient identification details described above (see later).

- **Documentation of the transfusion in the clinical record** should include:
  - the reason for transfusion including relevant clinical and laboratory information;
  - the risks, benefits and alternatives discussed with the patient, and the consent documented;
  - the components to be transfused and their dose/volume and rate;
  - any special requirements;
  - identification details of the member of staff starting the transfusion;
  - date and time the transfusion was started and completed;

- donation number of the blood component;
- record of observations made before, during and after the transfusion;
- management and outcome of any transfusion reactions or other adverse events;
- whether the transfusion achieved the desired outcome, e.g. improvement in symptoms, desired blood count increment.

- **Excellent communication.** Good communication is essential to avoid misunderstanding, especially at times of staff handover both in the wards and in the laboratory; it can be enhanced by a standardised and documented process. Verbal communication between clinical and laboratory staff is a particular risk, and written or electronic communication should be used wherever possible. Urgent requests should be supplemented by telephone discussion with the laboratory and these should be documented.

How to prevent errors

Efforts to reduce error have primarily relied on implementing the procedures for good practice described above, learning from previous incidents and training programmes [10]. This approach has not been effective in eliminating ABO incompatible red cell transfusions, which are described as 'never events' when they cause morbidity (27% of cases) or mortality (6%) [3].

There are considerable barriers to further improving the safety of transfusion practice in hospitals, but they can be overcome by 're-engineering' the process with the support of a multidisciplinary team with shared, achievable and measurable objectives, engaging with senior hospital management, and having a determination to see the development of a new process through to completion and its implementation as routine practice.

Several groups have taken advantage of new technology, and developed electronic transfusion management systems for safe transfusion practice [11-13]. All healthcare professionals are familiar with barcode technology from its use in commerce, and blood products have been barcoded for many years. It is surprising that it is not more widely used for patient identification and the bedside checking process for transfusion.

The general principles of these electronic transfusion procedures are (Figure 5) [11]:

- Redesign of the transfusion process incorporating barcode patient identification and handheld computers at the bedside to prompt staff through each step of the blood sample collection and administration of blood procedures to ensure that the blood sample is correctly collected and labelled and that the right blood is transfused.
- Positive patient identification is conducted in the same way as the non-electronic process by first asking the patient to state their first and last name and date of birth, wherever possible, and checking the details match those on the wristband. In addition, the wristband barcode is scanned with a handheld computer and the details are checked to ensure they match the verbally stated identification and the eye readable information on the wristband.
- A portable printer taken to the bedside is used to print blood sample labels, stickers of documentation of each step of the process to be placed in the paper patient records, and 'pick up' slips to be taken to the blood fridge for blood collection using an automated process.
- Vital signs are recorded using the handheld computer before, during and after the transfusion.
- Staff are required to identify themselves by scanning barcodes on their identity badges.
- All data are transferred to the laboratory information system enabling accurate blood tracking and a complete audit trail.

These systems have improved both the safety and the efficiency of transfusion by minimising blood sample mislabelling, poor patient identification, and mismatched transfusions, and reducing staff time in carrying out pre-transfusion checks [14]. Electronic monitoring of every step in the transfusion process permits compliance with regulations for the traceability of every blood unit, and national recommendations for the training and competency assessment of staff without the need for establishing additional procedures [15].

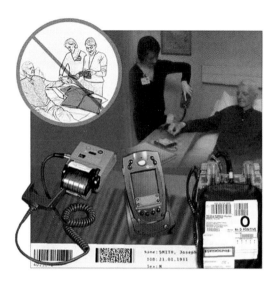

Figure 5. Bedside checks. The traditional method of pre-transfusion bedside checking requires two nurses and checks of multiple items of written documentation. With barcode technology, a handheld computer reads a barcode on the patient wristband containing full patient details. The handheld computer checks that the patient details on the wristband barcode match those on the barcode (in the red box) on the compatibility label attached to the unit after pre-transfusion testing. This barcode also contains the unique number of the unit, and is matched with the barcode number of the unit (top left of the bag) to ensure that the blood bank has attached the right compatibility label. *(This figure was originally published as the front cover of the September 2003 issue of Transfusion. Reproduced with permission from Wiley-Blackwell.)*

The National Patient Safety Agency (NPSA) in England recommended that hospitals appraise the use of barcode patient identification as a transfusion safety measure in 2006 [15], and electronic transfusion systems were one of the first recommended interventions in the National Health Service Quality, Innovation, Prevention and Productivity (QIPP) programme [16]. However, surveys carried out by the National Blood Transfusion Committee in England have found that very few hospitals in England are using barcode or other electronic systems for patient identification for blood transfusion.

These systems also allow 'electronic remote blood issue'. This is an extension of electronic issue enabling the issue of blood under electronic control at blood refrigerators remote from the blood transfusion laboratory to facilitate the rapid delivery of blood particularly to hospitals with no blood transfusion laboratory [17].

Centralised transfusion databases enhance patient safety

A centralised transfusion service (CTS) involves the operation of the transfusion services of several hospitals. Typically, the centralised service standardises clinical and laboratory procedures and practices, laboratory equipment, and information technology between the hospitals.

One of the most important patient safety enhancements inherent in a CTS is that each patient's entire serological and transfusion history is maintained in a centralised electronic database available at all hospitals within the CTS network. Thus, if the patient has ever had an ABO group or an antibody identified at one of the hospitals within the CTS, this crucial information will be available should the patient attend not only that hospital but any other within the CTS network [18].

Supporting and educating the prescriber when deciding if a patient needs to be transfused

Transfusion safety not only requires delivering the right product to the right patient, but also ensuring that the transfusion is clinically indicated. The use of computerised physician order entry (CPOE) systems, whereby the prescriber enters their order using a computer system that is linked to both the laboratory database and the blood transfusion laboratory, provides an opportunity to help educate the prescriber about evidence-based transfusion indications at the time the decision to order a transfusion is being made. Thus, the CPOE can function as a clinical decision support system (CDSS).

A CDSS is any process that helps the prescriber make an informed decision when ordering tests, making a diagnosis, or ordering interventions. In relation to transfusion medicine, a CDSS can range from the most manual and labour intensive such as a prescriber speaking directly with a transfusion medicine specialist before ordering blood to a sophisticated electronic on-screen warning that appears on a CPOE system when a prescriber attempts to order products on a patient whose laboratory results do not suggest that the transfusion is indicated. This latter type of CDSS helps to improve patient safety by drawing the prescriber's attention to a potentially overlooked laboratory value that indicates that the patient does not require the transfusion, or that the relevant laboratory test was not ordered at all and should be done before proceeding with the order for blood products. Information about transfusion, or weight-based dose adjustments can also be provided. Significant blood reduction has been found through the implementation of CDSS in some hospitals [19].

The general principles of a CDSS incorporated in a CPOE is that it allows:

- Electronic tracking of all blood product orders, which permits the blood transfusion laboratory and hospital transfusion/blood management committee to know which clinical services are ordering the most products.
- Rapid identification and re-education of prescribers whose ordering practices frequently generate alerts.
- Audits of transfusion practice by permitting the rapid identification of transfusions that do not meet the hospital guidelines, i.e. the order generated an alert.
- Benchmarking between hospitals or groups of hospitals, and the ability to evaluate the effect of focused education or other interventions to reduce non-evidence-based transfusion practice.

Conclusions

Good clinical and laboratory practice contribute to safe and effective transfusion through the avoidance of errors leading to 'wrong blood transfusion', appropriate decision-making about the correct use of blood based on assessment of the patient's clinical findings and laboratory parameters, and the monitoring of patients for adverse effects of transfusion and their management if they occur. Technology can be used to improve recipient safety at many stages in the transfusion process, and improve decision-making about the use of blood.

Implementing electronic enhancements of patient safety including barcode and remote issue technologies, CDSS within a CPOE, and centralisation of transfusion services takes dedication, time and considerable teamwork between transfusion medicine and information technology specialists. The benefits of these enhancements have already been demonstrated, and they will continue to evolve as clinical care changes and expands.

Checklist summary [9]

✓ 'Wrong blood transfusions' are nearly always caused by error and are avoidable; they may be fatal due to ABO incompatibility.

✓ Most 'wrong blood transfusions' are caused by errors in patient identification occurring at the time of blood sample collection, laboratory testing and handling of samples, blood retrieval from blood transfusion refrigerators and during the pre-transfusion bedside check.

✓ The pre-transfusion identity check between the patient and the blood component is the crucial final opportunity to avoid a wrong transfusion.

✓ The key elements of patient safety in the transfusion process are positive patient identification, excellent communication and good documentation. These can be enhanced by the use of electronic blood transfusion systems.

✓ Hospitals should develop local transfusion policies based on national guidelines and ensure that all staff involved in the clinical transfusion process are appropriately trained and competency assessed.

✓ Where possible, patients should give consent for transfusion based on appropriate information and discussion.

✓ Unnecessary transfusions should be avoided. Clinical decision support systems (CDSS) may help to minimise inappropriate transfusions.

References

1.   AuBuchon JP, Kruskall MS. Transfusion safety: realigning efforts with risks. *Transfusion* 1997; 37: 1211-6.

2.   US Food and Drug Administration. Fatalities reported to FDA following blood collection and transfusion. Annual summary for fiscal year 2012. http://www.fda.gov/biologicsbloodvaccines/safetyavailability/reportaproblem/transfu siondonationfatalities/ucm346639.htm.

3.   Bolton-Maggs PHB, Poles D, Watt A, Thomas D, on behalf of the Serious Hazards of Transfusion Steering Group. The 2013 SHOT Annual Report, 2014. http://www.shotuk.org.

4.   Baele P, De Bruyere M, Deneys V, *et al*. Bedside transfusion errors. A prospective survey by the Begium SANGUIS group. *Vox Sang* 1994; 66: 117-21.

5.   Novis DA, Miller KA, Howanitz PJ, *et al*. Audit of transfusion procedures in 660 hospitals. *Arch Pathol Lab Med* 2003; 127: 541-8.

6.   Murphy MF, Casbard AC, Ballard S, *et al*, on behalf of the BEST Research Collaborative. Prevention of bedside errors in transfusion medicine (PROBE-TM) study: a cluster-randomised, matched-paired-clinical areas trial of a simple intervention to reduce errors in the pre-transfusion bedside check. *Transfusion* 2007; 47: 771-80.

7.   Serious Hazards of Transfusion. Annual Report, 2003. Manchester, UK: Serious Hazards of Transfusion scheme, 2004. http://www.shotuk.org.

8.   British Committee for Standards in Haematology (BCSH). Guideline on the administration of blood components, 2009. http://www.bcshguidelines.com.

9.   UK Blood Services. *Handbook of Transfusion Medicine,* 5th ed. Norfolk D, Ed. The Stationery Office, 2013. http://www.transfusionguidelines.org/transfusion-handbook.

10.   National Patient Safety Agency. Safer Practice Notice 14. Right Patient — Right Blood, 2006. http://www.npsa.nhs.uk/nrls/alerts-and-directives/notices/blood-transfusions/.

11.   Turner CL, Casbard AC, Murphy MF. Barcode technology: its role in increasing the safety of blood transfusion. *Transfusion* 2003; 43: 1200-9.

12.   Chan JCW, Chu RW, Young BW, *et al*. Use of an electronic barcode system for patient identification during blood transfusion: 3-year experience in a regional hospital. *Hong Kong Academy of Medicine* 2004; 10: 166-71.

13.   Askeland RW, McGrane S, Levitt JS, *et al*. Improving transfusion safety: implementation of a comprehensive computerized bar code-based tracking system for detecting and preventing errors. *Transfusion* 2008; 48: 1308-17.

14. Murphy MF, Staves J, Davies A, *et al.* How do we approach a major change program using the example of the development, evaluation, and implementation of an electronic transfusion management system. *Transfusion* 2009; 49: 829-37.

15. Murphy MF, Fraser E, Miles D, *et al.* How do we monitor hospital transfusion practice using an end-to-end electronic transfusion management system? *Transfusion* 2012; 52: 2502-12.

16. Murphy MF. Electronic blood transfusion: improving safety and efficiency of transfusion systems. NHS Evidence Quality, Innovation, Prevention and Productivity (QIPP), 2014. http://www.evidence.nhs.uk/ topic/blood-transfusion.

17. Staves J, Davies A, Kay J, *et al.* Electronic remote blood issue: a combination of remote blood issue with a system for end-to-end electronic control of transfusion to provide a 'total solution' for a safe and timely hospital blood transfusion service. *Transfusion* 2008; 48: 415-24.

18. MacIvor D, Triulzi DJ, Yazer MH. Enhanced detection of blood bank sample collection errors with a centralized patient database. *Transfusion* 2009; 49: 40-3.

19. Goodnough LT, Shieh L, Hadhazy E, *et al.* Improved blood utilization using real-time clinical decision support. *Transfusion* 2014; 54: 1358-65.

Chapter 7

NICE guidance and blood management

Bruce Campbell MS FRCP FRCS
Past Chair of the Interventional Procedures and Medical Technologies Advisory Committees, National Institute for Health and Care Excellence (NICE), London, UK

- "NICE produces several types of evidence-based guidance on safety, efficacy, good practice, and both clinical and cost effectiveness."

- "All NICE guidance can be found on its website: the different recommendations are brought together in its pathways."

- "Relevant to blood conservation are technology appraisals, clinical guidelines, interventional procedures and medical technologies guidance."

- "In November 2015, NICE published a guideline on blood transfusion."

Background

This chapter is about how NICE (the National Institute for Health and Care Excellence) evaluates techniques, devices, pharmaceuticals and the management of a wide range of conditions, to produce different types of guidance for the National Health Service (NHS) in the United Kingdom. NICE guidance has become influential throughout the world and other countries are exploring ways of creating similar systems: some even use NICE guidance for their own health services.

Until 2015, only a small number of pieces of NICE guidance had focused on blood conservation and blood management. They included evaluations by NICE of techniques and devices involved in transfusion practice. This chapter describes the different types of NICE guidance but then focuses on the NICE guideline (NG24) entitled "Blood transfusion", published in November 2015.

A brief history of NICE

NICE was established in 1999 with the aim of promoting similar access for patients in all geographical areas to effective drug treatments, procedures and healthcare management in general. It does this by publishing evidence-based guidance for the NHS, drafted by independent groups of clinicians, scientists, lay representatives and other relevant people. Important principles of the process are shown in Table 1. Some types of NICE guidance apply only to England (e.g. clinical guidelines) while others apply throughout the UK (e.g. interventional procedures guidance).

At the outset, NICE's guidance was limited to technology appraisals (which assess the clinical and cost-effectiveness of drugs and other technologies) and clinical guidelines (about the management of specific conditions). These continue to attract the most publicity and often dominate people's thinking of what NICE does. However, NICE has developed a variety of other important programmes, which produce guidance for the NHS: interventional procedures (in 2002), medical technologies and diagnostics (both in 2009), and most recently, NICE

Table 1. Principles of production of all NICE guidance.

- Evaluations based on:
  - published evidence (+ other sources such as registers);
  - expert advice from clinicians and other experts;
  - views of patients and carers;
  - information from manufacturers;
  - input from other relevant 'stakeholders'.
- Evaluations by independent advisory committees.
- Explicit processes and timelines.
- Transparency, including public attendance at committee meetings.
- A period of public consultation followed by review and revision of draft guidance.
- Opportunity for appeal/resolution.

quality standards for healthcare. Its purview now extends beyond the immediate confines of the primary and secondary healthcare into public health (since 2005) and social care (since 2013). In addition, NICE has developed other initiatives including the NICE evidence services — a powerful internet facility for information about a wide range of health-related evidence and guidance.

The fact that NICE now produces so many different types of guidance can lead to confusion. NICE has developed online pathways which help to show how different pieces of guidance apply to particular areas of care. The sections below explain the types of NICE guidance which have been used, or might readily be used in the future, to address technologies or practices involved in blood conservation and patient blood management.

Technology appraisals

This is perhaps the most widely known type of NICE guidance: it addresses the clinical and cost-effectiveness of 'technologies' [1]. The technologies are selected by agreement with the Department of Health and are appraised by independent advisory committees called Technology Appraisal (TA) Committees. The agendas of these committees (which have increased from one to four in number) tend to be dominated by expensive new pharmaceuticals, because these are generally the innovations with potential for the greatest financial impact on the NHS. However, any technology which may have a significant impact on the NHS may be selected for guidance, including devices (e.g. coronary stents, hip prostheses) and occasionally diagnostics (e.g. neuroimaging). With direct relevance to blood conservation, TA323 "Erythropoiesis-stimulating agents (epoetin and darbepoetin) for treating anaemia in people with cancer having chemotherapy"; this supports their use as a treatment option and recommends using the one with the lowest acquisition cost when more than one is suitable [2]. This technology appraisal was published in November 2014, replacing TA142.

When evaluating a technology for TA guidance, the independent advisory committee considers the evidence for both its clinical and cost-effectiveness. Cost-effectiveness is calculated by complex modelling, based on agreed assumptions. As a result of these considerations, NICE produces recommendations about whether or not the technology should be routinely funded by the NHS, and for whom. If it recommends the use of the technology in a particular group of patients, then the NHS throughout England must make it available to all those patients. If clinical and cost-effectiveness considerations result in a recommendation not to use a technology, it may produce high-profile media coverage, especially if it affects patients who may be influential or for whom there are a lack of treatments. NICE and those advising NICE on its advisory committees invest almost limitless energy into making the best and fairest decisions which are possible, but dissatisfaction is inevitable when patients cannot routinely get treatments they want from the NHS.

The cost modelling used in technology appraisals produces a cost per quality adjusted life year (QALY) with the aim of allowing decisions to be made across the whole range of conditions dealt with by the NHS. This 'cost per QALY' provides a way of trying to assess the benefit in human terms of spending money from the finite NHS budget on people presenting, for example, with severe anaemia, acute blood loss, chronic pain, cancer, or influenza. It has resulted in the recognition of an approximate 'threshold value' of cost per QALY which seems reasonable for the NHS to spend, in the light of its limited resources.

This approach has understandably raised intense debate about whether the same criteria should be applied, for example, to otherwise fit people with a painful joint, people with incurable cancer, children with severe disabilities and babies with life-threatening conditions. NICE has engaged in longstanding initiatives to address the many ethical and other issues, including advice from its Citizens Council (a specially selected group of people from across the matrix of society, which meets for 2-day facilitated discussions on specific questions), and the creation and review of its social value judgements for the development of NICE guidance [3, 4].

NICE TA guidance results in far more recommendations to use new technologies than recommendations not to use them, but the media tend to publicise the restrictive decisions. This is the main reason that NICE has become regarded in some quarters as a 'rationing body'. The system used by NICE to produce its TA recommendations continues to be a subject of considerable internal and external reflection and debate.

Clinical guidelines

These consist of recommendations about best practice for the management of particular conditions, which have now become the basis for practice throughout many areas of medical practice [5]. They are produced by Guideline Development Groups, specially appointed for each guideline. The groups meet over a period of many months and agree recommendations based as far as possible on the best available evidence, but also, where necessary, on expert consensus.

There are now about 180 different clinical guidelines. Blood transfusion has been an element of some, such as CG114 "Anaemia management in people with chronic kidney disease" [6], in which the detailed recommendations include ones about the use of erythropoiesis-stimulating agents. In November 2015, after a long period of preparation and consultation, NICE published NG24 "Blood transfusion — assessment and management of blood transfusion". The key points of this are summarised below [7].

Clinical guidelines are precisely what their title says — guidelines. They are not protocols or 'recipe books'. They are designed to describe good management, which is likely to be applicable to most patients, but not to all. There is a tendency among some clinicians to follow NICE guidelines slavishly, and sometimes thoughtlessly [8]. Some clinicians (doctors, nurses and others) are worried that if they do not follow NICE guidance to the letter they will be at risk of censure. However, circumstances arise not infrequently when strict application of NICE recommendations may not be best for a patient. That is a matter of clinical judgement, which simply needs to be thoughtfully made and clearly recorded.

Like all types of NICE guidance, clinical guidelines are reviewed at regular intervals and updated accordingly: this is considered, typically, at 3-yearly intervals. There is not the capacity to revise every guideline regularly and updating depends on the pace of change of the evidence and advice from specialist clinicians about the need for a major update.

Interventional procedures

Interventional procedures (IP) guidance is based on the safety and efficacy of procedures. There is no consideration of their cost implications. It deals mostly with new procedures, but those which have been used for many years may be considered if uncertainties arise about their safety or efficacy [9]. Most procedures are notified to NICE by clinicians who want to do a procedure they have not done before, but they can be notified by anyone, including manufacturers, patients, medical insurers and hospitals. Specialist societies are also encouraged to notify new procedures in their specialist areas and the NICE Interventional Procedures team also keeps a watching brief on medical publications and the popular press. Through these avenues it is hoped that most new procedures entering NHS practice will be identified. Since 2002, over 1000 notifications have been received and over 500 pieces of IP guidance have been published (including updates, as the evidence base has grown for some procedures).

Differentiating between new procedures and new devices is potentially problematic [10]. Many new devices involve a new procedure, and if they do then they should be the subject of IP guidance. However, guidance is always focused on a 'generic' procedure (the title never uses the name of a particular commercial device). This is because more than one device may exist or come into existence and it is not practical to produce separate guidance on each.

The main kinds of recommendation of IP guidance are shown in Table 2. Guidance may also include recommendations about patient selection (e.g. by a specified multidisciplinary team), about the training and experience required to do the procedure, about the facilities needed and what information should be reported from future research or data collection, to resolve uncertainties. Good, comprehensive data collection is an aspiration for all procedures with an inadequate evidence base, but achieving this remains a challenge [10].

Table 2. Main types of recommendations of interventional procedures guidance.

- *Do not use*. This is very unusual and only occurs when there is evidence that a procedure does not work or that it is harmful.

- *Use in research only*. When the level of uncertainty about safety or efficacy (or both) is such that patients need to be protected by the scrutiny of research ethics; and especially when there is a real need for good data to underpin the use of a procedure. This kind of recommendation ideally requires the existence (or imminent existence) of one or more research studies for patients to enter.

- *Use with 'special arrangements'* for (a) clinical governance, (b) consent and (c) audit/research. In simple terms this means (a) tell your hospital that you intend to do the procedure, (b) tell your patients that the procedure is new and what the uncertainties are, and (c) audit and review the outcomes (and/or conduct research). This is the most common type of recommendation and is used when there are substantial uncertainties, but not enough to restrict the procedure to research use.

- *Use with 'normal arrangements'* for clinical governance, consent and audit/research. The evidence is sufficient for the procedure to be used in normal, 'routine' clinical practice.

There has been IP guidance on intra-operative red blood cell salvage both in obstetrics (IPG144) and during radical prostatectomy or radical cystectomy (IPG258) [11, 12]. The guidance on cell salvage in obstetrics is one of the few examples which fall outside the categories of recommendations shown in Table 2. The guidance states that there are theoretical safety concerns and recommends reporting all complications to the MHRA (Medicines and Healthcare products Regulatory Authority). The guidance on radical prostatectomy and cystectomy is for use with normal arrangements in place for clinical practice, but it specifies provision of good information for patients about the procedure and the alternative of allogeneic transfusion.

Medical technologies

This is aimed at trying to identify devices and diagnostics that are likely to offer substantial advantages to patients and/or to the health service, and to encourage their adoption in a speedier manner than has occurred in the past [13]. It depends on manufacturers notifying their products to NICE, by way of a clearly formatted notification portal. This is designed to allow them to set out clearly the features of their technology and its claimed advantages over current practice. This information is presented to the NICE Advisory Committee as part of a detailed briefing note and the Committee then decides whether or not to select the technology for NICE evaluation. The main considerations in deciding whether to select a technology are shown in Table 3.

Table 3. Criteria used to select devices and diagnostics notified to the NICE Medical Technologies Programme for evaluation and for publication of NICE guidance.
Does the technology appear to have advantages compared with current management in:
• **Patient outcome or experience?** e.g. better clinical outcomes, longer survival, fewer visits to hospital, less pain.
• **Use of resources?** e.g. outpatient care rather than inpatient, reduced length of stay, less staff required, fewer complications to treat.
• **Cost?** Less costly for equivalent outcomes, equivalent cost for better outcomes, or both.
• **Sustainability?** less energy use, less waste.

When making claims for the advantages of any new technology, defining 'current management' is vital, because that will be the comparator for any discussion and for cost modelling. Advice from medical specialists and other experts (e.g. nurses, scientists) is fundamental for agreeing the best comparator and on a whole range of other issues. This is because the published evidence on devices and diagnostics is typically poor – a frequent problem for evaluation. The available evidence needs to be balanced against the apparent 'promise' of a technology in selecting it for evaluation [14].

If selected, costly new diagnostics (e.g. expensive imaging devices) or diagnostic tests with a range of alternatives are likely to be referred to the NICE Diagnostic Assessment Programme. This has the capability for multiple technology evaluations [15]. More often, technologies selected for evaluation remain within the remit of the Medical Technologies Advisory Committee (see Table 4).

Table 4. Some particular features of the remit of the NICE Medical Technologies Advisory Committee and its medical technologies guidance.

- *Single products only* (although the guidance stipulates that if similar products have adequate evidence then they should be considered for adoption in a similar way).
- *Value proposition*. This is the basis of any evaluation. It means a clear case for benefit in specified patients, alongside a plausible calculation of costs.
- *Cost modelling*. A cost comparison, through modelling, of the use of the new technology compared with current management. This can include all kinds of considerations, provided they are plausible. It is designed to produce cost consequences only: not cost per QALY.
- *Cost considerations for guidance*. Medical technologies guidance cannot recommend a technology which is more costly than current management, overall (see also Table 3). That would need to be via a different NICE programme (e.g. diagnostic assessment, technology appraisal).

Medical technologies guidance focuses on the "case for adoption" by the NHS. Typically it states that "The case for adoption is supported by the evidence". It describes the patients and circumstances in which use of the technology is recommended; it specifies what the advantages are for patients; and it describes the estimates of cost (saving) compared with current management.

If the evidence supports use of a technology in principle but there is uncertainty about aspects of its introduction into care pathways in the 'real world' or its clinical utility, then there may be a recommendation for further research. NICE has a facility to foster that research through academic centres under contract to the Institute. These centres can hone research questions and can make all the arrangements for research to be done, in collaboration with manufacturers, up to the point of funding the work. There is normally a 2-year timeframe for the delivery of answers to research questions, followed by review of the guidance.

This novel approach to identifying and evaluating new devices and diagnostics for their clinical and cost advantages has not yet resulted in medical technologies guidance for any product specifically related to blood conservation or patient blood management. However, it is ideally placed to do so if manufacturers wish to enhance the uptake of any kind of new device or diagnostic for which they can proffer a good value proposition. The Medical Technologies team at NICE is always pleased to enter into discussion with manufacturers who would like to consider a notification, but who need to know more.

NICE guideline on the assessment and management of blood transfusion

Like other NICE clinical guidelines, NG24 (November 2015) comprises sections on key priorities, recommendations, implementation and recommendations for research [7]. The key priorities reflect the recommendations which were considered to be the most important to introduce into current practice. These are summarised in Table 5.

Table 5. Summary of the key recommendations of NICE NG24 on blood transfusion.

Alternatives to blood transfusion for patients having surgery:

- Offer oral iron before and after surgery to patients with iron deficiency anaemia.
- Offer tranexamic acid when moderate blood loss (>500ml) is anticipated and consider intra-operative cell salvage with tranexamic acid when high-volume blood loss may occur.

Red blood cells:

- Consider a transfusion threshold of 70g/L and a target haemoglobin after transfusion of 70-90g/L. Consider transfusing single units of blood to adults who are not actively bleeding.

Platelets:

- Offer prophylactic platelet transfusions to patients with a count <10 x 10^9/L who are not bleeding, not having operations, and who have not got specified types of thrombocytopenia. Do not routinely transfuse more than a single dose of platelets.

Fresh frozen plasma transfusions:

- Do not offer these to patients who are not bleeding or who need reversal of a vitamin K antagonist.

Prothrombin complex concentrate transfusions:

- Offer these for emergency reversal of warfarin anticoagulation in patients with severe bleeding or who have a head injury with suspected intracerebral haemorrhage.

Patient information:

- Provide verbal and written information to patients and their families about the reason for transfusion, the risks, the transfusion process, the alternatives and the fact that they are no longer eligible to donate blood.

The guideline recommends research into the clinical and cost-effectiveness of:

- Restrictive compared with liberal red blood cell thresholds and targets for patients with chronic cardiovascular disease.
- An electronic decision support system compared with current practice in reducing inappropriate blood transfusions.
- Postoperative cell salvage and reinfusion in reducing red blood cell use and improving clinical outcomes for patients having cardiac surgery with a significant risk of postoperative blood loss, compared with existing practice.

It also recommends research into the dose of fresh frozen plasma that is most clinically effective at preventing bleeding in patients with abnormal haemostasis who are having invasive procedures or surgery.

Conclusions

The NICE guideline on "Blood transfusion — assessment and management of blood transfusion" offers recommendations and guidance across the whole range of blood transfusion practice — from considering whether to transfuse, through the alternatives, to the use of all types of blood components. Nevertheless, if new methods or technologies start to become available, it is important that clinicians (and manufacturers) tell NICE about them. That will enable NICE to seek expert advice, to evaluate them when appropriate, and to produce guidance about introducing them safely and most effectively into the UK health services.

Acknowledgement

I thank Laura Gibson and Elizabeth Adelanwa for their proof reading and assistance with references.

Checklist summary

✓ NICE publishes a range of different types of guidance, all based on the best possible evidence, and with input from clinicians, patients and other stakeholders.

✓ The processes NICE uses are explicit, transparent and open: all draft guidance is subjected to public consultation and review before it is published.

✓ There is a NICE guideline on blood transfusion — "Blood transfusion — assessment and management of blood transfusion" (NG24, November 2015) which provides detailed recommendations on practice.

✓ Other NICE guidance addresses specific agents and technologies used in transfusion practice. As new ones emerge it is useful for clinicians to tell NICE about them.

References

1.   NICE technology appraisal guidance. http://www.nice.org.uk/About/What-we-do/Our-Programmes/NICE-guidance/NICE-technology-appraisal-guidance.

2.   National Institute for Health and Clinical Excellence. Erythropoiesis-stimulating agents (epoetin and darbepoetin) for treating anaemia in people with cancer having chemotherapy, TA323. London, UK: NICE, 2014. http://www.nice.org.uk/guidance/TA323.

3.   NICE Citizens Council. http://www.nice.org.uk/Get-Involved/Citizens-Council.

4.   National Institute for Health and Clinical Excellence. Social value judgements: principles for the development of NICE guidance. London, UK: NICE, 2008. http://www.nice.org.uk/about/what-we-do/research-and-development.

5.   NICE clinical guidelines. http://www.nice.org.uk/About/What-we-do/Our-Programmes/NICE-guidance/NICE-guidelines/NICE-clinical-guidelines.

6.   National Institute for Health and Care Excellence. Anaemia management in people with chronic kidney disease, CG114. London, UK: NICE, 2011. http://www.nice.org.uk/guidance/CG114.

7.   National Institute for Health and Care Excellence. Blood transfusion - assessment and management of blood transfusion, NG24. London, UK: NICE, 2015. http://www.nice.org.uk/guidance/ng24.

8. Baker M. Clinical guidelines: too much of a good thing. *Ann R Coll Surg Engl* 2014; 96: 157-8.

9. NICE interventional procedures guidance. http://www.nice.org.uk/About/What-we-do/Our-Programmes/NICE-guidance/NICE-interventional-procedures-guidance.

10. Campbell B, Stainthorpe A, Longson C. How can we get high quality routine data to monitor the safety of devices and procedures? *Br Med J* 2013; 346: f2782

11. National Institute for Health and Care Excellence. Intraoperative blood cell salvage in obstetrics, IPG 144. London, UK: NICE, 2005. http://www.nice.org.uk/guidance/IPG144.

12. National Institute for Health and Care Excellence. Intraoperative blood cell salvage during radical prostatectomy or radical cystectomy, IPG 258. London, UK: NICE, 2008. http://www.nice.org.uk/guidance/IPG258.

13. NICE medical technologies guidance. http://www.nice.org.uk/About/What-we-do/Our-Programmes/NICE-guidance/NICE-medical-technologies-guidance.

14. Campbell B. How to judge the value of innovation. *Br Med J* 2012; 344: e1457

15. NICE diagnostics guidance. http://www.nice.org.uk/About/What-we-do/Our-Programmes/NICE-guidance/NICE-diagnostics-guidance.

Chapter 8

Consent for blood transfusion in adults

Andrea Harris RGN BSc MSc
Regional Lead, Patient Blood Management, NHS Blood and Transplant, Birmingham, UK
Catherine Howell RGN
Chief Nurse, Diagnostic & Therapeutic Services, NHS Blood and Transplant, Bristol, UK

- "Patient-centred care is widely recognised as a core dimension of a quality modern health service. Informed decision-making — a two-way dialogue between patients and their health practitioners about the benefits, risks and alternatives of treatment, taking into account the patient's personal circumstances, beliefs and priorities — is vital to truly patient-centred care." [1]
  Queensland Health, Australia, 2012

- "The doctor is... under a duty to take reasonable care to ensure that the patient is aware of any material risks involved in any recommended treatment, and of any reasonable alternative or variant treatments. The test of materiality is whether, in the circumstances of the particular case, a reasonable person in the patient's position would be likely to attach significance to the risk, or the doctor is or should reasonably be aware that the particular patient would be likely to attach significance to it." [2]
  Montgomery v Lanarkshire Health Board, 2015

Background

To consent is to agree to, or allow someone, to do something. In healthcare, valid or informed consent is the process of obtaining permission before conducting an intervention on a person, after having provided information about the risks and benefits of the intervention, and whether there are any alternative interventions (including doing nothing). The basic difference between consent and informed consent is the patient's knowledge behind the consent decision [3]. For consent to be valid it must also be voluntary, without influence or pressure from anyone, including healthcare professionals, friends or family.

Consent may be given verbally, for example, by stating that they are happy to have an X-ray, or in writing, for example, by signing a consent form prior to surgery. Patients may also passively agree to treatment taking place, for example, by holding out an arm to show they are happy to have a blood sample taken. However, none of these examples are informed consent if the benefits, risks and alternatives of the intervention have not been explained and understood.

These key principles of consent are an important part of medical ethics. The four main principles of medical ethics are justice, non-maleficence, autonomy and beneficence [4]. Sellinger describes how autonomy is the main ethical consideration underlying informed consent, with honesty and truthfulness required to make the process of consent valid, and the need for a patient's right to make a decision to be respected [3].

Blood transfusion has often been considered as part of the patient's overall treatment and care, and consent for transfusion generally implied through the patient's consent to medical treatment. However, there has been considerable debate internationally about whether separate informed consent for blood transfusion should be obtained [5, 6]. In 2008, the European Blood Alliance performed a survey of member country practices to better understand approaches to consent for blood transfusion [7]. Nineteen countries participated, and the results highlighted mixed practices ranging from no national consent requirement to full written informed consent.

An allogeneic blood transfusion involves taking blood from one person (the donor) and administering it to another person (the patient). It is, therefore, akin to a 'liquid transplant', and so it would seem perfectly reasonable to ask a patient's valid informed consent before performing such an intervention. However, Davis *et al* found that only 55% of patients recalled consenting to transfusion, with the majority only being told that "they needed a transfusion" [8]. Only 1 patient (n = 110) recalled having a full discussion about the risks and the benefits of transfusion.

In 2010, the UK National Comparative Audit (NCA) of Blood Transfusion performed an audit of patient information and consent [9]. One hundred and sixty-three hospital sites participated in various aspects of the audit, which included an organisational survey, a case note audit, and a patient and a staff survey. Table 1 provides a summary of the results, which indicate a clear discordance between hospital policy and actual practice, in particular around the provision of written information to patients.

The World Health Organisation reminds us that patients' rights vary in different countries and in different jurisdictions, often depending upon prevailing cultural and social norms [10]. This has led to the development of different models of the patient-physician relationship with varying rights to which patients are entitled, and different professional obligations of the physician toward the patient. As communities become increasingly multi-cultural, this may lead to additional healthcare consent challenges.

This chapter focuses on consent in adults. An important issue to consider is when does a child (or young person) become an adult? There are important differences in who is defined an 'adult' in different countries, and an interpretation of the term 'adult' needs to be considered by healthcare professionals in the country in which they practice. This is also discussed in Chapter 9.

Table 1. NCA consent for blood transfusion — summary of results.

Audit/survey question	Yes	To a certain degree	No	Can't remember	Not stated
Organisational survey (141 sites)					
Do you have a policy on consent?	85%	-	-	-	-
Do you have a policy on the provision of patient information?	89%	-	11%	-	-
Are patients routinely given written information as part of the consent process?	77%	-	22%	-	1%
Case note audit (164 sites/2784 cases)					
Is the indication for transfusion documented?	81%	-	18%	-	1%
Is consent documented?	43%	-	57%	-	
Is it documented that written information was given to the patient?	19%	-	77%	-	5%
Patient survey (162 sites/2243 patients)					
Were you involved with the decision-making process about if you should receive a blood transfusion?	56%	18%	21%	5%	0.1%
Did anyone talk to you about blood transfusion?	76%	-	17%	6%	0.5%
Did you receive any written information about blood transfusion (e.g. leaflet)	28%	-	82%	9%	0.6%
Did you understand the information you were given?	71%	-	9%	-	20%
Were the possible benefits of having a transfusion discussed with you?	68%	-	19%	11%	1%

Continued

Table 1 *continued*. NCA consent for blood transfusion — summary of results.

Audit/survey question	Yes	To a certain degree	No	Can't remember	Not stated
Were the possible risks associated with a blood transfusion explained to you?	38%	-	44%	15%	2%
Were you offered alternatives to blood transfusion?	8%	-	76%	12%	3%
Were you given the opportunity to ask questions?	73%	-	16%	10%	1%
Were you asked to give your consent to have a blood transfusion?	59%	-	23%	16%	2%
Did you feel you had received enough information about having a blood transfusion?	75%	-	15%	8%	2%
Staff survey (163 sites/1663 staff members)					
Did you explain the rationale for transfusion to the patient?	85%	-	14%	-	1%
Did you document this rationale?	63%	-	34%	-	3%
Did you provide the patient with written information on blood transfusion?	18%	-	80%	-	1%

Evidence (best practice)

It is not the intention of this chapter to provide definitive guidance on how consent for transfusion should be obtained. Different countries will have different legislation which must be considered as part of this process. We will, however, provide a summary of issues which should be considered, regardless of the country in which you practice.

Who can obtain consent for transfusion?

It is generally considered best practice that the healthcare practitioner who decides that a transfusion is (or may be) needed should obtain the patient's consent. Whereas the decision to transfuse has generally been seen as the responsibility of a doctor, there are now extended multi-disciplinary practices being developed. Non-medical registered professionals (especially nurses and midwives) are increasingly making these decisions (under appropriate legislation and guidance) and are therefore more integrally involved in patient consent. It is the responsibility of a healthcare organisation to define which registered professionals are able to undertake this activity, and it is important that non-medical practitioners are provided with appropriate governance frameworks and policies to support them in this advanced additional role.

Regardless of professional background, it is important that individuals involved in the consent for transfusion process have sufficient transfusion-related knowledge (including alternatives to transfusion) to be able to discuss all relevant issues with the patient. O'Brien *et al* and Friedman *et al* both reported marked knowledge deficits in transfusion for recently graduated medical students and clinicians working in various specialties [11, 12]. Increased education is necessary to improve knowledge of transfusion indications, benefits and risks, which may lead to more meaningful discussion with patients [12].

Patient capacity to consent

This is the ability to understand and process information to make a decision and to communicate any decision made. Any lack of capacity may be permanent or temporary.

In England and Wales, the Mental Capacity Act 2005 is designed to protect and empower adults (over the age of 16) who may lack the mental capacity to make their own decisions about their care and treatment [13]. Scotland has its own law, the Adults with Incapacity (Scotland) Act 2000 [14].

According to the Mental Capacity Act 2005, the following principles apply:

- A person must be assumed to have capacity unless it is established that he lacks capacity.
- A person is not to be treated as unable to make a decision unless all practicable steps to help him to do so have been taken without success.
- A person is not to be treated as unable to make a decision merely because he makes an unwise decision.
- An act done, or decision made... must be done, or made, in [the person's] best interests.
- Before the act is done, or the decision is made, regard must be had to whether the purpose for which it is needed can be as effectively achieved in a way that is less restrictive of the person's rights and freedom of action.

It is important to remember that to deem a patient as not having capacity is to remove an individual's right to make decisions for themselves. This is a complex area of healthcare, and individuals must ensure that they follow legal frameworks appropriate for the country in which they practice.

Patient refusal of consent

An important aspect of valid consent is that no healthcare professional should force or coerce a competent adult to accept any treatment, even if their decision appears to be irrational. It is important that you document any decisions clearly, seeking additional advice as appropriate in a timely manner, and fully explore alternative treatment options.

Patients who refuse transfusion is discussed elsewhere in this book.

Advanced decisions (or directives)

Competent adults who understand the implications of their choices can state in advance how they wish to be treated if they later suffer loss of mental capacity, including the advanced refusal of medical procedures or treatments recommended by health professionals [15]. This again is discussed in more detail elsewhere, but it is important to remember that any person may have an advanced decision, not just those who refuse transfusion on the grounds of religious belief.

A refusal of any recommended medical treatment can result in deterioration in the patient's condition or even death. The British Medical Association states that if an individual intends specifically to refuse life-sustaining procedures, they must:

- Clearly indicate that it is to apply even if life is at risk and death will predictably result.
- Put the advanced decision in writing.
- Ensure it is signed and witnessed [15].

It may be prudent to seek legal advice. In England and Wales, if there is doubt about the validity of an advance decision, an application may be made for a declaration from the Court of Protection.

The provision of information

Information may be provided to patients both verbally and in writing. Both of these have their merits, and an approach that combines the two is generally considered best practice. What is vitally important is that the information provided is up-to-date and correct, and for this reason it is important that healthcare professionals maintain their own transfusion knowledge and competence. Within the UK, the UK Blood Services provide patient information leaflets, which are regularly reviewed by expert groups to ensure accuracy. However, despite these being freely available, their use has been found to be variable and often limited. Court et al found that only 27% of surveyed patients were aware of these patient information leaflets [16], and the National Comparative Audit of Blood Transfusion found that only 28% recalled receiving any written information [9].

It is important that information is given to the patient, wherever possible, in a timely manner prior to the transfusion, allowing patients the time to digest, to read any written information, and to ask questions.

In order to ensure consent is informed, the following key areas must be discussed with the patient: the risks of transfusion, benefits of transfusion and alternatives to transfusion.

Risks of transfusion

The risks of transfusion will differ internationally. The current infectious risks of transfusion in the UK are shown in Table 2. Whilst many patients and healthcare professionals focus on the infectious risks of transfusion, there are also non-infectious risks which need to be considered for each individual patient. These include risks related to human error (wrong blood to patient), transfusion reactions, transfusion-associated circulatory overload, post-transfusion purpura and transfusion-associated acute lung injury. For patients requiring irradiated blood components, there is also the risk of transfusion-associated graft-versus-host disease, and for long-term multi-transfused patients, additional factors such as iron overload, allo-immunisation and platelet refractoriness (human leukocyte antigen [HLA] antibodies). It is important to discuss the risks of *not* receiving a transfusion, which will be fully dependent on the patient's individual clinical

Table 2. Infectious risks of transfusion in the UK. *Adapted from NHSBT (2013) Patient Information Leaflet 'Will I Need a Blood Transfusion?'.*

Infection	Estimated Infectious Risk
HIV	1 : 6.5 million donations
Hepatitis C	1 : 28 million donations
Hepatitis B	1 : 1.3 million donations
variant Creutzfeldt-Jakob Disease (vCJD)	Unquantifiable (classed extremely low risk)

condition, the indication for the transfusion, and whether any alternatives are available or suitable.

There is evidence that some patients may overestimate the actual risks of transfusion, especially in relation to infectious risks [17]. The process of consent may therefore also have the benefit of allaying any misconceptions about transfusion, reducing unnecessary concerns or fears.

Benefits of transfusion

These will be largely dependent on the individual patient's clinical condition and the indication(s) for the transfusion. It is essential that the transfusion is clinically appropriate, and any benefits must outweigh the risks.

It is important that the benefits of transfusion are not misconstrued. Friedman *et al* looked at what medical residents tell patients as part of informed consent for the blood transfusion process, and found that the benefits cited were not always true benefits, or that they were overestimated [12].

Alternatives to transfusion

There are a number of alternatives to transfusion, which may be appropriate depending on the patient's clinical condition and indication(s) for transfusion. These are discussed in detail in other chapters. The use of alternatives to blood transfusion may not be suitable for all patients, and some organisations may not have access to some of these. It is important that as a healthcare clinician, you are conversant with the various options that may be available and suitable to each individual patient.

How much information to give?

This question can leave many healthcare professionals in a dilemma. Some patients may have a multitude of underlying conditions or treatment requirements which have significant risks associated with them in addition to the need to have a transfusion. Consider these three scenarios:

- A patient who has been diagnosed with an acute form of leukaemia who will require regular multiple blood component transfusions as a mainstay of their treatment regime.
- A patient who is consenting for total hip replacement surgery, who, according to audit data for their surgeon, faces a 10% chance of needing a transfusion intra-operatively.
- A patient who is consenting for liver resection surgery, whose surgical prognosis is poor, and who has multiple additional significant risk factors which warrant discussion as part of the consent for surgery process.

Whilst a clinician may determine on behalf of the patient how much information should be given to each of these patients, is this right? How does the clinician know what a patient's pre-conceived perceptions of a blood transfusion are, how much information that a patient may (or may not) want or need, or how significant a transfusion may be to that patient?

In the UK, following the judgement in the case Montgomery v Lanarkshire Health Board (2015), the law relating to informed consent has changed [2]. The previous Bolam test (which asks whether a doctor's conduct would be supported by a reasonable body of medical opinion) no longer applies to the issue of consent. UK law now requires a doctor to take "reasonable care to ensure that the patient is aware of any material risks involved in any recommended treatment, and of any reasonable alternative or variant treatments". This decision reinforces principles already included in the General Medical Council consent guidance [18]. Sokol warns that a "pro forma approach to consent — repeating a memorised script — is a common but ethically and legally dubious practice", and states that doctors must ask themselves three questions [19]:

- Does the patient know about the material risks of the treatment I am proposing? What sort of risks would a reasonable person in the patient's circumstances want to know, and what sort of risks would this particular patient want to know?

- Does the patient know about reasonable alternatives to this treatment?
- Have I taken reasonable care to ensure the patient actually knows this?

Key factors here are 'material risk' with a focus on 'this particular patient'.

Patient choice also means that patients will differ in the amount of information they wish to receive. Some patients may state that they do not wish to receive any information. Reasons for this can be varied and multifactorial. It is generally accepted that no one else can make a decision on behalf of an adult who has capacity. The GMC states that in such cases, you should try to find out why they do not want to receive information, but if they are adamant, you should respect their wishes as far as possible [18]. However, you must still give them the information they need in order to give their consent, including what the treatment aims to achieve, what it will involve (e.g. whether the procedure is invasive) and if it involves any serious risks. You must document that the patient has declined any additional information.

Has the patient understood the information I have given?

In order for consent to be informed and valid, the patient needs to have understood what they have been told. This is again a difficult area where clinical judgement in needed. Sellinger suggests that patients are often giving consent without being truly informed because the information provided is often poorly understood or retained [3].

In 2011, Court *et al* looked at patient recall of the consent process and found that only 59% could recall discussing the need for transfusion [16]. Cheung *et al* also looked at patient recall following informed consent [20]. Whilst 100% of patients could recall being told a reason for the transfusion, only 85% recalled discussing the benefits, 33% the risks, and 24% recalled discussing any alternatives. Only 54% could remember discussing potential reactions during/after the transfusion. 33% stated that they had concerns or worries about the transfusion.

How to do it

Within the UK, the Advisory Committee on the Safety of Blood, Tissues and Organs (SaBTO) produced a series of recommendations for consent for blood transfusion [21]. These are summarised in Table 3.

Focusing on 'competent' patients, or patients in an emergency situation, there are four key clinical patient groups to consider.

Patients where a transfusion has been determined clinically necessary as a 'one-off' procedure

In this situation, after making the clinical decision to transfuse, the healthcare professional (ideally the same healthcare professional who has made that clinical decision) should inform the patient of the reasons why a transfusion is clinically indicated (including what components are required), the risks and the benefits of the transfusion, the expected outcomes, and discuss any potential alternatives to the transfusion. Written information should also be provided where possible. Their right to refuse transfusion, along with the risks inherent in this choice, should also be discussed. Wherever possible, patients should be given the time and opportunity to assimilate this information and to ask questions. Depending on relevant legislation or guidance, best practice would be that this discussion and subsequent patient decision is recorded in the patient's clinical notes, or on a dedicated consent form, with or without the patient's signature (depending on local requirements). An example flowchart checklist provided by SaBTO can be found in Figure 1 [22].

Patients requiring long-term multiple transfusion episodes over an extended period of time (e.g. a patient with thalassaemia)

In this situation, an important question to consider is how often should recurrently transfused patients be asked to provide consent? Should this be for every transfusion episode, for every admission, or should the consent cover a set period of time (e.g. relevant for 1 year)? There are no clear answers to this question. What is important is that patients

Table 3. Summary of UK SaBTO (2011) consent for transfusion recommendations.

Clinical recommendations:

- Valid consent for blood transfusion should be obtained and documented in the patient's clinical record by the healthcare professional.
- There should be a modified form of consent for long-term multi-transfused patients, details of which should be explicit in an organisation's consent policy.
- There should be a standardised information resource for clinicians indicating the key issues to be discussed by the healthcare professional when obtaining valid consent from a patient for a blood transfusion (available at: www.transfusionguidelines.org/transfusion-practice/consent-for-blood-transfusion-1).
- There should be a standardised source of information for patients who may receive a transfusion in the UK (leaflets provided by NHS Blood and Transplant (England) are available at: http://hospital.blood.co.uk/patient-services/patient-blood-management/patient-information-leaflets/).
- Patients who have received a blood transfusion and who were not able to give valid consent prior to the transfusion should be provided with information retrospectively.
- SaBTO good practice guidance to help identify the most effective way of providing information retrospectively when patients were unable to give prior consent is available at: www.transfusionguidelines.org/transfusion-practice/consent-for-blood-transfusion-1.

Educational recommendations:

- UK Blood Services should have an ongoing programme for educating patients and the public about blood transfusion.
- Use of the www.learnbloodtransfusion.org.uk e-learning package should be promoted by the UK Blood Services and Royal Colleges for all staff involved in the blood transfusion process.
- Consent for blood transfusion should be included in the undergraduate curriculum as part of the learning objectives outlined for the principles of consent.

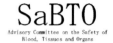

GUIDANCE FOR CLINICAL STAFF

TO SUPPORT PATIENT CONSENT FOR BLOOD TRANSFUSION

Patient may require Blood / Blood Component Transfusion

Patients receiving a blood transfusion (red cells, platelets or plasma) whether for a medical or surgical cause should be informed of the indication for the transfusion including risks, benefits and alternatives. A record of this discussion should be documented in the patient's clinical records.

Ideally the decision to transfuse should be made with the patient or parent/carer in advance of any planned transfusion.

In the emergency setting, the information will need to be given retrospectively.

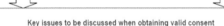

Prospective Information	Retrospective Information
Valid consent* should be obtained prior to any planned transfusion and documented in the patient's clinical record.	Patients treated in emergency setting where it was not possible to obtain valid consent pre-transfusion.
*Valid consent entails the provision of information on risks, benefits and alternatives available before asking the patient to give consent. This does not have to include a signature from the patient.	Patients who were told pre-procedure (e.g. pre-operatively) that they *might* require a transfusion then need to be informed whether they did/did not receive a transfusion.

Key issues to be discussed when obtaining valid consent

1. The following information should be discussed:
   o Type of blood / blood component
   o Indication for transfusion
   o Benefits of the transfusion
   o Risks of transfusion
   o Possible alternatives to transfusion
   o How the transfusion is administered and the importance of correct patient identification
   o Inform patient that following a blood transfusion they can no longer be a blood donor.
2. Provide written information.
3. Check if patient needs time to consider or requires further information.
4. Document the discussion in the patient's clinical records.

At discharge

1. If patient has had a transfusion, ensure that they have been informed.
2. Record information about the transfusion in the discharge summary, also stating that the patient has been informed.

Figure 1. SaBTO (2011) guidance for clinical staff to support patient consent for blood transfusion.

understand that they can ask questions at any time throughout their treatment. If there are known changes to the risks, benefits or available alternatives, this should be a key consent trigger point.

Patients where it is thought that a transfusion may be required as part of a procedure, e.g. during surgery, but is not definite at the time of pre-procedure consent

Where a procedure carries a possibility that a transfusion may be needed, but the patient will be incapacitated (e.g. anaesthetised) during the procedure, they will not be able to consent at the point that the transfusion is deemed necessary. These patients therefore need to consent to the prospect of a transfusion pre-procedure. They should be given the same information as any other patient consenting for transfusion, and this should be documented in the same way.

Post-procedure, and before being discharged home, the patient should be given confirmation as to whether or not they received a transfusion. Apart from the ethical considerations that any patient should know whether they actually did or did not receive another person's blood, in the UK this has particular importance. Since 2004, any person in the UK who has received a blood donation is excluded from donating in future. This measure was introduced as a means of restricting the potential spread of variant Creutzfeldt-Jakob disease (vCJD). During their review of consent for transfusion, SaBTO identified that patients who are unaware whether they have received a blood transfusion may go on to donate blood when they should not [23].

Emergency situations where it is not possible to consent the patient pre-transfusion

In an emergency situation where a patient may be temporarily incapacitated and unable to provide consent, it is generally deemed acceptable (and indeed expected) for healthcare professionals to act in the best interests of the patient and to provide the immediate treatment that is necessary to preserve life.

However, any *known* previously held beliefs must be taken into account. If the patient has clearly given an advanced directive while still competent, treating physicians are bound to respect this [3].

Within the UK, when a patient lacks capacity, the GMC states that you must consider[18]:

• Whether the patient's lack of capacity is temporary or permanent.
• Which options for treatment would provide overall clinical benefit for the patient.
• Which option, including the option not to treat, would be least restrictive of the patient's future choices.
• Any evidence of the patient's previously expressed preferences, such as an advance statement or decision.
• The views of anyone the patient asks you to consult, or who has legal authority to make a decision on their behalf, or has been appointed to represent them.
• The views of people close to the patient on the patient's preferences, feelings, beliefs and values, and whether they consider the proposed treatment to be in the patient's best interests.
• What you and the rest of the healthcare team know about the patient's wishes, feelings, beliefs and values.

When the patient regains capacity, they must be informed what treatment they have received and why, and this discussion should be documented in the patient's clinical records.

An example retrospective information flowchart checklist provided by SaBTO can be found in Figure 2 [24].

Conclusions

Informed decision-making and valid consent is an essential part of patient-centred care, and healthcare professionals have a responsibility to ensure that patients are aware of the decisions for, and any associated material risks, benefits and alternatives, of blood component transfusion.

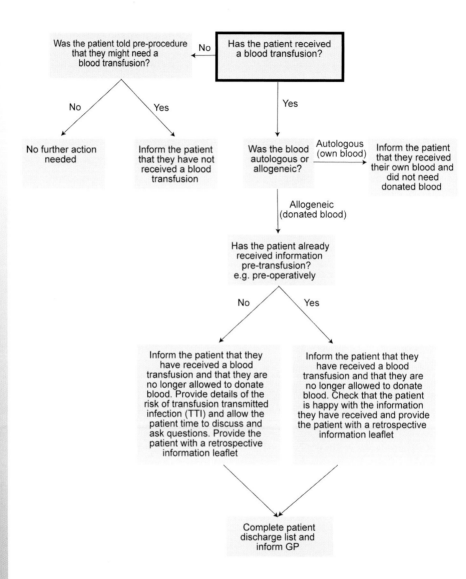

Figure 2. SaBTO (2011) consent for blood transfusion: retrospective patient information — good practice guidance.

The first step is to ensure the decision to transfuse is appropriate, based on best practice guidelines and individual patient assessment. It is vital that all healthcare professionals involved in the consent for transfusion process are knowledgeable and competent in appropriate blood transfusion practices, and the use of available alternatives to transfusion.

Checklist summary

Ensure that:

✓ You are aware of your responsibilities for consent for transfusion, and national/local requirements regarding documentation of consent.

✓ You maintain your own transfusion knowledge and competency, and knowledge of any alternatives to transfusion.

✓ All your decisions to transfuse are appropriate, based on individual patient clinical assessment and indications (risk vs. benefit), and having considered any alternatives to transfusion.

✓ Patients are provided with sufficient information for them to make an informed decision, allowing time (wherever possible) for them to assimilate the information and to ask questions.

✓ You use written patient information to supplement verbal discussions.

✓ Following an informed discussion, accept a (competent) patient's right to refuse treatment, even if their decision appears irrational to you. Document any decisions clearly, seek additional advice as appropriate in a timely manner and fully explore alternative treatment options.

✓ Patients who have consented to a possible transfusion pre-procedure, or who were transfused during an emergency (and the patient is therefore unaware of the transfusion) are provided with retrospective confirmation that they have received a transfusion when they have regained capacity and prior to discharge home.

References

1. Queensland Health. Health informed decision-making in healthcare policy. Brisbane: Queensland Health, 2012.

2. Montgomery (Appellant) v Lanarkshire Health Board (Respondent) (Scotland) (2015) UKSC 11.

3. Sellinger CP. The right to consent: is it absolute? *Br J Med Pract* 2009; 2(2): 50-4.

4. Gillon R. Medical ethics: four principles plus attention to scope. *Br Med J* 1994; 309: 184-8.

5. Williams FG. Consent for transfusion. *Br Med J* 1997; 315: 380-1.

6. Farrell AM, Brazier M. Patients should consent to blood transfusion. *Br Med J* 2010; 341: c4336.

7. European Blood Alliance Member Consultation: consent to transfuse. Unpublished internal report. Latvian Blood Service, 2008.

8. Davis R, Vincent C, Sud A, *et al.* Consent to transfusion: patients' and healthcare professionals' attitudes towards the provision of blood transfusion information. *Transfus Med* 2012; 22: 167-72.

9. National Comparative Audit of Blood Transfusion. 2014 Audit of Patient Information and Consent. http://hospital.blood.co.uk/media/27580/2014-audit-of-patient-information-consent.pdf.

10. World Health Organisation. Patients' rights, 2015. http://www.who.int/genomics/public/patientrights/en/.

11. O' Brien KL, Champeaux AL, Sundell ZE, *et al.* Transfusion medicine knowledge in postgraduate year 1 residents. *Transfusion* 2010; 50: 1649-53.

12. Friedman M, Arja W, Batra R, *et al.* Informed consent for blood transfusion: what do medicine residents tell? What do patients understand? *Am J Clin Pathol* 2012; 138: 559-65.

13. The Mental Capacity Act 2005. The Stationery Office. http://www.legislation.gov.uk/ukpga/2005/9/contents.

14. Adults with Incapacity (Scotland) Act 2000. http://www.legislation.gov.uk/asp/2000/4/contents.

15. British Medical Association. Advance decisions and proxy decision-making in medical treatment and research, 2007. http://www.bma.org.uk/.

16. Court EL, Robinson JA, Hocken DB. Informed consent and patient understanding of blood transfusion. *Transfus Med* 2011; 21: 183-9.

17. Ngo LT, Bruhn R, Custer B. Risk perception and its role in attitudes toward blood transfusion: a qualitative systematic review. *Transfus Med Rev* 2013; 27(2): 119-28.

18. General Medical Council. Consent: patients and doctors making decisions together, 2008. http://www.gmc-uk.org/static/documents/content/Consent_-_English_1015 .pdf.

19. Sokol DK. Update on the UK law on consent. *Br Med J* 2015; 350: h1481.

20. Cheung D, Lieberman I, Callum J. Consent for blood transfusion: do patients understand the risks and benefits? *Transfus Med* 2014; 24: 269-73.

21. Advisory Committee on the Safety of Blood, Tissues and Organs (SaBTO). Patient consent for blood transfusion, 2011. https://www.gov.uk/government/publications/ patient-consent-for-blood-transfusion .

22. Advisory Committee on the Safety of Blood, Tissues and Organs (SaBTO). Guidance for clinical staff to support patient consent for blood transfusion, 2011. www.transfusionguidelines.org/transfusion-practice/consent-for-blood-transfusion-1.

23. Howell CA, Forsythe JLR. Patient consent for blood transfusion - recommendations from SaBTO. *Transfus Med* 2011; 21: 359-62.

24. Advisory Committee on the Safety of Blood, Tissues and Organs (SaBTO). Consent for blood transfusion: retrospective patient information - good practice guidance, 2011. www.transfusionguidelines.org/transfusion-practice/consent-for-blood-transfusion-1.

Chapter 9

Patient consent in children

Olugbenga Akinkugbe LLB MA MRCPCH
Specialty Registrar in Paediatrics, Imperial College Healthcare NHS Trust, London, UK
David Inwald FRCPCH FFICM PhD
Consultant and Honorary Senior Lecturer in Paediatric Intensive Care, Imperial College
Healthcare NHS Trust, London, UK
Helen New PhD FRCP FRCPath
Consultant in Paediatric Haematology and Transfusion Medicine, Imperial College
Healthcare NHS Trust/NHS Blood and Transplant, London, UK

- "... childhood is entitled to special care and assistance." [1]

- "According to the World Health Organization a significant proportion of patients who receive blood transfusions are children [2]. As for adults, blood transfusion in children is a medical procedure associated with risks so consent should be obtained for this procedure."

- "Obtaining consent in children raises specific social, ethical and legal issues, and requires special consideration of the principle of 'best interests'. These all have implications both for a child's ability to give consent to and refuse medical treatment."

Background

The United Nations Convention on the Rights of the Child [1] is an international treaty that outlines the social, economic and health rights of children. Currently, 194 countries are signatories but the principles may be applied in all countries. The Convention articles relevant to consent in children include:

- Article 12 which concerns the importance of children being allowed to express their views:

"... Parties shall assure to the child who is capable of forming his or her own views the right to express those views freely in all matters affecting the child, the views of the child being given due weight in accordance with the age and maturity of the child" [1].

- Article 14 which highlights the role of parents and legal guardians:

"... Parties shall respect the rights and duties of the parents and, when applicable, legal guardians, to provide direction to the child in the exercise of his or her right in a manner consistent with the evolving capacities of the child" [1].

Several countries have enacted laws that promote the principles outlined in the Convention. In England and Wales, the Children Act of 1989 [3] places obligations upon parents, local authorities, courts and other organisations to safeguard children and promote their welfare. In the UK, professional guidance from the General Medical Council and the Nursing and Midwifery Council also requires doctors and nurses to safeguard and protect the health and well-being of children and young people [4, 5].

Obtaining consent for blood transfusion or any other medical procedure is a legal and ethical requirement. If a medical treatment were performed without consent it might be considered an assault on the person [6]. The views of young people should be taken into account and respected when making decisions that affect them [7].

Best interests

The 'best interests' of children must always be the primary concern when making decisions that affect them [1].

The principle of best interests is used in many countries including the UK [7], the USA [8], South Africa [9] and Australia [10]. There is no standard definition for determining best interests and it will vary according to the child's individual situation. Table 1 contains some important factors to consider when determining best interests.

Table 1. Summary of 'best interests' considerations.

- The child's views and wishes including any previously expressed preferences.
- The views of parents and others close to the child or young person.
- Religious, cultural or other beliefs and values relevant to the child or parents.
- Safety and well-being.
- Enabling the child to develop and fulfil their potential [7].

The concept of best interests is frequently applied when making decisions on behalf of patients (children and adults) who are unable to make decisions [11]. For example, in an emergency situation where a blood transfusion may be necessary to save life or prevent serious illness, treatment can be given on the basis of the child's best interests. In unclear situations or where there is a disagreement about the best interests of the child, it may be necessary to seek legal advice.

Competence

Background to competence in children

Competence is the ability to perform a particular task or duty [12]. A person's competence is relative to the task or decision to be made and in the context of this chapter it refers specifically to the ability to make decisions about blood transfusion. Another way to describe competent individuals is to say they have capacity. Competence is an important component of consent for all patients but it is particularly significant for children and young people for two reasons:

- Adults are generally presumed to be competent to make medical decisions but this cannot be presumed in children because of young age or neurological disability (although the latter may also be relevant in adults).
- Whereas in adults the issues of consent and refusal of treatment are treated in the same manner, a child's capacity to refuse treatment is treated differently to the capacity to consent.

In relation to children and young people, age is often the main factor affecting the capacity to both give consent and refuse treatment.

Age, childhood and the threshold of adulthood

A child is defined by the United Nations in its Convention on the Rights of the Child as a human being below the age of 18 years [1]. The legal threshold of adulthood varies worldwide between administrative divisions but the stated age is 18 in England and Wales [13] and many other jurisdictions.

This threshold is of significance to the ability to give consent because, as we have seen, adults are generally presumed competent to consent or refuse medical treatment. In practice a child may develop the maturity to consent to medical treatment before the age of 18. This is because autonomy develops and progresses with the child's age so the ability to make decisions often occurs before the age at which the law considers them to be adults [14].

Parental responsibility

In some situations children and young people under 18 will be unable to give consent. If a child lacks capacity, for example, because of immaturity, learning disability or illness, consent may be obtained from an individual with parental responsibility.

The law on parental responsibility differs between countries so practitioners should be aware of the applicable guidance in their area. In England and Wales, the Children Act [3] states that the following individuals automatically have parental responsibility (Table 2):

- A child's biological mother.
- A father who is married to the mother when the child is born.
- A father who is not married to the mother but is registered on the child's birth certificate (applies to children born after 1 December 2003) [15].

Fathers outside of the above situations and civil partners can legally acquire parental responsibility in accordance with the Children Act [16]. Parents do not lose parental responsibility if they divorce. In some situations legal guardians and other individuals who provide care for the child, such as teachers, may give consent for medical procedures.

Table 2. Summary of those with parental responsibility (England & Wales).

- Biological mother.
- Father married to mother at time of child's birth.
- Father registered on child's birth certificate (if child born after 1 December 2003).
- Individuals who legally acquire parental responsibility.
- Guardians and other carers in accordance with the child's best interests [3, 15, 16].

Consent between the ages of 16 and 18

Individuals from the age of 16 up to 18 are considered as having the same capacity to give consent for medical treatment as those aged 18 and over [13]. Therefore, the process of obtaining consent for blood transfusion in children between 16 and 18 should be performed as for those aged 18 and over.

Consent in children under 16

The position for children under 16 is more complex. This was considered in the case of Gillick [17]. Gillick, a mother of four children, sought a court declaration that doctors should not offer contraceptive advice to children under 16 without the consent of their parents. The House of Lords held that any child with sufficient understanding can consent to treatment. However, the young person must be able to demonstrate 'Gillick competence' [17] (see Table 3).

Table 3. Summary of factors required to demonstrate 'Gillick competence' (children under 16).

The child must be able to:

- Understand information.
- Retain information.
- Use and weigh information.
- Communicate their decision.

In addition they must be able to understand:

- What the treatment is.
- Why it is proposed.
- Its benefits and risks.
- The consequences of not proceeding with it [17].

It is important to re-emphasise that competence is relative to the nature of the decision being made. As such a 16-year-old who is competent to consent to a blood transfusion may not be competent to consent to another procedure, such as a heart transplant. Healthcare professionals should consider the child's maturity and understanding in relation to the specific situation. Provision of information about the procedure should therefore be given in an age-appropriate format.

Refusal of treatment

In England and Wales the law in relation to children considers the child's ability to consent to medical treatment differently to the ability to refuse (Figure 1). In several cases, courts have held that the right of a minor to refuse treatment is not absolute and can be overridden by an individual with parental responsibility or by a court [18, 19].

When faced with such decisions courts have generally favoured an outcome that is in the best interests of the child. A refusal of treatment, for example, refusal of blood transfusion in a child with life-threatening anaemia, is unlikely to be upheld by a Court [6].

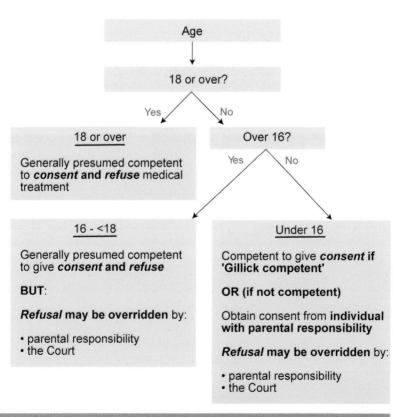

Figure 1. Assessing a child's competence to give consent and refuse medical treatment.

Clinical context of consent for blood transfusion in children

A recent national survey of blood transfusion practice in children in the UK showed that the majority of red cell transfusions for those in non-neonatal wards were for patients with underlying haematologic or oncologic diagnoses (53%). Surgical patients (including cardiac surgery) accounted for the second largest transfused group (26%) [20].

The survey also showed that transfusions take place in a range of settings:

- General paediatric wards.
- Day-care wards.
- Haematology/oncology/bone marrow transplant wards.
- Operating rooms.
- Paediatric intensive care units.
- Neonatal units.

Given the variety of clinical conditions and settings in which children receive blood transfusions, the approach to consent will involve different considerations depending on the context. Healthcare professionals caring for children who receive blood transfusions should be aware of the general considerations for children outlined above as well as specific issues for their patient, and should be able to discuss them with the patient, parents or guardians as appropriate and provide information in an age-appropriate format. Discussion of these issues is often an integral part of the care in paediatric haematology, oncology and cardiac units but should be regarded as no less important for patients transfused in other clinical areas.

Neonates and blood transfusions

"Children transfused in fetal or neonatal life have the longest potential lifespan in which to develop late adverse effects of transfusion"
Transfusion Handbook (UK) [21].

In the UK and many other countries several measures are taken to minimise the risks of blood transfusion to neonates. These include providing additional safety features for neonatal blood components [22] and reducing the need for blood transfusion by decreasing blood sampling, iron supplementation and adopting restrictive blood transfusion policies for stable neonates.

In this patient group the same principles apply as for older children. It is important that the decision to give a blood transfusion is made in the best interests of the baby and that consent is obtained from a person with parental responsibility following provision of appropriate information.

Emergencies and the incapacitated patient

In emergencies and other situations where it is not possible to obtain consent, decisions about blood transfusions should be taken on the basis of the child's best interests, as outlined above.

Situations where blood transfusions may be refused

A competent young person or parent may refuse a blood transfusion for several reasons. One of the most well-recognised reasons is on the grounds of religious beliefs. For example, Jehovah's Witnesses decline transfusions of whole blood, red cells, white cells, platelets and unfractionated plasma [21]. The donation of blood is also contrary to the religious beliefs of many Jehovah's Witnesses. However, many will accept autologous blood transfusions (for concurrent procedures) and fractions of blood such as albumin, immunoglobulin, cryoprecipitate and clotting factors [21].

There have been numerous occasions where the conflict between deeply held religious beliefs and life-saving blood transfusion has been placed before the courts. In these situations English courts have been reluctant to support decisions both from competent children [23] and parents [6] when they have refused life-saving transfusions on the basis of their religious beliefs. Decisions by Canadian [24] and German [25] courts have been consistent with this.

Jehovah's Witnesses have established Hospital Liaison Committees to provide information to hospitals and clinicians. These Liaison Committees are available to offer support in individual cases in both emergency and elective situations. Negotiations may be facilitated by the adoption of techniques that aim to minimise transfusion requirements, including the use of erythropoietin in neonates and cell salvage in elective surgical procedures and multidisciplinary input is likely to be required (see Chapters 14-20 for further details of strategies to minimise the need for blood transfusion).

In situations where there are differences of opinion between professionals and the patient or those with parental responsibility, the priority must always be to safeguard the best interests of the child. If it is not possible to reach a consensus it may be necessary to seek a court order.

Documenting consent

Guidance on documentation of consent has been provided by The Advisory Committee on the Safety of Blood, Tissues and Organs (SaBTO) [26, 27] endorsed by the British Committee for Standards in Haematology [28] and by the UK Transfusion Handbook [21].

In the United Kingdom there is currently no requirement to obtain written consent for blood transfusion. Documented verbal consent is adequate and considered to be valid by SaBTO [26]. However, there are variations in practice so local policies should be followed. In all cases, good communication, using sources of age-appropriate information [29], is essential and it is important to document the following in the patient's record:

- The discussions, indications, decision-making process leading to transfusion.
- Consent (written or verbal, and by whom).

Practical guidance and information

A key component of competence is the ability to understand information. In order to provide valid consent the child and/or person with parental responsibility must be given all the information required to make an informed decision regarding a blood transfusion. (The use of 'parent' below includes those with parental responsibility.)

Practical guidance when obtaining informed consent for blood transfusion has been given by SaBTO [30] and is summarised here, modified for paediatric transfusion recipients:

- Children and/or parents of children receiving a blood transfusion (red cells, platelets or plasma) whether for a medical or surgical indication should be informed of the reason for the transfusion including risks, benefits, consequences and alternatives. Other key issues to discuss include:
  - type of blood/blood component;
  - mode of administration and the importance of correct patient identification;
  - inform them that following a blood transfusion they can no longer be a blood donor.
- Ideally the decision to transfuse should be made with the child or parent in advance of any planned transfusion and valid consent documented in the patient's clinical record. Some hospitals may require signed written consent.
- In the emergency setting where it is not possible to obtain valid consent pre-transfusion, the child or parent will need to be given information retrospectively. This must also be documented in the patient's clinical record.
- If, prior to a procedure, a child or their parent were told the child might require a transfusion, they should subsequently be informed whether the child did or did not receive a transfusion.
- Children and parents should be offered information, including a standardised information leaflet in a form that is age-appropriate and easy for them to understand. They should be given time to consider the information and an opportunity to ask questions.

Conclusions

Practitioners undertaking blood transfusions in children should be aware of the special considerations that differentiate this group of patients from adults. Where possible, the autonomy of children should be promoted but practitioners must also be able to identify those with parental responsibility when working with children who lack capacity. Older children cannot be presumed to have capacity to make decisions about medical treatment so it may be necessary for their competence to be demonstrated. It should also be appreciated that a child's refusal of treatment has different legal implications to consent. The overriding consideration must always be the best interests of the child.

Checklist summary

✓ Decisions affecting children must be made in their best interests.

✓ Children and young people should be involved in decisions about blood transfusion where possible.

✓ Maintain good communication and provide information in a form that is easy for children and parents/guardians to understand.

✓ Assess capacity for consent and refusal using the flowchart in Figure 1.

✓ Young people age 16-18 can give consent.

✓ Those under 16 can give consent if they are 'Gillick' competent.

References

1. United Nations General Assembly. United Nations Convention on the Rights of the Child, November 1989. http://www.unicef.org.uk/Documents/Publication-pdfs/UNCRC_PRESS200910web.pdf.

2. World Health Organization Blood Safety and Availability, Fact sheet No 279, June 2014. http://www.who.int/mediacentre/factsheets/fs279/en/.

3. Children Act 1989. http://www.legislation.gov.uk/ukpga/1989/41/contents.

4.   General Medical Council. Good medical practice: duties of a doctor, 2013. www.gmc-uk.org.

5.   Nursing and Midwifery Council. Working with young people, 2012. www.nmc-uk.org.

6.   Mason JK, Laurie GT. Consent to treatment. In: *Mason and McCall Smith's Law and Medical Ethics*, 8th ed. Oxford, UK: Oxford University Press, 2011.

7.   General Medical Council. Good medical practice: 0-18 years: guidance for all doctors. www.gmc-uk.org.

8.   Child Welfare Information Gateway. Determining the best interests of the child, 2012. Washington DC, USA: US Department of Health and Human Services, Children's Bureau.

9.   South African Constitution Act No 108 of 1996, s28(2) from Dausab Y. The best interest of the child. In: *Childrens Rights in Namibia*. Ruppel OC, Ed. Windhoek, 2009. www.kas.de/upload/auslandshomepages/namibia/Children.../children_h.pdf.

10.   Australian Law Reform Commission. The best interest principle in seen and heard: priority for children in the legal process (ALRC Report 84), 1997. Canberra, Australia: Australian Government. www.alrc.gov.au/publications/16-childrens-involvement-family-law-proceedings/best-interests-principle.

11.   Mental Capacity Act 2005, ss. 3-4. http://www.legislation.gov.uk/ukpga/2005/9/contents.

12.   Beauchamp T, Childress J. *Respect for Autonomy in Principles of Biomedical Ethics*, 6th ed. Oxford, UK: Oxford University Press, 2009.

13.   Family Law Reform Act 1969. http://www.legislation.gov.uk/ukpga/1969/46.

14.   Bridgeman J. Because we care? The medical treatment of children. In: *Feminist Perspectives on Health Care Law*. Sheldon S, Thomson M, Eds. London, UK: Cavendish, 1998: 97-114.

15.   Children Act 1989, ss. 2-6. http://www.legislation.gov.uk/ukpga/1989/41/contents, as amended by the Adoption and Children Act s111. http://www.legislation.gov.uk/ukpga/2002/38/contents.

16.   Gheera M. Parental responsibility. Standard Note SN/SP/2827.

17.   Gillick v West Norfolk and Wisbech. AHA [1996] 3 All ER 402.

18.   Re: R (A Minor) [1991] 4 All ER 177 CA.

19.   Re: W (A Minor) (Medical Treatment) [1992] 4 All ER 627.

20.   New HV, Grant-Casey J, Lowe D, *et al*. Red blood cell transfusion practice in children: current status and areas for improvement? A study of the use of red blood cell transfusions in children and infants. *Transfusion* 2014; 54: 119-27.

21.   Norfolk D, Ed. *Handbook of Transfusion Medicine*, 5th ed. United Kingdom Blood Services, 2013. http://www.transfusionguidelines.org.uk/transfusion-handbook.

22.   New HV, Stanworth SJ, Engelfriet CP, *et al*. Neonatal transfusions. *Vox Sang* 2009; 96: 62-85.

23. Re: E (A Minor) [1993] 1 FLR 386.

24. A.C. v. Manitoba (Director of Child and Family Services), 2009 SCC, [2009] 2 S.C.R. 181.

25. Decision of the German Federal Constitutional Court: [1] BVerfG, 1 BvR618/93 vom 2.8.2001.

26. The Advisory Committee on the Safety of Blood, Tissues and Organs (SaBTO). Guidance for clinical staff to support patient consent for blood transfusion (version 1.1). SaBTO, 2011.

27. The Advisory Committee on the Safety of Blood, Tissues and Organs (SaBTO). Patient consent for blood transfusion. SaBTO, 2011. https://www.gov.uk/government/uploads/system/uploads/attachment_data/file/2165 86/dh_130715.pdf.

28. British Committee for Standards in Haematology. Guideline on the administration of blood components. Consent for blood transfusion addendum, 2012. http://www.bcshguidelines.com/documents/BCSH_Blood_Admin_-_addendum_August_2012.pdf.

29. NHS Blood and Transplant Patient information leaflets. http://hospital.blood.co.uk/patient-services/patient-blood-management-resources/patient-information-leaflets/.

30. The Advisory Committee on the Safety of Blood, Tissues and Organs (SaBTO). Guidance for clinical staff to support patient consent for blood transfusion, 2011. http://www.transfusionguidelines.org.uk/transfusion-practice/consent-for-blood-transfusion-1.

Chapter 10

Using clinical audit to improve transfusion practice

John Grant-Casey BSc RN
Programme Manager, National Comparative Audit of Blood Transfusion, NHS Blood and Transplant, Oxford, UK

- "We cannot solve our problems with the same thinking we used to create them."
  Albert Einstein

- "Insanity is doing the same thing over and over again and expecting different results."
  Albert Einstein

- "Quality is not an act — it is a habit."
  Aristotle

- "There is only one corner of the universe that you can be certain of improving, and that is yourself."
  Aldous Huxley

- "Quality is doing it right when no one's looking."

Background

Clinical audit is the systematic critical analysis of healthcare delivery comparing outcomes and practice against defined, evidence-based guidance. It enables care providers and patients to know where their service is doing well, and where there could be improvements.

With its origins in medical audit in the mid 1980s, audit has evolved to now include the work of many healthcare professionals, which in the context of hospital-based blood transfusion can include transfusion laboratory staff, nursing staff, operating department staff and those staff who decide to use blood as part of clinical management.

Typically, clinical audit comprises a number of process steps, set out in Figure 1.

Let's look at these steps in more detail in the context of blood transfusion.

A. Decide on a topic for audit

There are four good reasons for auditing an aspect of transfusion practice: high risk, high cost, high volume and local interest.

High risk

If the management of a particular clinical situation can pose a high risk, you can manage that risk by auditing the practice. For example, there are metabolic consequences and complications of performing a massive neonatal red cell transfusion [1], and so auditing each episode can confirm that practice is optimal or reveal areas for improvement, hence reducing the number of times that the risk translates to harm.

A. Decide on a topic for audit.

B. Agree the clinical behaviours to be audited, based on evidence-based guidance where possible.

C. Agree what data should be collected, any data cleaning necessary, and how the data will be analysed and presented so that data is transformed into information that will help practitioners to understand why practice needs to be improved and how they can achieve that improvement.

D. Practice the data collection, cleaning, analysis and reporting by conducting a pilot audit with a limited number of clinical areas. In one healthcare setting this might be a few patients in a select number of areas, but for audits conducted at a countrywide level the audit will be piloted in a number of hospitals.

E. Evaluate the pilot data — that is, was it easy to collect and are the responses valid, or in other words, did the questions return the kinds of answers you were expecting? Did the cleaning, analysis and reporting of the data go as planned?

F. Make any necessary changes to the dataset to be collected and the plans for processing the data, and then run the audit.

G. Process and report the data and provide feedback reports to the appropriate people.

H. Allow some time for the information to be absorbed by healthcare practitioners and for any recommendations to be implemented, and then re-audit to see if the anticipated improvements in care have been delivered.

Figure 1. Eight steps in conducting a clinical audit.

High cost

A procedure can be expensive because of the cost of the blood products, equipment and human resources involved in carrying it out. Auditing a high-cost event can help to ensure that value for money is being obtained, either by demonstrating that the event proceeds without waste or that the desired outcome has been achieved.

High volume

Many things are done repeatedly in transfusion practice, such as the taking of blood samples for testing prior to the administration of blood. If the sampling or labelling practice reveals errors, then there is the possibility that those errors can affect many patients, so systematically checking a sample of phlebotomy practice helps to provide assurance that quality control procedures are effective.

Local interest

Sometimes an event may have occurred that does not fit into the above categories but it is something that has generated local concern. For example, audit can reveal that patients awaiting an exchange transfusion during a painful crisis have to wait for treatment because of the length of time it takes to establish a central line *in situ*. Performing this earlier in the patient journey or having more staff trained in the process can shorten that wait, helping to resolve the painful crisis sooner.

B. Agree the clinical behaviours to be audited, based on evidence-based guidance where possible

In transfusion medicine, as in many other areas of healthcare, there is often a shared agreement about what constitutes the best way to treat a particular patient. These agreements are often issued in the form of guidelines by various professional bodies or by government health departments. Practice is also influenced by published research, but for some areas of practice there simply is neither agreement on nor evidence to support one particular way of managing a patient.

For the purposes of clinical audit, though, it is important to decide what evidence is to be used to judge the quality of healthcare given. The audit will eventually collect data on how a healthcare professional has acted, and so needs to define its measures: what constitutes good practice and where is the evidence to support the claim that it is practice that should be universally adopted?

Standards

Clinical audits most commonly are 'criterion-based audits', where clinical performance is measured against one or more criteria. These can be quantitative, qualitative or both. For example, a healthcare provider may set a standard that 100% of patients who attend a pre-operative assessment clinic have a blood sample taken for a full blood count, in order to assess if the patient is anaemic and if that anaemia can be corrected. An audit may show that this is only being achieved in 80% of patients, so efforts are made to improve practice. Auditing over time will hopefully show an upward trend. The standard here is *100% of patients attending the pre-operative assessment clinic have a full blood count performed to assess them for anaemia.* While that provides information about the quantity of patients being assessed, it does not say anything about the quality of the process. Suppose, for example, you wanted the healthcare professional to also give the patient information about blood transfusion and explain the risks, benefits and alternatives. You could still count the number of times this happened, but that would not tell you if that information or explanation was provided appropriately. The standard, therefore, changes to become one in which behaviour is described. For example, *The physician gives the patient, during the pre-operative assessment, the leaflet "Do I need a blood transfusion?" and tells the patient why they need a transfusion and how they will benefit, explains what the risks are and if there are alternatives.* This is a standard that contains three important points: **What** is done, **when** and **who** does it. There is a useful acronym to use when writing standards for a clinical audit — standards must *RUMBA!* — see Table 1.

Table 1. Writing standards for audit.

	X	✓
Relevant	Patients must be seen within 10 minutes of their appointment time — not *relevant to the quality of transfusion practice.*	Patients are given the leaflet that explains the need for blood transfusion.
Understandable	Patients must be told of the importance of following instructions — *not universally understandable: can be interpreted in different ways.*	A blood sample is taken and a full blood count requested.
Measurable	All patients must be completely satisfied after their visit — *not easy to measure: who will define what equates with complete satisfaction and how can it be objectively measured?*	The healthcare professional records the patient's previous medical history in the care record.
Behavioural	Pre-transfusion Hb must not be higher than 130g/L for men — *there is no indication of who does what.*	The physician only requests platelets if the platelet count falls below the agreed level.
Achievable	All iron-deficient patients have their anaemia corrected through the use of oral therapy — *not achievable because some patients cannot tolerate oral iron and so are given it parenterally.*	The date and start time of unit of red cells transfused is documented in the care record.

Standards should be written in the present tense: not *A post-transfusion Hb should be/ought to be/must be taken after each unit of blood transfused,* but *A post-transfusion Hb **is** taken after each unit of blood transfused.* The standard is unequivocal — the Hb either is or is not taken.

C to G. Agree what data should be collected/fed back to appropriate people

Having set standards you now know what clinical behaviour you are trying to measure, and so the next step is to agree what data will best inform you about current practice. Such data are often collected from the written care record; for example, evidence that a procedure was carried out or a clinical test result used to support a decision. Besides these data, healthcare staff and service users can be surveyed for their opinions, and systems and processes can be observed to check if the expected actually occurs. Data can be collected by recording it on paper and then keying it into computers for analysis, or can be drawn from existing electronic sources. It is useful to trial data collection on a small sample or records or people, and this serves two purposes: it enables a sense check to see that everyone understands what is being asked and allows a validity check so you can see that the information you get is the information you were expecting.

Once your data collection questionnaires are ready, you can plan how to analyse and report the data you collect, and how you will turn that data into useful and relevant information for those who will receive the report. Remember that there may be more than one audience and so you may need to tailor your analysis and feedback accordingly. Analysis can be descriptive, when you use the data to represent a snapshot of the current situation: how many patients seen, age groups, average amount of blood transfused, and so on. Analysis is most useful when it is qualitative — when it compares the current situation to best practice, identifies the reasons for any deficiencies and suggests remedies.

Making a difference

Many audit reports are informative but not useful — they paint a problematical picture but do not provide solutions, and the power of clinical audit soon wanes if your report criticises without putting forward constructive recommendations. A good recommendation is one that is based on the data you collect, which itself has been used to measure practice against some agreed benchmark. Suggesting who should do what, when and how, and how the reader will know that doing that has made a difference, is much more likely to be useful to a reader than merely presenting a report that highlights problems without analysing why they occur or what might be done to improve things.

H. Allow some time for the information to be absorbed

Having reported your audit you need to allow time for the report to be read, its contents absorbed, debated and discussed. Change is sometimes very difficult to achieve and healthcare professionals can be quite defensive about their practice, especially when they are accustomed to a degree of autonomy. It is useful to structure some time to discuss the report and create an action plan for change, and this can be done about 1 month after the report is issued. As part of these discussions, it is good practice to plan to audit the topic again — what is known as "closing the audit loop" (Figure 2).

Your audit can show that practice is acceptable or that change is required, but unless you re-audit you will not know if the acceptable level of practice is maintained or if the changes put in place have improved practice. The healthcare environment is a dynamic one. Staff and patients change, as does treatment which is moderated by such things as academic research, new drugs and techniques, the socioeconomic environment and emerging disease. Continuous audit allows you to measure change over time and to demonstrate consistent if not improving quality of care.

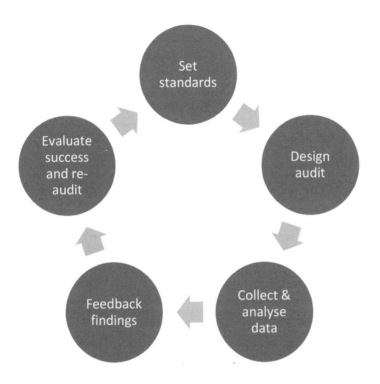

Figure 2. The audit loop.

Clinical audit and clinical governance

Clinical audit, then, is a mechanism for agreeing best practice and collecting information to assess if local practice is the best it can be. It is the systematic, critical evaluation of healthcare against a pre-defined, evidence-based standard.

Clinical governance goes wider in that it is a systematic approach to maintaining and improving the quality of patient care within a health system. The English Department of Health defines clinical governance as "A framework through which NHS organisations are accountable for continually improving the quality of their services and safeguarding high

Table 2. Clinical governance themes.

Theme	Examples of issues that are covered by each theme
Accountabilities and structures	• Clarity and effectiveness of committee responsibilities. • Clarity and effectiveness of staff responsibilities at all levels of the organisation (board, top management team, directorate teams). • Adequacy of monitoring and reporting arrangements.

Strategies and plans	• Extent to which there is a coherent strategy for the activity...
	• ...that is broken down into actionable plans and is resourced (staff, budget).
	• Extent to which strategies and plans for different clinical governance activities are connected to wider quality improvement programmes.
	• Involvement in the development of strategies and plans by:
	  - patients and the public;
	  - stakeholder organisations.
	• Resources (staff and budget) to support the implementation of the strategy.

Application of policies, strategies and plans	• Extent to which systems are implemented and operational.
	• Effectiveness of communication to staff, and their understanding of their responsibilities.
	• Extent of:
	  - staff involvement in the activity;
	  - multidisciplinary involvement;
	  - team-based involvement;
	  - cross-team involvement;
	  - cross-organisation involvement.

Continued

Table 2 _continued_. Clinical governance themes.

Theme	Examples of issues that are covered by each theme
Quality improvements and learning	• Extent to which information from the activity is considered systematically and is acted upon. • Extent to which use of the information has led to quality improvements. • Dissemination of lessons learnt and whether organisation-wide improvements have resulted.

Resources and training for staff and patients	• Access to, and use of, resources to support essential processes and systems, e.g.:
	   - information and means of accessing it;
	   - human and financial resources to support systems.
	• Uptake of training by staff.

standards of care by creating an environment in which excellence in clinical care will flourish" [2].

This definition is intended to embody three key attributes: recognisably high standards of care, transparent responsibility and accountability for those standards, and a constant dynamic of improvement. In short, clinical governance describes the structures, processes and culture needed to ensure that healthcare organisations — and all individuals within them — can assure the quality of the care they provide and are continuously seeking to improve it. Since the term was first introduced, it has been recognised that these structures and processes should be fully integrated with other aspects of the governance of healthcare organisations, including their financial, information and research governance. Table 2 illustrates some of the clinical governance themes that can be used in a clinical governance programme.

Conclusions

All the elements discussed so far can be in place and yet practice could still remain unchanged. Clinical audit and clinical governance takes time and consumes valuable resources, and to become a worthwhile investment certain structures need to be in place. There needs to be a *shared vision* of what constitutes good-quality healthcare, and that vision has to encompass the views of many stakeholders, including those who commission it, those who consume it and those who deliver it. There also has to be a *shared belief* that change and improvement is possible as well as desirable.

The measures used to assess quality of care must be agreed by those whose practice will be audited, and sufficient data must be collected to demonstrate a representative sample of practice. Failure to engage healthcare professionals will almost certainly lead to a failure to change. Results should be fed back in a meaningful way so that those considering the report can see how it relates to their day-to-day practice, and understand why change is important to achieve. Healthcare professionals are seldom motivated by bad news but have a genuine desire to give of their best, so audit feedback which describes what needs to be changed, why and how, and how a practitioner can tell when things become better, are all important parts of any report.

Monitoring the quality of healthcare is challenging because new pressures, new evidence, new research and new patient demands constantly change the environment, but those who use health services expect, and should get no less than, the highest level of care that can be provided. Clinical governance provides the structure in which that care can be overseen and clinical audit provides the means to monitor and improve it.

Checklist summary

✓ Clinical audit is a legitimate inquiry into the quality of work performed by healthcare practitioners, and if done correctly, can lead to consistent improvement in care.

✓ Deciding what and when to audit can be based on high cost, high volume, high risk or local concern. If something is not done well, then resources are wasted, many patients are affected and patients are harmed by the manifestation of risk.

✓ Healthcare professionals are taught to use evidence to inform practice but also to be autonomous. Audit design must be based on a sound evidence base for good practice, or a consensus of best practice if no formal evidence exists, otherwise why should they change?

✓ When deciding on what data to collect, ask yourself how those data will help you to comment on the quality of practice. If they don't do that, don't collect the data. Audit is not cheap research.

✓ Practice operating your audit in a pilot phase, engaging actual healthcare professionals in the pilot. Their experience, observations and advice will be invaluable in running the real thing. Plan and timetable the various stages of activity.

✓ Behaviour change theory strongly supports giving feedback in a timely way, as close to the measured behaviour as possible. Report your audit in weeks rather than in months. Tell people how their practice compares to good practice, what they need to do to change and when they need to do it. Audit again to see if you have made a difference.

References

1. Bharadwaj A, Khandelwal M, Bhargava SK. Perioperative neonatal and paediatric blood transfusion. *Indian J Anaesth* 2014; 58(5): 652-7.

2. Scally G, Donaldson LJ. Clinical governance and the drive for quality improvement in the new NHS in England. *Br Med J* 1998; 317: 61-5.

Chapter 11

Who needs transfusion?

Jonathan Wallis BA MB BS FRCP FRCPath
Consultant Haematologist, Freeman Hospital, Newcastle-upon-Tyne, UK

- "States of the body really requiring the infusion of blood into the veins are probably rare: yet we sometimes meet with cases in which the patient must die unless such operations can be performed."
  James Blundell, often regarded as the "Father of blood transfusion".
  Lancet, June 13th 1828 [1].

- "Accidents following transfusion have been sufficiently frequent to make many medical men hesitant to advise transfusion except in desperate cases." [2]

- "A restrictive strategy of red-cell transfusion is at least as effective as and possibly superior to a liberal transfusion strategy in critically ill patients." [3]

Background

James Blundell's original trials of clinical transfusion in the early 1800s were not followed up for many years not least because of frequent occurrence of acute haemolysis. In 1901, Karl Landsteiner speculating on the clinical implications of his discovery of the A, B and O blood groups wrote: "Finally, it must be mentioned that the reported observations allow us to explain the variable results in therapeutic transfusions of human blood" [4]. A few years later in New York, Ottenburg described the use of a serological test, the cross-match, to match donor with patient before transfusion [2]. These critical advances paved the way for the safer transfusion of red cells than Blundell had been able to achieve. Blood transfusion slowly became an established clinical intervention for the treatment of surgical, traumatic or obstetric blood loss. In the second half of the 20th century, blood transfusion really accelerated. Improved donor collection, red cell storage and matching procedures, together with the stimulus of a growing number of surgical procedures such as joint replacement and cardiac surgery, saw a dramatic increase in the clinical use of blood transfusion.

The value of red cell transfusion to keep the haemoglobin level near normal was perhaps not initially questioned and the main disadvantages were considered to be infection and haemolysis, but during the 1980s and 1990s clinicians began to ask whether red cell transfusion was always beneficial. In 1990, Blair *et al* suggested that transfusion for upper gastrointestinal (GI) haemorrhage actually increased the risk of rebleeding and a poor outcome [5]. Evidence from renal transplant centres suggested that prior transfusion increased survival of kidney allografts [6]. The mechanism was hypothesised to be some form of immunosuppression or modulation. This raised the possibility that in other circumstances this might have adverse effects, such as on tumour growth or infection after surgery. In 1999, the influential Canadian TRICC trial (Transfusion Requirements In Critical Care) demonstrated that in the small subgroup of haemodynamically stable patients on intensive care units receiving top-up transfusions, a more conservative approach to transfusion was as good and possibly better than a liberal approach [3]. The results of these trials chimed with clinicians' growing concerns about the cost and efficacy of liberal transfusion and since the turn of the last century we have witnessed a steady fall in the use of red cell transfusion for surgical indications. Medical use, however, is stable or increasing in part due to the ageing population with their specific clinical needs [7].

We are now fortunate to have an increasing body of good-quality clinical trials to drive a more evidenced approach to red cell transfusion (Table 1). This chapter will set out why we transfuse red cells, when red cell transfusion is likely to be of benefit to the patient, and where it is of no value or possibly harmful.

Table 1. Some important randomised controlled trials of red cell transfusion thresholds.

Trial and year of publication	Patient group	Patient number	Low threshold	High threshold	Result
Blair et al, 1986 [5]	Acute severe GI bleeding	50	80g/L	All transfused	Liberal transfusion associated with increased rebleeding
TRICC trial, 1999 [3]	Haemodynamically stable patients on intensive care	838	70g/L	100g/L	Restrictive group had non-significantly better outcomes than liberal group
TRIPICU, 2007 [34]	Haemodynamically stable children on paediatric intensive care ward	637	70g/L	95g/L	Identical outcomes in both groups
TRACS trial, 2010 [22]	Unselected cardiac surgery patients	502	Hct 24% (80g/L)	Hct 30% (100g/L)	Primary outcome equal. Liberal group had non-significantly better survival
FOCUS trial, 2011 [21]	Patients with fractured hip requiring surgery and known or high risk of cardiovascular disease	2016	Symptoms of anaemia or Hb <80g/L at physician's discretion	100g/L	No differences in any pre-specified outcome

Table 1 *continued*. Some important randomised controlled trials of red cell transfusion thresholds.

Trial and year of publication	Patient group	Patient number	Low threshold	High threshold	Result
Transfusion Strategies for Acute Upper Gastro-intestinal Bleeding, 2013 [18]	Acute and subacute GI bleeding	921	70g/L	90g/L	Better survival and reduced rebleeding in restrictive group
Womb trial, 2014 [35]	Postpartum anaemia (48-79g/L)	521	48g/L	79g/L	No clinically significant differences in quality of life parameters
TRISS study, 2014 [27]	Patients with anaemia and septic shock	1005	70g/L	90g/L	No difference in mortality or other specified outcomes
TITRe2 trial, 2015 [23]	Cardiac surgery patients at high risk of transfusion	2003	75g/L	90g/L	No difference in primary specified composite outcome Significantly fewer deaths at 30 days and lower incidence of acute kidney injury in liberal group

What do red cells do?

Red cells carry oxygen from the lungs via the body's blood circulation to tissues. All cells require oxygen for aerobic metabolism but cardiac muscle and brain are particularly dependent on plentiful oxygen supplies. The brain extracts about 30% of the oxygen from the cerebral blood supply but cardiac muscle extracts 50-60% of bound oxygen. Exercising skeletal muscle has a high demand for oxygen but usage depends entirely on activity. Anaemia reduces the viscosity of blood compensating in part for the reduced oxygen content of the blood through increased blood flow through the microcirculation. However, if insufficient oxygen is supplied to the heart it will fail to pump sufficient blood to maintain adequate perfusion of other tissues. The result is cardiac failure and peripheral organ dysfunction. Increased cardiac demand is normally met by increasing coronary blood flow. Patients with coronary artery disease with stenosed vessels are therefore at particular risk of developing cardiac failure due to anaemia. When additional demands for oxygen come from exercise, anaemia will limit both the cardiac response and also reduce the endurance of the skeletal muscle. Evidence in animal studies and humans confirms that at rest anaemia as low as 50g/L can be well tolerated in health, but that coronary artery disease reduces this leeway considerably [8-11]. Evidence from doping in athletics and from physiological testing shows that higher haemoglobin increases physical endurance [12].

The response to anaemia, the need for correction and any thresholds for possible transfusion will therefore depend on factors such as the patient's cardiac status, the activity expected of them (whether recovering in bed or pursuing an active life) and also if and when the anaemia will correct without transfusion.

Red cells have other functions including modulation of microcirculation and a role in haemostasis, but oxygen carriage is the principal function.

Why do we transfuse red cells?

There are five main indications for transfusing red cells:

* **Acute blood loss/uncontrolled haemorrhage**. The aim is to prevent death from massive blood loss. This might be due to trauma, surgery, childbirth or internal bleeding such as from a ruptured aneurysm or gastric ulcer.
* **Recoverable anaemia in a haemodynamically stable patient**. The aim is to improve short-term outcomes from surgical and other causes of anaemia. This might be after blood loss during elective surgery or

due to a treatable haematinic deficiency. The anaemia will recover in time but transfusion is given with the intention of improving or speeding up recovery and rehabilitation.

- **Bone marrow failure**. The aim is to improve longer-term quality of life in patients whose bone marrow is unable to make enough red cells to maintain a satisfactory haemoglobin level. The typical case might be a patient with myelodysplasia or thalassaemia whose everyday activities, without transfusion, are severely curtailed by marked anaemia.

- **Exchange transfusion**. The aim is to replace the patient's own red cells that are causing damage. This might be in infants at risk of kernicterus from maternal antibody-induced haemolysis or due to sickle cell haemoglobin causing an acute life-threatening crisis or more chronic cerebral damage.

- **Radiotherapy**. The aim is to improve response to cancer treatment. There is observational evidence to suggest that a Hb >100g/L is associated with a better response to radiotherapy for cervical cancer.

Acute blood loss (Table 2)

During a period of rapid blood loss the circulating blood volume falls from the normal average of 70ml per kg lean body mass, but the haemoglobin concentration does not immediately change. With time there is a movement of extravascular fluid into the circulation, and/or intravenous fluids are given causing haemodilution and anaemia. For patients not receiving intravenous fluid the rate of haemodilution is probably related to the amount of blood lost. Blood donors giving a single unit of blood show relatively little change over 24 hours especially if not bedbound. Bedbound patients show slightly more rapid haemodilution. After major acute blood loss the rate of haemodilution is much faster and quite large falls in haemoglobin may be seen in a short period [13]. Nevertheless, the Hb level should not be used as a primary indication of the amount of blood lost not least because the pre-bleed haemoglobin level is not necessarily known. Blood volume loss in acute haemorrhage is therefore better judged by physiological factors such as blood pressure, pulse rate/pressure and skin perfusion, allied where possible to other interventional measurements such as left atrial filling. These physiological measures may also be difficult to interpret. Patients with 'clean' trauma such as stab wounds may behave very differently, with hypotension and a relative bradycardia, to patients with blunt trauma and tissue damage who typically have a marked tachycardia and vasoconstrictor response. Patients who are anaesthetised or who have had a spinal anaesthetic may also have a poor vasoconstrictor response to hypovolaemia. Therefore, observed blood loss, physiological measurements and laboratory measures all need to be considered. A blood loss of 20-30% will in general lead to marked hypotension and, where bleeding is continuing, urgent red cell transfusion, either allogeneic or autologous (if cell salvage is underway), should be considered.

Acute blood loss of 50% or more is life-threatening. The use of major haemorrhage packs/protocols in these settings may be life-saving. Appropriate use of a one-to-one ratio of plasma and red cells has been shown to be beneficial in reducing early haemorrhagic deaths in both retrospective and in prospective studies [14, 15].

Two other factors need to be considered during resuscitation from acute haemorrhage. Haemostasis as judged by the skin bleeding time is increased when the haemoglobin falls below 100g/L [16]. It has been hypothesised that platelets are pushed to the periphery of small blood vessels by red cells and that at lower haematocrits this effect is lost. Maintenance of an adequate haemoglobin of around 90-100g/L may therefore improve haemostasis, though there is no randomised study evidence to support this contention. Secondly, in major trauma, before surgery to halt the bleeding, and in some elective surgical operations, a policy of permissive hypotension is recommended to lower arterial and more especially capillary and venous filling and so reduce the rate of bleeding. Red cell transfusion and other intravenous fluid replacement must therefore be used judiciously to maintain a reasonable haematocrit without overly increasing the blood pressure in keeping with these policies. The effect of transfusion on arterial, venous and capillary pressures may be particularly important in GI bleeding. An early randomised study in acute upper GI blood loss found that liberal blood transfusion was associated with more rebleeding and poorer outcome [5]. Retrospective evidence [17] and a more recent and larger randomised study [18] have both confirmed this finding. It is suggested that increased pressures in the splanchnic circulation following red cell transfusion leads to further bleeding, and that splanchnic hypotension as in permissive hypotension in surgery reduces bleeding. Both prospective studies in GI bleeding excluded patients with haemodynamic instability and neither study included sufficient patients with known cardiovascular disease to decide if this subgroup should be treated differently.

Table 2. Examples of severe blood loss.

- A 28-year-old male motorcyclist involved in a road traffic accident is admitted within 1 hour with abdominal pain and distension, a blood pressure of 80/40mmHg and a pulse of 120/minute. Haemoglobin done at the bedside is 110g/L. He is bleeding internally and the haemoglobin is a poor indicator of acute blood loss. Call for the major haemorrhage pack and transfuse appropriately to maintain blood pressure whilst arranging urgent imaging or surgery.

- A 37-year-old multiparous mother with epidural anaesthesia delivers at term with a poorly contracting uterus. She has approximately 1L of visible blood loss with ongoing bleeding per vagina. Blood pressure is 80/50mmHg with a pulse of 120. Haemoglobin is 80g/L after 2L of crystalloid over 1 hour. Although the epidural anaesthesia may be contributing to the hypotension, she is bleeding actively and at serious risk. Do not delay calling for the major haemorrhage pack. Start transfusing red cells and plasma according to the major haemorrhage protocol. Arrange urgent testing of coagulation whether by bedside devices such as rotational viscoelastometry or by conventional laboratory tests.

- A 54-year-old man with a history of alcohol abuse is admitted with a 4-day history of malaena. He has a blood pressure of 110/60mmHg with a pulse of 90. Haemoglobin is 80g/L. He has sub-acute blood loss but is haemodynamically well compensated. He has already haemodiluted. Do not transfuse red cells while he is haemodynamically stable. Arrange for an urgent endoscopy for active treatment of likely variceal bleeding. Red cell transfusion may increase splanchnic venous pressure and increase the risk of rebleeding and mortality.

Recoverable anaemia in a haemodynamically stable patient (postoperative and other anaemias in patients without bone marrow failure) (Table 3)

Patients who are haemodynamically stable with new anaemia perhaps due to blood loss associated with surgery will, if otherwise healthy, show little change in haemoglobin for about 7 days, after which time there will be a fairly rapid erythroid response with a recovery of about two-thirds of the Hb deficit by 28 days assuming iron stores or supplies are adequate [19]. No association with speed of rehabilitation, time in hospital or quality of life measures has ever been demonstrated for moderate postoperative anaemia (>80g/L) [20, 21].

Table 3. An example of a recoverable anaemia in a haemodynamically stable patient.

- A 40-year-old female patient has a pre-operative Hb of 140g/L, loses a little more than a third of her blood volume during spinal surgery and on day 1 postoperatively has a Hb of 80g/L. The level will not change much for a week but by day 28, assuming the patient is not iron depleted or in renal failure, her Hb will have recovered to just over 120g/L. She will not benefit from red cell transfusion. Ensure adequate iron stores or dietary iron. Increased erythropoietin levels due to the anaemia will increase absorption from oral iron supplements postoperatively.

Following the TRICC trial of liberal versus conservative transfusion in stable patients in the intensive therapy unit (ITU) [3], a move towards lower postoperative transfusion trials has been followed worldwide. There were concerns that this threshold might not be suitable for elderly and frail patients especially those with cardiovascular disease. The Focus trial looked at just such patients who had suffered a hip fracture with emergency operative repair [21]. The trial found that despite being high-risk patients, there was no difference in any outcome whether they were given a transfusion threshold of 80g/L or 100g/L Hb. It should be noted that those in the more liberal transfusion arm did not fare any worse than those in the conservative arm, unlike the TRICC trial, and this may be due to the type of red cell units used (low-volume residual plasma and largely leuco-reduced units). Nor did patients with more transfusion suffer more infections or other adverse effects. In other words transfusion was not bad for you, but neither was it good for you down to a trigger of 80g/L either to prevent medical problems or to promote rehabilitation. Most patients in the restrictive transfusion arm of this study had a lowest haemoglobin of around 85g/L. The patients either had documented cardiac disease or had significant risk factors for such disease. They did not have acute cardiac decompensation or ischaemia. The place of transfusion in these patients remains uncertain. Two recent prospective randomised studies of transfusion policy in patients undergoing cardiothoracic surgery had similar results but came to slightly different conclusions. Hajjar et al in the TRACS trial reported no significant difference in overall outcomes with a trigger for transfusion of 24% haematocrit (Hb of 80g/L) as compared to 30% haematocrit (Hb of 100g/L) both intra-operatively and postoperatively in a total of 502 patients mainly having coronary artery grafting [22]. The TITRe2 study compared a transfusion trigger of 75g/L with 90g/L in the postoperative period only in 2003 patients with more valve replacements than coronary artery grafts alone. The pre-specified composite outcome was not different between the groups, but in sub-analyses showed an increased incidence of acute kidney injury and an increased incidence of death at 90 days in the restrictive group [23]. The absence of harm from blood transfusion and the possible early benefits of a higher postoperative haemoglobin level in the latest study suggest that we should remain cautious about allowing too great a degree of anaemia in patients with known cardiac compromise.

How low can we safely go before transfusing in the cardiovascularly fit patient? Studies of patients who refuse blood transfusion have shown that remarkable degrees of anaemia may be tolerated. Morbidity increases once the Hb falls below 50g/L and mortality increases when the Hb is less than 30g/L[11], but again there is evidence that those with coexisting cardiac disease do less well [10]. Anecdotal reports, liable to publication bias, do report survival with nadir haemoglobin levels as low as 10g/L; however, these patients require intensive support. Guidelines from various professional bodies around the world recommend a threshold of 60-70g/L for younger fitter patients and a threshold of 70-80g/L for the older less fit patients. The available evidence supports these guidelines. For those with poorly controlled heart failure or acute coronary syndrome, the evidence, from large retrospective surveys, is contradictory [24, 25]. A threshold of 90g/L is prudent and some have argued for the use of fresh blood with preserved 2,3-diphosphoglycerate (2,3-DPG) and thus immediate oxygen delivery if available (blood of 7 days' storage or less). However, in a large and diverse population of patients on intensive care and requiring ventilation, the use of fresher blood gave no improvement in outcome [26].

Easily treatable causes of red cell production failure, e.g. iron deficiency or vitamin B12 deficiency, should be treated without transfusion. Patients who have become anaemic slowly may tolerate profound anaemia with little complaint. A normal response to adequate oral iron is, like the response to postoperative anaemia, prompt, with a 50% recovery of the haemoglobin deficit in 21 days. Patients with vitamin B12 deficiency may present with very profound anaemia. Transfusion for compensated pernicious anaemia has in the past been associated with catastrophic heart failure. This may have been due to a mixture of volume overload, the provision of old blood with initially poor oxygen delivery and possible effects on myocardial function of severe vitamin B12 deficiency. Transfusion in such patients should be avoided, or if felt clinically vital, be given as a single unit at a time (with freshest blood available), transfused as slowly as possible, with diuretic cover.

Another specific group of patients are those with sepsis. Following the TRICC trial there remained concern that this subgroup might be better served by a higher haemoglobin. However, a large prospective study found no difference in outcome between those randomised to a liberal or restrictive trigger for transfusion [27].

The division between acute bleeding and stable anaemia is not always precise. Over reliance on transfusion should be avoided but patients must not be allowed to die or suffer morbidity because of irrational patient or physician fear of blood transfusion.

Medical patients with infective or inflammatory disease may have marked secondary anaemia and are sometimes transfused. Anaemia in such patients is due both to a reduction in red cell production and an increased rate of red cell destruction (a shortened red cell life span). The clinical response to transfusion is often limited, and because of the shortened red cell life span the anaemia usually recurs fairly rapidly. It is better to treat the underlying cause and manage any symptoms of anaemia via other means. There are no trials of note to support practice in these patients. Transfusion before an operation may be considered but consideration may then be given to the use of erythropoietin as an alternative.

Bone marrow failure

Possible causes are outlined in Table 4.

Table 4. Commoner causes of marrow failure requiring red cell transfusion.

Inherited causes:

- Thalassaemia.
- Haemoglobinopathies, e.g. sickle cell disease.
- Diamond-Blackfan syndrome.
- Fanconi's anaemia.
- Red cell functional defects, e.g. hereditary spherocytosis.

Aquired non-clonal causes:

- Pure red cell aplasia.
- Immune and other forms of acquired haemolysis.
- Aplastic anaemia.

Clonal causes:

- Acute leukaemias.
- Myelodysplasia.
- Myelofibrosis.
- Myeloma.
- Lymphoma.
- Non-haemopoietic marrow infiltration.

In patients where blood loss or breakdown exceeds the marrow's capacity to replace (e.g. chronic GI loss), treatment should primarily be aimed at treating the cause. This is not always possible and then transfusion must be tailored to maintain a level at which the patient's everyday function is not overly impaired (Table 5).

Table 5. An example of chronic blood loss exceeding marrow production capacity.

- A 75-year-old man with a mechanical mitral valve has a paravalvular leak. He requires prophylactic anticoagulation that cannot be stopped other than for short periods but has evidence of chronic GI blood loss. Investigation reveals no clear site of bleeding and it is thought he has angiodysplasia affecting either the small or large bowel. His iron stores are severely depleted despite previous transfusion and his endogenous erythropoietin level is appropriately high. He is unable to maintain his Hb with oral iron alone. He is given regular intravenous iron which maintains his haemoglobin at around 90g/L with a good quality of life. Transfusion is avoided but is an option if his quality of life suffers due to worsening anaemia.

The total body haemoglobin (rather than the absolute venous level) has a direct and linear effect on the maximal oxygen consumption and expenditure of physical energy. Endurance athletes in particular are aware of this. The optimal level of haemoglobin depends on the individual patient and the activities he/she undertakes (Table 6). Although response to anaemia varies considerably most patients feel short of breath when climbing stairs or a small hill when the Hb falls below 100g/L. Shopping becomes more of a chore. Many remark on a tendency to fall asleep during the day when the level is below 80g/L. When down to 60g/L, some, though not all, feel profoundly weary and fatigued undertaking relatively minor tasks such as dressing. Symptoms of cardiac failure are much increased. Activities that require significant energy expenditure become impossible. Oddly, angina symptoms are often not increased or prominent, perhaps due to the better flow characteristics of blood with a low haematocrit. There are very few studies on the effects of chronic

Table 6. Transfusion thresholds in marrow failure.

- An elderly bed-bound patient with myelodysplasia finds attending hospital difficult. She has few symptoms with a Hb of between 70 and 100g/L. Avoid transfusion if possible. Only transfuse if her quality of life is demonstrably impaired by the anaemia.
- A young mother with aplastic anaemia struggles to perform normal domestic chores when her Hb falls to 90g/L. She is better served by an active transfusion regime to maintain her Hb between 90-120g/L with active iron chelation therapy to prevent transfusional iron overload.
- A 55-year-old cycling enthusiast with myelodysplasia plans to follow a Tour de France stage, the etap. Agree to maintain his haemoglobin at 140g/L prior to the competition.

transfusion on adult patients and as such there is little evidence to guide us. That will hopefully be addressed soon. In the meantime practice is largely based on established custom and clinical experience.

Although it may be tempting to transfuse patients to maintain a minimum Hb of, say 10g/dL, this must be balanced against the long-term iron accumulation, and the cost, potential risks and inconvenience of transfusion.

Thalassaemia

Patients with thalassaemia and similar conditions represent a special group with different requirements. Most of these patients will require life-long transfusion and thus are particularly at risk of iron overload. At the same time they develop anaemia early in life when physical growth and cerebral development may be critically affected by anaemia, and when excessive marrow activity may result in bony deformities such as frontal 'bossing' of the skull. Transfusion therefore has a number of indications unique to the disease phenotype. Recommendations come from specialist groups that suggest maintaining the pre-transfusion Hb between 90 and 105g/L and the post-transfusion Hb at <145g/L. The typical transfusion interval should be 2-3 weeks [28].

There are at present few prospective studies to guide transfusion thresholds or patterns. Some patients have found that regular transfusions of one or two units, with less fluctuation on the Hb level, is preferable to having 4 units every 4 weeks.

Exchange transfusion

Exchange transfusion is indicated in a small number of specific clinical conditions:

* Allo-immune neonatal haemolysis with dangerous levels of hyperbilirubinaemia.
* As an emergency for sickle cell crisis with certain clinical features or stroke.
* As part of a chronic programme of transfusion for sickle cell anaemia to reduce sickle cell haemoglobin and to minimize iron overload.
* To remove inadvertently transfused mismatched ABO red cells.

The use of exchange transfusion for adjuvant treatment of very heavy *Falciparum* malarial infection is no longer recommended [29].

The detailed indications and protocols for exchange transfusions are outside the remit of this chapter.

Radiotherapy

Observational studies have suggested that patients having radiotherapy for cancer of the cervix had a better long-term outcome with fewer relapses if their Hb was above 100g/L at the time of treatment [30]. This benefit was seen both in those whose Hb was in any case well maintained and in those whose Hb was boosted by transfusion. It was hypothesised that the better Hb level improved oxygenation of the tumour and so increased the effect of radiotherapy (which works by creating oxygen radicals which then damage DNA). A subsequent study, with this mechanism in mind, looked at the outcome from radiotherapy when using exogenous erythropoietin to maintain the Hb level. Contrary to expectations this resulted in a poorer outcome with higher rates of cancer progression [31]. Similar studies in head and neck cancer and breast cancer all found that use of administered erythropoietin was unexpectedly associated with a greater risk of relapse and tumour progression [32]. Erythropoietin may have protected tumours by inducing heat shock proteins or increasing blood vessel growth within the tumour. It is arguable that the clinical benefit of a higher Hb as observed by Grogan *et al* may have been by suppression of endogenous erythropoietin excretion rather than effects on tumour oxygenation. Transfusion to a Hb of 10-11g/dL remains a standard practice in many units and without contrary evidence remains a valid indication for red cell transfusion whether it is working through increased oxygen delivery to the tumour, or by suppressing endogenous erythropoietin levels.

Risks of blood transfusion

Many initiatives have improved the safety of blood transfusion over the years, ranging from Landsteiner's critical elucidation of the ABO blood group system to the more recent development of haemovigilance systems. In developed health systems the safety of individual components is now very high. There remain risks associated with how the components are used. Of these, perhaps the chief residual risk is of cardiac overload (TACO: transfusion-related cardiac overload) [33]. The majority of red cell transfusions are now given to haemodynamically stable patients, that is patients with normal circulating blood volumes. Some of these patients may be small and may have pre-existing cardiac failure. TACO has emerged as a significant cause of morbidity and mortality. Red cell transfusion should be prescribed in volumes appropriate to the patient's size and cardiac status whatever the indication. The questions to ask when considering transfusion for any patient are outlined in Table 7.

Table 7. Questions to ask when considering transfusion for any patient.

- Is the anaemia acute or chronic?
- Is the patient symptomatic of their anaemia?
- Does the patient have cardiovascular or respiratory disease?
- Is the patient septic or actively bleeding?
- Is the anaemia correctable or not by means other than transfusion?
- What is the quality of the red cells available for transfusion?
- What activity is expected of the patient?

Conclusions

Over the last 15 years there has been a 50% reduction in red cell use for surgical patients in the UK, despite an increase in numbers of patients and complexity of operations. This change has been echoed in many other countries. Even with this fall there remains room for further reduction in these patients. Medical use has remained stable but is expected to increase given the ageing demographic of most western populations. More than 60% of blood transfusions are now given for medical indications. Erythropoietin has proved helpful in a minority of cases but may carry risks. There is a need for more evidence-based guidance on optimum transfusion regimes in the chronically transfused medical patient. Until then we should transfuse red cells dependent on the patient, their condition, comorbidities and exercise requirements, and their future prospects of recovery of anaemia. Transfusion should be avoided where sensible alternatives exist.

Checklist summary

Active bleeding and haemodynamically unstable:

✓ Manage the source of the bleeding.

✓ Transfuse to maintain circulation and a haemoglobin of >90g/L.

✓ Use cell salvage if practical.

Sub-acute anaemia/bleeding (e.g. postoperative anaemia or GI bleeding):

✓ Transfuse sparingly according to age and cardiac status.

✓ Ensure adequate availability of iron.

Chronic correctable anaemia (e.g. iron deficiency):

✓ Avoid transfusion unless there are overriding clinical indications.

Bone marrow failure:

✓ Transfuse to maintain an adequate quality of life with a view to minimizing iron loading.

Exchange transfusion:

✓ Follow expert guidance/protocols.

Radiotherapy:

✓ Maintain haemoglobin at 110g/L by transfusion or haematinic replacement.

✓ Do not use erythropoietin.

References

1. Blundell J. The after management of floodings and on transfusion. *Lancet* 1828; 13: 673.

2. Ottenberg R, Kaliski DJ. Accidents in transfusion: their prevention by preliminary blood examination: based on an experience of one hundred twenty-eight transfusions. *JAMA* 1913; 61(24): 2138-40.

3.   Hébert PC, Wells G, Blajchman MA, *et al*. A multicenter, randomized, controlled clinical trial of transfusion requirements in critical care. Transfusion requirements in critical care investigators, Canadian Critical Care Trials Group. *N Engl J Med* 1999; 340: 409-17.

4.   Landsteiner, K. Agglutination phenomena in normal human blood. *Wien Klin Wochenschr* 1901; 14: 1132-4.

5.   Blair SD, Janvrin SB, McCollum CN, Greenhalgh RM. Effect of early blood transfusion on gastrointestinal haemorrhage. *Br J Surg* 1986; 73(10): 783-5.

6.   Opelz G, Graver B, Terasaki P. Induction of high kidney graft survival rate by multiple transfusion. *Lancet* 1981; 317(8232): 1223-5.

7.   Tinegate H, Chattree S, Iqbal A, *et al*. Ten-year pattern of red blood cell use in the North of England. *Transfusion* 2013; 53(3): 483-9.

8.   Geha AS, Baue AE. Graded coronary stenosis and coronary flow during acute normovolemic anaemia. *World J Surg* 1978; 2: 645-52.

9.   Weiskopf RB, Feiner J, Hopf H, *et al*. Fresh blood and aged stored blood are equally efficacious in immediately reversing anemia-induced brain oxygenation deficits in humans. *Anesthesiology* 2006; 104: 911-20.

10.   Carson JL, Duff A, Poses RM, *et al*. Effect of anaemia and cardiovascular disease on surgical mortality and morbidity. *Lancet* 1996; 348: 1055-60.

11.   Carson JL, Noveck H, Berlin JA, Gould SA. Mortality and morbidity in patients with very low postoperative Hb levels who decline blood transfusion. *Transfusion* 2002; 42(7): 812-8.

12.   Wright SE, Pearce B, Snowden CP, *et al*. Cardiopulmonary exercise testing before and after blood transfusion: a prospective clinical study. *Br J Anaesth* 2014; 113(1): 91-6.

13.   Wallace J, Sharpey-Schafer EP. Blood changes following controlled haemorrhage in man. *Lancet* 1941; 238(6162): 393-5.

14.   Borgman MA, Spinella PC, Perkins JG, *et al*. The ratio of blood products transfused affects mortality in patients receiving massive transfusions at a combat support hospital. *J Trauma* 2007; 63(4): 805-13.

15.   Holcomb JB, Tilley BC, Baraniuk S, *et al*. Transfusion of plasma, platelets, and red blood cells in a 1:1:1 vs. a 1:1:2 ratio and mortality in patients with severe trauma: the PROPPR randomized clinical trial. *JAMA* 2015; 313(5): 471-82.

16.   Valeri CR, Cassidy G, Pivacek LE, *et al*. Anemia-induced increase in the bleeding time: implications for treatment of nonsurgical blood loss. *Transfusion* 2001; 41(8): 977-83.

17.   Hearnshaw SA, Logan RF, Palmer KR, *et al*. Outcomes following early red blood cell transfusion in acute upper gastrointestinal bleeding. *Aliment Pharmacol Ther* 2010; 32(2): 215-24.

18.   Villanueva C, Colomo A, Bosch A, *et al*. Transfusion strategies for acute upper gastrointestinal bleeding. *N Engl J Med* 2013; 368(1): 11-21.

19.   Wallis JP, Wells AW, Whitehead S, Brewster N. Recovery from postoperative anaemia. *Transfus Med* 2005; 15(5): 413-8.

20.   So-Osman C, Nelissen R, Brand R, *et al.* Postoperative anemia after joint replacement surgery is not related to quality of life during the first two weeks postoperatively. *Transfusion* 2011; 51(1): 71-81.

21.   Carson JL, Terrin ML, Noveck H, *et al.* Liberal or restrictive transfusion in high-risk patients after hip surgery. *N Engl J Med* 2011; 365(26): 2453-62.

22.   Hajjar LA, Vincent JL, Galas FR, *et al.* Transfusion requirements after cardiac surgery: the TRACS randomized controlled trial. *JAMA* 2010; 304(14): 1559-67.

23.   Murphy GJ, Pike K, Rogers CA, *et al.* Liberal or restrictive transfusion after cardiac surgery. *N Engl J Med* 2015; 372(11): 997-1008.

24.   Rao SV, Jollis JG, Harrington RA, *et al.* Relationship of blood transfusion and clinical outcomes in patients with acute coronary syndromes. *JAMA* 2004; 292: 1555-62.

25.   Wu WC, Rathore SS, Wang Y, *et al.* Blood transfusion in elderly patients with acute myocardial infarction. *N Engl J Med* 2001; 345(17): 1230-6.

26.   Lacroix J, Hébert PC, Fergusson DA, *et al.* Age of transfused blood in critically ill adults. *N Engl J Med* 2015; 372(15): 1410-8.

27.   Holst LB, Haase N, Wetterslev J, *et al.* Lower versus higher hemoglobin threshold for transfusion in septic shock. *N Engl J Med* 2014; 371(15): 1381-91.

28.   Cappellini MD, Cohen A, Eleftheriou A, *et al.* Guidelines for the clinical management of thalassaemia [internet]. Nicosia (CY): Thalassaemia International Federation, 2008: 5-7.

29.   Tan KR, Wiegand RE, Arguin PM. Exchange transfusion for severe malaria: evidence base and literature review. *Clin Infect Dis* 2013; 57(7): 923-8.

30.   Grogan M, Thomas GM, Melamed I, *et al.* The importance of hemoglobin levels during radiotherapy for carcinoma of the cervix. *Cancer* 1999; 86(8): 1528-36.

31.   Thomas G, Ali S, Hoebers FJ, *et al.* Phase III trial to evaluate the efficacy of maintaining hemoglobin levels above 12.0g/dL with erythropoietin vs. above 10.0g/dL without erythropoietin in anemic patients receiving concurrent radiation and cisplatin for cervical cancer. *Gynecol Oncol* 2008; 108(2): 317-25.

32.   Henke M, Laszig R, Rübe C, *et al.* Erythropoietin to treat head and neck cancer patients with anaemia undergoing radiotherapy: randomised, double-blind, placebo-controlled trial. *Lancet* 2003; 362(9392): 1255-60.

33.   Piccin A, Cronin M, Brady R, *et al.* Transfusion-associated circulatory overload in Ireland: a review of cases reported to the National Haemovigilance Office 2000 to 2010. *Transfusion* 2015; 55(6): 1223-30.

34.   Lacroix J, Hébert PC, Hutchison JS, *et al.* Transfusion strategies for patients in pediatric intensive care units. *N Engl J Med* 2007; 356: 1609-19.

35.   Prick BW, Jansen AJG, Steegers EAP, *et al.* Transfusion policy after severe postpartum haemorrhage: a randomised non-inferiority trial. *Br J Obstet Gynaecol* 2014; 121(8): 1005-14.

Chapter 12

Blood stock management from a laboratory perspective

Julie Staves BSc FIBMS

Transfusion Laboratory Manager, Oxford University Hospitals NHS Foundation Trust, Oxford, UK

- "The ordering of the blood products is usually managed within the laboratory and this is a key step in the management of stock."

- "The rotation of blood stocks is relevant in all laboratories."

- "Reviewing blood stocks and wastage is an important part of ensuring products are not wasted."

- "Many hospitals use the percentage of O RhD negative red cells used as a key performance indicator."

- "Many consider stock management as an art form rather than a science."

Background

The blood transfusion laboratory plays a key role in the management of blood stocks within an establishment or group of hospitals. The ordering of the blood products is usually managed from within the laboratory and this is the key step in the management of stocks. The ideal stock is a fine balance between ensuring that products are available to meet patient requirements with minimal delays whilst ensuring that there is no wastage by time expiry. This chapter will look at the issues encountered by the laboratory and how to work towards the perfect balance between stock and wastage.

Determining stock levels

There are many factors which should be considered when trying to determine a suitable stock level of products. These may be broken down into five groups:

- The size and type of the establishment.
- The medical/surgical specialties which use the service.
- The blood group distribution of the local population.
- If the laboratory is within a network of laboratories or standalone.
- Other factors.

The size of the establishment is important, as it is usually an indication of the number of patients being treated. The type of establishment is a term used to mean the complexities of organisations; for example, are there services on multiple sites, is the laboratory distant from the operating theatres or emergency department or other large-use areas?

The medical and surgical specialties using the service are possibly the key factor, as there is such a wide spread of requirements between specialties; for example, an ophthalmic department is unlikely to require blood product support, whilst the presence of a major trauma centre (MTC) will require a large amount of support.

The type of products which also need to be stocked may also be related to the specialties present; for example, the presence of a haematological transplant unit will mean that gamma-irradiated and *Cytomegalovirus* (CMV) products will probably be required regularly [1, 2].

The blood group distribution of the local population being served is important to know but may be difficult to obtain. Most laboratory IT systems will be able to calculate the blood group distribution of the group and save samples processed by the laboratory which is a good representation. The Blood Stocks Management Scheme in the UK undertook a national survey in 2008 which showed considerable variation in some blood groups across regions of the UK; for example, 13.5% of patients in the London region are group B RhD positive, whilst in the South West region this group only makes up 7.7% of the patient population. (This report is available on the BSMS website www.bloodstocks.co.uk [3].)

The importance of a laboratory being part of a network should not be underestimated. Sharing stock between sites can be important and may prevent undue wastage. This may also allow a stock to be warranted in a small-usage laboratory so improving rapid access to products with minimal risk of wastage. This stock sharing may not necessarily be limited to establishments within the same legal operation although a Service Level Agreement (SLA) will need to be in place to cover the legal and technical aspects of the arrangements. There have been a number of reports demonstrating that stock sharing between establishments can lead to a reduction in the time expiry of blood products [4].

'Other factors' is a term which covers factors which may vary in establishments but which are difficult to quantify. Some may be related to the personnel in the establishment. Although the laboratory may ultimately decide on a product stock level, the demands made by medical personnel can be a big influence. The ordering patterns will be individual to services and may depend on any number of factors (including personal preference). Other factors include things such as the availability of an electronic blood transfusion management system or if the establishment has employed new technologies such as the implementation of electronic remote issue. The distance from the supplier is frequently quoted as a factor in calculating blood stocks. If you compare establishments which are similar, then it is likely that the establishment close to the supplier may well carry a lower stock then the one further away.

The final factor which must be discussed is how comfortable the laboratory feels about a stock level. It is important that the staff feel that they have sufficient stocks for potential requirements and that they can order more as required. A lack of confidence that additional supplies can be obtained in a specific time frame is important and because of this the stock levels at locations further away from the supplier are likely to be higher than one nearby.

It is extremely difficult to be prescriptive on how to determine an ideal stock level even for what appears to be the most simple establishment.

The experience of the laboratory staff and their knowledge of the establishment and ordering patterns should not be underestimated.

Despite all the difficulties in determining what a stock level should be, it is extremely important that ideal levels are decided upon. Without this, less experienced laboratory staff would find it difficult to know when to reorder stocks and may allow levels to drop to a level which may place the service at risk.

Ordering blood products

The way blood products are ordered is dependent upon the supplier, and timings will be different for every establishment. The number and frequency of routine deliveries is a key factor but usually this is related to the volume of products used in an establishment.

Laboratories which receive more frequent deliveries are likely to settle on a lower stock level than laboratories having fewer, less frequent deliveries. Although hospitals always have the ability to order additional supplies, these may (depending on supplier) be charged separately and so most suppliers and hospitals are keen to keep additional orders to a minimum.

The NHS Blood and Transplant (NHSBT), the national blood supplier for England and North Wales, has undertaken a pilot programme looking at vendor managed inventory (VMI). In this pilot, four hospital trusts (13 separate hospital sites) have pre-agreed stock levels for routine products with NHSBT. An electronic link between the product stock levels within the laboratories has been established such that NHSBT receives information on stock levels every 30 minutes.

A snapshot of the stock is taken 90 minutes before every routine delivery and NHSBT replenishes the laboratory with the stock required to return the stock level of each product back to an ideal level.

This pilot has enabled each hospital trust to reduce the stock level of red cells in variable amounts up to 28%, but by 8% overall across all sites. Four hospital laboratories have actually increased their stock holding of platelets. The number of additional deliveries required has reduced considerably (30% reduction), whilst the overall wastage of products has also reduced (30% in red cells, 25% in platelets).

All hospital sites reported that they have found having a replenishment service has standardised stock levels. This is because it has removed a lot of interpersonal variability which all laboratories experience, and which is seen because staff have different 'comfort' zones on what ideal levels are.

Rotating of blood stocks

The rotation of blood stocks is relevant in all laboratories, although it holds increased importance in laboratories who have stock sharing arrangements with other laboratories.

In order to minimise wastage, a laboratory should issue products in a manner such that patients who are most likely to receive the requested blood product are issued with the unit(s) which are closest to going out of date. This is only possible when the laboratory is provided with good and relevant clinical information.

It should be noted that whilst some medical staff feel that fresher red cell products are better for patients, there is no supporting evidence for this [5].

Electronic remote blood issue is a system whereby non-laboratory staff issue red cells from a specific electronically controlled blood fridge as units are required by the patients. This means that laboratories may have blood stocks stored in a fridge or fridges away from the laboratory. The rotation of stocks in these fridges could go out of date without ever being issued to a patient and as such they should be rotated back to the laboratory in time such that it may be issued and transfused to a patient in another area. The lifespan at which these units should be returned will need to be determined by the managing laboratory and may vary by blood group.

Issuing of blood products

The appropriateness of a request for a blood product should not be a factor influencing whether or not a blood product is wasted. In an ideal situation, all requests would be appropriate and all blood issued would always be transfused. However, it must be recognised that not all requests for products will lead to a transfusion and as such it is important that if it is likely that a product will not be transfused, that it is returned to routine stock for reallocation as soon as possible.

The laboratory staff should also look at each request for a product and before selecting a product to issue consider if the request is likely be transfused or be returned at a later date.

To prevent expiry of the products a number of tools can be used:

- Only issue the product when it is about to be transfused. This may not always be possible if the patient has atypical antibodies or is at a distant site.
- Allow units to be reserved for patients for a minimum length of time — this will usually be 24 hours, although in the UK, 52% of hospitals in 2012 still used a 48-hour reservation period. (UK Transfusion Collaborative personal communication.)

A potentially contentious issue may be the issuing on non-ABO/Rh D identical blood products. There is much variation in practice and some laboratories would not issue a compatible, although non-identical, blood product to patients. There is no evidence that the issue of compatible, although non-identical, blood group red cells has any detrimental impact on the patient or on the survival of the transfused cells, and as such the issue of a shorter dated compatible unit of a different ABO group is a useful tool that many laboratories use to ensure red cells close to time expiry are transfused. Apart from the recommendation not to transfuse group O platelets to non-group O paediatric patients [6], the issue of non-group identical platelets is an essential option in most large hospitals. To only match ABO group would result in an increase of the stock level units of each group. This would almost certainly result in an increase in product wastage.

Returning of allocated units to stock

The returning of non-transfused allocated units to routine stock is important, as not only does it ensure units are recycled quickly and made available for another patient, it also ensures that units which may no longer be suitable for a patient are deallocated promptly and cannot be transfused.

Although most hospitals only return blood products once a day, some return untransfused units on a number of occasions each day. This allows the rapid reissuing of products and may well reduce wastage. It is, however, recognised that this may not be possible for laboratories with multiple remote fridges.

Audit

Reviewing blood stocks and wastage is an important part of ensuring products are not wasted.

In the UK, most hospitals take park in the Blood Stocks Management Scheme (BSMS). The scheme was established in 2001 and has provided help and information to participating hospitals (http://www.bloodstocks.co.uk).

Hospitals and blood services enter data into the data collection tool on products received (or issued from the blood service), products in stock and wastage.

A hospital transfusion team (HTT) can then produce a graphical representation of their stock levels and wastage over time so that the effectiveness of an intervention can be judged. It is also possible to benchmark levels/wastage against hospitals of a similar size, local to the NHSBT and specialties present.

Laboratories should consider and review stock levels at least annually as part of the laboratory annual management review. This will ensure that an appropriate level for the services in the hospital is maintained and wastage kept to a minimum. Examples are outlined in Figures 1, 2 and 3.

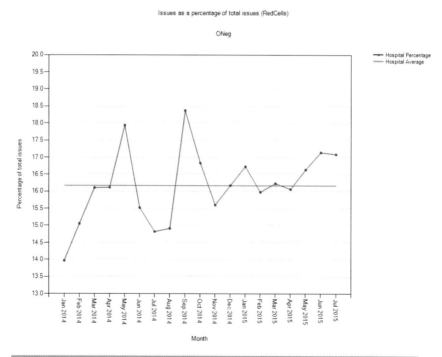

Figure 1. O RhD negative issued displayed as a percentage of the total.

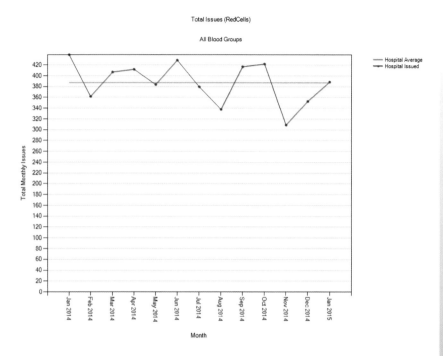

Figure 2. Example of red cell issues monthly and the moving average.

It is recognised that many hospitals use the percentage of O RhD negative red cells and the percentage of red cells wasted as key performance indicators and as such monitor these monthly. Whilst this is a recognised way of monitoring stocks and performance, it may not be such a useful tool for laboratories holding only a small volume of stock, as the effect of one patient may cause the figures to 'jump' considerably, and as such each laboratory should agree a system of monitoring which is appropriate for them. This may mean monitoring over a longer period of time to offset the effects of individual patients.

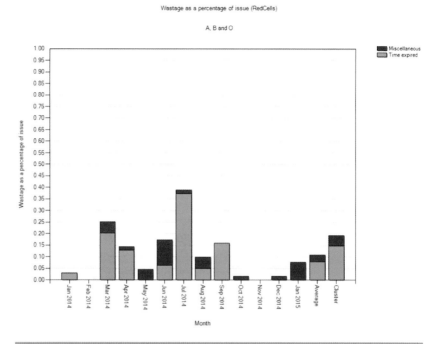

Figure 3. Example of wasted red cells as a percentage of the total issues.

Specific considerations

O negative red cells

It is well recognised that in the UK 12.5% of red cells transfused to patients is O RhD negative, whilst only 8.5% of the population are O RhD negative. This disparity in numbers is due to the fact that O RhD negative units are used as units suitable for use in an emergency when there is no time available to complete pre-compatibility testing.

Hospital laboratories frequently provide emergency stock in blood fridges remote from the transfusion laboratory, to ensure all patients may receive red cells in an emergency [7]. The National Patient Safety Agency issued a rapid response report in 2010 regarding the availability of emergency blood products, which may have led to an increase in the volume of emergency blood stored in blood fridges away from the main laboratory.

Having this stock away from the laboratory increases the risk that it may time expire before it can be transfused to a patient. The rotation of emergency stock back to the laboratory is critical as this will prevent time expiry and ensure units are not wasted [8, 9].

It is well recognised that clinical staff frequently request as much emergency stock as available in a laboratory, and as such a suitable risk assessment as to the most appropriate level of emergency stock should be undertaken before any increase. The usage of emergency stock should be audited to ensure it is being used appropriately.

The use of O RhD positive units for male and female patients beyond child-bearing potential is now becoming more common. This can only be introduced with clinical staff training as most show an initial reluctance to use O RhD positive units as emergency stock.

Frozen components

Frozen components in the UK have a shelf life of 2 years. Stock sharing should be considered for laboratories who use small numbers of units. Very small users will probably only stock A and AB units which can be used to cover all blood groups.

The largest wastage in frozen components is units being ordered and not transfused. The short post-thaw shelf life currently in the UK (4 hours for cryoprecipitate and 24 hours for FFP) means that unless a laboratory is large or provides products for a trauma unit, it is unlikely that smaller laboratories will be able to reassign thawed unused products. Units being thawed and that are not transfused are unlikely to be able to be reissued to another patient. As such ensuring that all requests are appropriate is critical to prevent wastage.

Wastage of products

Getting the stock levels in a laboratory agreed and undertaking appropriate stock selection and rotation helps to prevent wastage due to units exceeding their expiry date.

There is wastage which occurs for other reasons, some (but probably not all) of which can be influenced by the laboratory.

A big cause of wastage is over-ordering of products either because it may be needed or because the clinical situation of the patient changes, the latter of which is probably beyond the control of the laboratory. The ordering of products on a 'just in case' basis should be actively discouraged. It is well recognised that clinical areas remote from the laboratory (potentially even on a different site) order products 'just in case' more frequently than those that are close to the laboratory services. The reason for this is usually the confidence in the clinical staff that they will have access to blood products when they are required. This may not be a lack of confidence in the laboratory service but may be related to transportation services.

It is important that laboratory management works with the clinical teams to improve confidence that products can be made quickly available and transported to the correct location when needed. The implementation of remote electronic blood issue (REBI) is an option. This is whereby a stock of red cells and potentially thawed FFP is available in a specialised blood fridge nearby, and trained clinical staff issue the products as they are required for the patients. This has been shown [10] to improve confidence of the clinical staff in the availability of red cells and reduces pre-ordering by up to 52%.

REBI needs to be implemented and monitored carefully as it can also contribute to the wastage of red cells. As the products are stored away from the laboratory, stock management is not straightforward, especially on remote sites. A clear and monitored policy on stock rotation is critical to ensure that stock close to expiry can be returned to the laboratory with sufficient time remaining to allow for it to be issued to a patient who maybe requires an urgent transfusion or at least who is likely to have the blood administered when requested.

Clinical areas also waste blood products for a number of reasons. These reasons include:

- The unit is 'spiked' — whereby the giving set is not placed into the unit properly, so compromising the integrity of the unit.
- The unit is ordered to be taken to the clinical area before the patient is prepared for the transfusion. This increases the risk that the unit will be wasted if the transfusion is not able to go ahead and should be discouraged.
- The patient's clinical requirements change which means the transfusion is no longer required.
- Clinical staff order more products than they can transfuse at once and 'forget' to return it to the blood storage.
- Units can be placed in ward drug fridges, which are not suitable for storage of blood products.

With regard to wastage it is important for medical and nursing staff to be aware of this problem and to recognise that blood products are a precious resource that must not be wasted. As such the importance of training and competency assessment of clinical staff is key in this area as well as the safe administration of products.

Conclusions

There are many and very varied factors which are related to the management of blood product stocks within the laboratory. The setting of ideal stock levels is important but complicated in itself. All aspects in the cold chain of ordering, receipting, issue and returning of blood products are key to ensuring that wastage due to time expiry is kept to an absolute minimum.

The experience and teaching skills of the senior laboratory staff are critical within the entire process and it is important that these skills are taught to junior laboratory staff from the point they enter the laboratory so that good practices are built up and maintained for future generations of laboratory staff.

It is almost impossible to set out a regimental process which will ensure no blood stocks are wasted because of the differences between establishments and the medical/surgical specialties that are using the service. Although laboratories are run by well-qualified scientists it is often said that stock management is an art form rather than a science.

Checklist summary

✓ The importance of stock management within the laboratory should not be underestimated.

✓ The setting of an ideal stock level, although difficult, facilitates good stock management and allows for vendor-managed replenishment where available.

✓ A policy and audit process on the issuing of blood products is required to limit the amount of products issued and not transfused.

✓ Special considerations for the use of O RhD negative red cells should be given.

✓ The knowledge and experience of the laboratory staff should not be underestimated.

References

1. National Patient Safety Agency (NPSA). Safer Practice Notice: right patient, right blood, 2006. http://www.nrls.npsa.nhs.uk/resources/type/alerts.

2. The British Committee for Standards in Haematology (BCSH). Guidelines on the use of irradiated components, 2010. http://www.bcshguidelines.com.

3. Blood Stocks Management Scheme (BSMS). Distribution of ABO groups report, 2008. http://www.bloodstocks.co.uk.

4. Stanger SHW, Cotton S, Wilding R, Yates N, BBTS 2011. Reduction of time expiry wastage in the blood supply chain by sharing stock. http://www.bloodstocks.co.uk.

5. Lacroix J, Hébert PC, Fergusson DA, *et al*. Age of transfused blood in critically ill adults. *N Engl J Med* 2015; 372: 1410-8.

6.   The British Committee for Standards in Haematology (BCSH). Transfusion guidelines for neonates and older children, including 2005 and 2007 amendments, 2004.. http://www.bcshguidelines.com.

7.   National Patient Safety Agency (NPSA). The transfusion of blood and blood components in an emergency, 2010. NPSA/2010/RRR017. http://www.nrls.npsa.nhs.uk.

8.   National Comparative Audit of Blood transfusion. 2010 Re-audit of the use of group O RhD negative red cells. http://hospital.blood.co.uk/media/26868/nca-re-audit_of_the_use_of_group_o_rhd_negative_red_cells_doc_2010.pdf.

9.   The National Blood Transfusion Committee (NBTC). The Chief Medical Officer's National Blood Transfusion Committee - The appropriate use of group O RhD negative red cells, 2009. http://www.transfusionguidelines.org.uk/uk-transfusion-committees/national-blood-transfusion-committee.

10.   Staves J, Davies A, Kay J, et al. Electronic remote blood issue: a combination of remote blood issue with a system for end-to-end electronic control of transfusion to provide a 'total solution' for a safe and timely hospital blood transfusion service. Transfusion 2008; 48: 415-24.

Chapter 13

Prehabilitation

Ben Clevenger MBBS BSc MRCP FRCA
Clinical Research Associate, Division of Surgery and Interventional Science, University College London, London, UK
Toby Richards BSc FRCS MD
Professor of Surgery, Division of Surgery and Interventional Science, University College London, London, UK

- "I warn you against shedding blood, indulging in it and making a habit of it, for blood never sleeps."
  Saladin

- "Success depends upon previous preparation, and without such preparation there is sure to be failure."
  Confucius

- "A pint of sweat will save a gallon of blood."
  George S. Patton

- "The best preparation for tomorrow is to do today's work superbly well."
  William Osler

- "To the worn out or languid blood it [iron] gives a spur or fillip whereby the animal spirits which lay prostrate and sunken under their own weight are raised and excited."
  Thomas Sydenham

Background

Prehabilitation is the process of improving a patient's functional capacity to enable them to better withstand the stress of surgery. Developed initially as part of enhanced recovery programmes, prehabilitation includes physical and psychological preparation for surgery, and the pre-optimisation of comorbidities such as hypertension, diabetes, and respiratory disease, as well as anticipation, identification and management of surgical risks including renal dysfunction and venous thromboembolism.

Pre-operative anaemia and blood transfusion is a risk in surgical patients. Patient blood management (PBM) focuses upon three 'pillars' of care in the surgical patient:

- Detection and treatment of pre-operative anaemia.
- Reduction of peri-operative blood loss.
- Harnessing and optimising the physiological reserve of anaemia (including restrictive haemoglobin transfusion triggers).

Each pillar is relevant in the patient's prehabilitation in preparation for surgery (Table 1).

Table 1. Prehabilitation components of patient blood management.

	Pillar 1 Optimise erythropoiesis	Pillar 2 Minimise blood loss	Pillar 3 Manage anaemia
Pre-operative	• Diagnose anaemia. • Identify, evaluate and treat anaemia. • Treat absolute or functional iron deficiency. • Refer for further evaluation as necessary.	• Identify and manage bleeding risk (past medical and family history). • Review medications (antiplatelet, anticoagulation therapy). • Minimise iatrogenic blood loss (e.g. venepuncture). • Procedure planning and rehearsal.	• Compare estimated blood loss with patient-specific tolerable blood loss. • Decide upon appropriate transfusion thresholds. • Assess and optimise the patient's physiologic reserve, e.g. pulmonary and cardiac function. • Formulate a patient-specific management plan using appropriate blood conservation modalities.

In order for prehabilitation to be effective, good communication between patients and clinicians, including primary care, surgeons, haematologists and anaesthetists is paramount. To the patient, prehabilitation improves information delivery and empowers them to be involved in decisions about their care, improving understanding and reducing uncertainty and anxiety. Patient blood management similarly engages patients in the discussion of risk and the plan of action to be implemented peri-operatively. Recommendations have now been released for the implementation of PBM in the NHS with the aim of decreasing inappropriate transfusion of blood and blood products to optimise patient care.

Pre-operative anaemia

Anaemia is common. Defined as an insufficient circulating red blood cell (RBC) mass with a haemoglobin (Hb) concentration of <130g/L for men and <120g/L for women, the population prevalence of anaemia varies with age and comorbidity. With an average age of adult patients who required transfusion peri-operatively in the UK of 76 years from national audit data, approximately a quarter of patients in this population will have anaemia. As well as an increased prevalence with age, anaemia is more common with increasing frailty.

There is a clear association between pre-operative anaemia and surgical morbidity and mortality. In 227,435 surgical patients undergoing non-cardiac surgery, pre-operative anaemia was strongly predictive of both mortality and morbidity[1] (Figure 1). Even mild anaemia increased relative risk (RR) by 30-40%, with the additional effect of a relationship between anaemia severity and outcome. A further series of 39,309 non-cardiac surgical patients in the European Surgical Outcomes Study (EuSOS) demonstrated that patients with severe or moderate anaemia had higher in-hospital mortality than those with a normal pre-operative Hb (odds ratio [OR] 2.28 [95% CI 2.06-3.85] versus OR 1.99 [95% CI 1.67-2.37]), respectively [2].

Prehabilitation should aim to correct anaemia pre-operatively, to reduce the risk of intra-operative transfusion, improve functional capacity in preparation for surgery and to aid recovery and rehabilitation postoperatively.

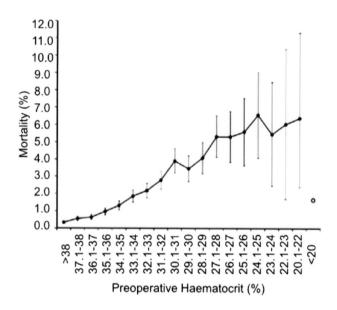

Figure 1. The percentage of patients with mortality outcome per fractional, 1-unit (%) pre-operative haematocrit drop from the normal baseline (>38%). (Error bars represent 95% CI; the shaded circle represents data that are too minimal to be analysed). *This graph (previously unpublished) represents data presented in Musallam KM, Tamim HM, Richards T, et al. Pre-operative anaemia and postoperative outcomes in non-cardiac surgery: a retrospective cohort study. Lancet 2011; 378(9800): 1396-407* [1].

Maintaining tissue oxygen delivery

Tissue oxygen delivery is greatly influenced by haemoglobin concentration. Symptoms of fatigue, dyspnoea and tachycardia develop as Hb falls below two-thirds normal (to less than 90-100g/L). The body responds to anaemia by increasing cardiac output, vasodilation, increasing minute ventilation, and optimising the oxygen saturation of haemoglobin in the lung and its extraction at the tissues. Cardiovascular stability can be maintained in healthy individuals with an Hb as low as 50g/L. However, even in the healthy population, mild anaemia leads to impaired functional capacity, poorer physical performance and a reduced quality of life. The impact of anaemia is thought to have a similar effect on health in the population to that of diabetes and cardiovascular disease.

The causality between anaemia and outcome has not been proven but surgery, like exercise, places metabolic demands on the patient. Cardiopulmonary exercise testing (CPET) is now routinely used to assess fitness for major surgery. CPET can be used to determine exertional oxygen uptake (VO_2) at the anaerobic threshold (AT) and peak oxygen consumption (VO_2 peak) as measures of the ability to meet increasing oxygen demands. The degree of surgical insult and the ability to meet the additional postoperative oxygen demand are key determinants of surgical outcome. Patients with poor CPET results (reduced VO_2 peak and AT) are at greater risk of adverse outcomes. Whilst cardiac output is recognised as a parameter limiting exertional VO_2, the impact of anaemia and reduced concentration of haemoglobin is less recognised. Anaemia is associated with lower exertional VO_2 and impaired exercise performance [3], therefore anaemia may be associated with reduced fitness for surgery.

Iron is an essential component of myoglobin, required for oxygen storage within muscle tissues, and is a component of oxidative enzymes and respiratory chain proteins within mitochondria. Iron deficiency can therefore precipitate reduced exercise endurance through failure of these pathways, in addition to the reduction in tissue oxygen delivery from the reduction in circulating haemoglobin. Even in the context of iron deficiency without anaemia, endurance capacity can be reduced when tissue oxygen stores are reduced.

Nutrition and physical training

Central to most prehabilitation programmes are pre-operative physical training programmes to improve exercise capacity and muscle strength in order to improve the patient's physical reserve to withstand the stress of surgery and recovery. Within 6 weeks of implementing a pre-operative exercise regimen, significant improvements in physical function can be seen compared to controls. Regular physical training improves the body's adaptation to the stress of exercise and patients can utilise a greater proportion of their physiologic reserve.

In addition, nutritional programmes optimise nutritional status pre-operatively to prevent the loss of lean body mass during the postoperative period, when a catabolic state is induced in response to surgical stress. Deficits of iron, vitamin B12 and folate are all common causes of anaemia. Nutritional deficits are common pre-operatively, particularly in the context of malignancy, chemotherapy and other chronic comorbidities, leading to protein, carbohydrate, lipid, vitamin and trace element deficiencies. Nutritional supplementation, including protein and iron can improve tissue oxidative capacity and muscular function.

Defining pre-operative anaemia

Whilst identification of anaemia is easy, this task is rarely performed in the surgical clinic at the time a patient is listed for operation. Within the process of pre-assessment for surgery, the recognition and diagnosis of anaemia is often too late. 'Mild' anaemia often goes unrecognised, with staff only raising a query when a patient has significant anaemia, usually a Hb of <100g/L.

The recognition of anaemia pre-operatively is not merely an indication only to cross-match the patient, but an opportunity to review the patient's overall fitness. It is the responsibility of all clinicians to review the appropriateness of their hospital's anaemia management strategy. In some centres, patients for primary joint replacement are not listed for operation unless they have a normal haemoglobin concentration; in those patients with a short timeline to operation, it is possible to delay surgery [4].

The next step is to define the aetiology of the anaemia. The main causes of anaemia in the population — iron, folate and vitamin B12 deficiency, haemoglobinopathy and renal failure — are rarely newly diagnosed at pre-operative assessment. Surgical patients may have an established or treated cause of anaemia, but may also suffer from anaemia due to the condition for which they are undergoing surgery. This could either be directly related, for example, due to gastrointestinal blood loss in colorectal cancer, or indirectly as a consequence of chronic disease. The latter has traditionally been regarded as the "anaemia of chronic disease", which is the most common type of anaemia seen in hospitalised patients.

The definition of iron deficiency anaemia refers to depletion of the body's iron stores due to dietary deficiency or chronic blood loss, resulting in an absolute iron deficiency (AID), characterised by a plasma ferritin <16μg/L [5]. It is now recognised that several disease states, and in particular inflammation, have a direct effect on the pathway of iron absorption and metabolism leading to a state of iron deficiency and anaemia (Figure 2). Consequently, those patients previously diagnosed with anaemia of chronic disease are now recognised to have iron deficiency anaemia, despite the presence of normal, or even increased, body iron stores. A state of functional iron deficiency is the result of the inability to mobilise these stores.

Hepcidin and functional iron deficiency

Hepcidin, predominantly produced by the liver, is the key iron regulatory hormone [6]. Hepcidin is regulated by feedback from iron stores and erythropoietic activity, becoming upregulated in response to increased iron stores. Hepcidin acts upon ferroportin, a transmembrane iron transporter found in duodenal enterocytes and macrophages. The binding of hepcidin degrades ferroportin, preventing iron absorption from the gut by inhibiting transport of iron from the duodenal enterocyte. Iron is sequestered within hepatocytes and macrophages as ferritin (the main iron storage protein) because transport of stored iron into the plasma is inhibited. Less iron is then available in the plasma to be bound to transferrin, the main plasma iron transport protein, for transport to the bone marrow for erythropoiesis.

Inflammation activates and increases hepcidin expression and ferritin synthesis. Thus, in response to the effects of inflammatory mediators, a state of functional iron deficiency is created as a consequence of the sequestration of iron. Meanwhile, hepcidin upregulation in the presence of inflammation blocks the absorption of dietary iron, including oral iron supplementation, compounding this state of iron-restricted erythropoiesis

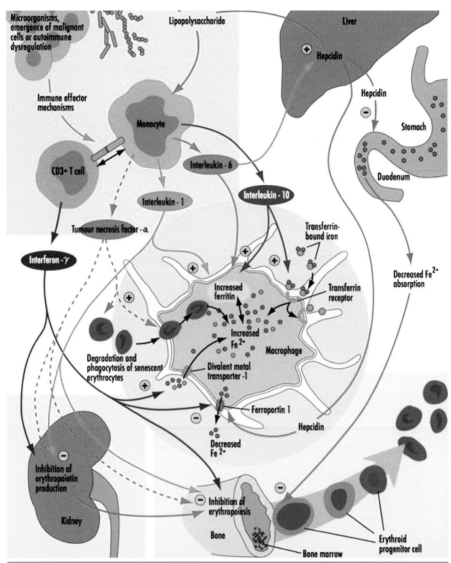

Figure 2. Iron homeostasis and inflammation. Inflammation caused by infection, malignant cells or autoimmune mechanisms, activates T cells and monocytes, triggering a cascade that alters the homeostasis of iron and limits its availability. Inflammation and increased iron levels upregulate hepcidin inhibiting duodenal absorption. Macrophages are stimulated by inflammatory mediators to take up ferrous iron (Fe^{2+}). They upregulate expression of transferrin receptors, increasing transferrin-bound iron uptake into the

macrophage. Transferrin can be functionally blocked by increased hepcidin. Activated macrophages phagocytose ageing red blood cells permitting the recycling of iron. The transmembrane iron transporter ferroportin is downregulated by hepcidin, reducing iron transport from macrophages and duodenal enterocyte. Thus, functional iron deficiency is created by the sequestration of iron within the duodenum and macrophages. Tumour necrosis factor alpha (TNF-α) can induce macrophages and damage red cell membranes, leading to early phagocytosis. Inflammatory mediators also reduce erythropoietin production by the kidney. *Adapted from: Clevenger B, Richards T. Pre-operative anaemia. Anaesthesia 2015: Suppl 70(1): 20-8, e6-8* [7].

driven by inflammatory mediators (Figure 2) [7]. Functional iron deficiency is well recognised in renal and cardiac disease and is now increasingly recognised as a cause for anaemia in the general surgical patient as a consequence of inflammation, malignancy and other chronic diseases.

Diagnosis of anaemia and iron deficiency

Guidelines for the diagnosis and management of anaemia have been issued by several bodies, including the National Institute for Health and Care Excellence (NICE) [8]. The European Society of Anaesthesiology guidelines recommend that patients at risk of bleeding should be assessed for anaemia 4-8 weeks before surgery. However, in current surgical pathways, the time between surgical review and the scheduled operation is often shorter. For example, for colorectal cancer surgery, the average time from listing to operation in the UK is less than 3 weeks, providing challenges to the detection and adequate treatment of anaemia.

NICE guidelines for the use of routine pre-operative tests in elective surgery exist in order to guide the appropriate use of resources [9]. Guidance for full blood count (FBC) testing is based upon grade of surgery, patient age and the presence of comorbidities. The diagnosis of anaemia should lead to investigation of the cause, including assessment for nutritional deficiency, chronic renal insufficiency and chronic inflammatory disease.

Measurement of the reticulocyte count indicates bone marrow activity. This can distinguish between high turnover of red cells, with the reticulocyte count rising to compensate for red cell loss, destruction (e.g. haemolysis), or poor bone marrow function. Decreased reticulocyte count is seen in iron deficiency anaemia and the anaemia of chronic disease, vitamin B12 and folate deficiency, and bone marrow failure. Mean cell volume (MCV) and mean cell haemoglobin (MCH) values are useful to make a diagnosis of iron deficiency, and can assess the trend over weeks or months. Most patients with anaemia of chronic disease have a normochromic, normocytic anaemia. Red cell distribution width (RDW) measuring the variation in RBC size can be used along with MCV values to determine the cause of anaemia.

Serum tests of haematinic factors, including iron concentration, total iron-binding capacity (TIBC), transferrin saturation (TSAT) (measuring the ratio of serum iron to TIBC) and ferritin are used to distinguish the differing types of iron deficiency. Serum ferritin is essential in the measurement of iron stores. One µg/L of ferritin in serum is equivalent to 8-10mg of iron in stores. However, ferritin is also an acute phase protein, confounding its use as a marker of iron stores in the presence of infection and inflammation.

For patients with low red cell haemoglobin indices (low MCH and mean cell haemoglobin concentration [MCHC]) and microcytic anaemia indicating acquired iron deficiency anaemia, algorithms exist for the investigation of coeliac disease and gastrointestinal cancer. Similarly, anaemia in patients with chronic kidney disease is usually managed as part of their illness. However, diagnosis of anaemia due to functional iron deficiency remains under appreciated.

Local hospital transfusion committees should set definitions based on recent evidence, national guidelines and the availability of tests. The authors recommend a serum ferritin <100µg/L and TSAT <20% as an acceptable definition of functional iron deficiency and serum ferritin <16µg/L to indicate absolute iron deficiency. Current guidelines do not give a recommendation for the highest serum ferritin concentration beyond which it is unsafe to give a trial of intravenous iron therapy, but suggest that a serum ferritin <100µg/L in non-dialysed patients and <200µg/L in chronic haemodialysis patients indicate a high likelihood of iron deficiency and the potential to respond to intravenous iron.

Pre-operative management of anaemia

A cut-off risk of bleeding of 10% is useful in determining those patients in whom elective surgery should be postponed if anaemic (Figure 3) [10].

Oral iron is a well established and inexpensive treatment for anaemia. The total body stores of iron in a healthy adult are 3-4g. The bioavailability of ferrous iron is 10-15%, and ferric iron a third to a quarter of this. However, oral iron may be poorly absorbed due to the downregulation of duodenal absorption by inflammation, infection and chronic disease under the influence of hepcidin, further reducing its bioavailability. Oral iron is absorbed at a rate of 2-16mg per day, and for a 1000 to 2000mg replenishment of body stores, 3-6 months of treatment may be required. Reduced uptake is one of the main reasons why oral iron often fails to improve anaemia in surgical patients. Poor compliance is frequent due to common side effects including abdominal pain, diarrhoea and constipation.

Intravenous iron has been shown to be effective in correcting anaemia in iron-deficient patients. There are several intravenous iron preparations available, including iron dextrans, iron polymaltose, ferumoxytol, ferric carboxymaltose, iron sucrose, ferric gluconate and iron isomaltoside. Parenteral preparations have historically been associated with high rates of adverse events including anaphylaxis. Many reactions were related to dextran-containing preparations, often because antibodies to dextran are produced following exposure to dental caries. Modern preparations are effective, with improved safety profiles, allowing total dose infusions of iron to be administered in as little as 15 minutes. There is now good evidence for the safety and efficacy of modern parenteral iron preparations in a range of conditions, including the peri-operative setting. A systematic review by Litton *et al* demonstrated an increase in haemoglobin concentration and relative risk reduction in red cell transfusion with intravenous iron when compared to oral iron or no iron supplementation (RR 0.74, 95% CI 0.62 to 0.88) [11].

Intravenous iron can be used throughout the pre-operative period but, ideally, treatment should take place 10 days pre-operatively in order to

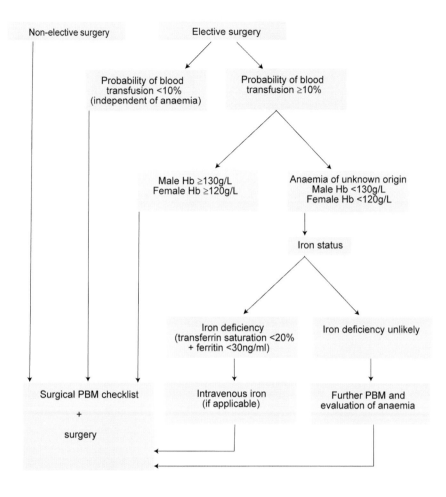

Figure 3. Pre-operative patient blood management algorithm (PBM). *Adapted from Meybohm P, Fischer DP, Geisen C, et al; the German PBM Study Core Group. Safety and effectiveness of a patient blood management (PBM) program in surgical patients — the study design for a multicentre prospective epidemiologic non-inferiority trial. BMC Health Serv Res 2014; 14: 576 [10].*

allow erythroid cell maturation and haemoglobin accumulation. However, there has been a lack of good-quality trials to show an effect on mortality or quality of life in adults with anaemia undergoing surgery.

Minimisation of bleeding risk

Medical pre-optimisation of coagulation, bleeding and thrombotic risk is essential. Pre-operative assessment including the patient's past medical history, particularly that of bleeding and previous surgical complications or challenges, a family history of bleeding disorders and a drug history, including antiplatelet agents and anticoagulants, should be undertaken. The use of a standardized bleeding questionnaire in all patients to stratify this risk has been advocated. This can help to stratify bleeding and thrombotic risk of stopping anticoagulation, and plan requirements for bridging anticoagulation therapy. In patients with a negative history, it is not necessary to perform a routine coagulation screen.

Patients increasingly must continue antiplatelet and anticoagulant therapy into the peri-operative period to reduce their peri-operative cardiovascular and thrombotic risk, or have bridging therapy instituted by the substitution of long-acting anticoagulation such as warfarin with shorter-acting drugs, and this must be balanced with the risk of bleeding on an individual patient basis. Evidence-based guidelines such as the American College of Cardiology/American Heart Association guidelines exist to facilitate the risk assessment that must be made for the individual patient's thrombotic and bleeding balance. Liaison with a haematologist is recommended for patients with known haemostatic derangements, including anticoagulant drug therapies, presenting for surgery [12].

Novel oral anticoagulant drugs (NOAC) including direct thrombin inhibitors (dabigatran) and direct factor X10a inhibitors (rivaroxaban and apixaban) are increasingly used due to their predictable pharmacokinetics without the requirement for regular laboratory monitoring, as is needed with warfarin, particularly for those with poor control. These require pre-operative discontinuation depending upon the risk of bleeding, restarting according to bleeding and thrombotic risk after surgery.

For patients taking antiplatelet agents, particularly in the context of coronary artery stents, and especially drug-eluting stents, peri-operative planning can be complicated by the high risk of myocardial infarction if discontinued, with the increased risk of bleeding if continued — sometimes leading to the cancellation of surgery. However, individual responses to antiplatelet agents are varied with wide-ranging degrees of inhibition between patients. Point-of-care platelet testing is now available using rotational thromboelastometry (ROTEM®) platelet modules or thromboelastography (TEG®) platelet mapping. TEG® platelet mapping uses the agonists adenosine diphosphate (ADP) (for clopidogrel) and arachidonic acid (AA) (for aspirin), measuring the inhibition of platelet function compared to baseline by measuring the reduction in maximum amplitude (MA). Platelet function testing aids the stratification of risk of bleeding whilst quantifying the level of platelet inhibition. Patients with high platelet inhibition have been shown to have a higher risk of intra-operative and postoperative transfusions, and redo surgery, with an ADP platelet receptor inhibition by clopidogrel of 34% providing a cut-off point above which bleeding risk was high [13].

As part of a patient's prehabilitation and pre-operative planning, attention should be given to the multimodal nature of bleeding and transfusion in surgical practice. Consideration of anaesthetic and surgical technique, pharmacological interventions and the use of cell salvage should be undertaken. The choice of surgical technique can reduce intra-operative blood loss, with laparoscopic and minimally-invasive surgical techniques, such as robotic urological surgery, associated with reduced bleeding. The position of the patient intra-operatively can also influence bleeding. Obstruction of venous return, leading to vessel engorgement and increased venous pressure at the operative site, increases bleeding. This is particularly true in lumbar spinal surgery where the patient is prone, increasing intra-abdominal compression and epidural vessel engorgement. Efforts should be made to ensure that venous drainage is maintained by careful positioning pre-operatively.

Neuraxial anaesthesia has been shown to reduce bleeding, most likely due to the sympathetic blockade reducing venous tone and systemic blood pressure. Avoidance of intra-operative hypervolaemia and hypertension reduces surgical bleeding, as well as improving operating conditions.

Conclusions

Prehabilitation combines many features to optimise patient fitness for surgery with the aim of improving recovery and postoperative outcome. Patient blood management has the same goals by reducing unnecessary transfusions in surgery. Physical training and nutritional supplementation improve the patient's functional reserve to tolerate the stress of surgery. The diagnosis and management of pre-operative anaemia both ameliorates a pre-operative risk factor but also can improve physical performance and quality of life. Recognition that chronic disease can cause anaemia due to a functional iron deficiency has improved treatment and potential risk reduction in surgical patients. Although the link between anaemia and adverse outcome is in general associative, this is demonstrated in most surgical specialties. In the UK, audits of transfusion rates by operation and hospital are planned, and pre-operative anaemia has been proposed as a key performance indicator, reinforcing the need for multidisciplinary planning. Individualised assessment of bleeding and thrombotic risk should be undertaken at an early point in the surgical pathway to prevent unnecessary delays to surgery whilst providing opportunity to optimise risk. In addition, prehabilitation increases patient involvement with their pre-operative planning and care, leading to both empowerment and a reduction in anxiety.

Checklist summary

✓ Prehabilitation aims to improve a patient's functional capacity prior to surgery to improve outcomes.

✓ Pre-operative diagnosis and management of anaemia, assessment of bleeding risk and physical fitness are facets of both prehabilitation and patient blood management.

✓ Physical training programmes and nutritional supplementation can improve patient fitness and physiological reserve.

✓ Shared decision-making between patients, surgeons, anaesthetists, haematologists and primary care providers can facilitate effective prehabilitation, empower patients and reduce their anxiety.

✓ All patients scheduled for surgery with >10% risk of bleeding should have their Hb checked when the procedure is booked.

✓ Patients found to be anaemic (Hb <120g/L in women and <130g/L in men) should have simple investigations (serum ferritin and haematinics) and receive oral iron (if >6 weeks before surgery) or intravenous iron if functional iron deficiency is demonstrated.

✓ Consideration of delaying elective surgery should be made if patients are anaemic at pre-assessment.

✓ Assessment of bleeding and thrombotic risk must be undertaken on an individual patient basis.

✓ Consideration of bridging anticoagulation should be made for those patients taking anticoagulant medications at a high risk of thrombosis and of intra-operative bleeding.

✓ Patients taking antiplatelet agents with minimal (<30%) platelet inhibition on platelet function testing are considered to not be at an increased risk of bleeding.

References

1.   Musallam KM, Tamim HM, Richards T, *et al*. Preoperative anaemia and postoperative outcomes in non-cardiac surgery: a retrospective cohort study. *Lancet* 2011; 378(9800): 1396-407.

2.   Baron DM, Hochrieser H, Posch M, *et al*; the European Surgical Outcomes Study (EuSOS) group for the Trials Groups of the European Society of Intensive Care Medicine and the European Society of Anaesthesiology. Preoperative anaemia is associated with poor clinical outcome in non-cardiac surgery patients. *Br J Anaesth* 2014; 113(3): 416-23.

3.   Otto JM, O'Doherty AF, Hennis PJ, *et al*. Association between preoperative haemoglobin concentration and cardiopulmonary exercise variables: a multicentre study. *Perioperative medicine* 2013; 2(1): 18.

4.   Kotze A, Carter LA, Scally AJ. Effect of a patient blood management programme on preoperative anaemia, transfusion rate, and outcome after primary hip or knee arthroplasty: a quality improvement cycle. *Br J Anaesth* 2012; 108(6): 943-52.

5.   Pratt JJ, Khan KS. Non-anaemic iron deficiency - a disease looking for recognition of diagnosis: a systematic review. *Eur J Haematol* 2015; Aug 8 [Epub ahead of print].

6.   Ganz T. Hepcidin and iron regulation, 10 years later. *Blood* 2011; 117(17): 4425-33.

7.   Clevenger B, Richards T. Pre-operative anaemia. *Anaesthesia* 2015; 70 Suppl 1: 20-8, e6-8.

8.   National Institute for Health and Care Excellence. Anaemia - iron deficiency; clinical knowledge. Summary. London, UK: NICE, 2013. http://cks.nice.org.uk/anaemia-iron-deficiency#!topicsummary.

9.   National Institute for Health and Care Excellence. Preoperative tests: the use of routine preoperative tests for elective surgery, CG3. London, UK: NICE, 2003. http://www.nice.org.uk/guidance/cg3.

10.   Meybohm P, Fischer DP, Geisen C, *et al*; the German PBM Study Core Group. Safety and effectiveness of a patient blood management (PBM) program in surgical patients - the study design for a multi-centre prospective epidemiologic non-inferiority trial. *BMC Health Serv Res* 2014; 14: 576.

11.   Litton E, Xiao J, Ho KM. Safety and efficacy of intravenous iron therapy in reducing requirement for allogeneic blood transfusion: systematic review and meta-analysis of randomised clinical trials. *Br Med J* 2013; 347: f4822.

12.   Fleisher LA, Fleischmann KE, Auerbach AD, *et al*. 2014 ACC/AHA guideline on perioperative cardiovascular evaluation and management of patients undergoing noncardiac surgery: a report of the American College of Cardiology/American Heart Association Task Force on practice guidelines. *J Am Coll Cardiol* 2014; 64(22): e77-137.

13.   Kasivisvanathan R, Abbassi-Ghadi N, Kumar S, *et al.* Risk of bleeding and adverse outcomes predicted by thromboelastography platelet mapping in patients taking clopidogrel within 7 days of non-cardiac surgery. *Br J Surg* 2014; 101(11): 1383-90.

Further reading

1.   NHS Improving Quality in Collaboration with NHS England. Enhanced Recovery Care Pathway. www.nhsiq.nhs.uk/download.ashx?mid=8808&nid=8846.

2.   The Preoperative Association: Prehabilitation. http://www.pre-op.org/useful-resources/prehabilitation.

3.   McGill University Peri Operative Programme. https://www.mcgill.ca/peri-op-program/patient-information/what-prehabilitation.

Chapter 14

Intra-operative cell salvage

John Thompson MS FRCSEd FRCS
Consultant Surgeon, Royal Devon and Exeter Hospitals, University of Exeter Medical School, Exeter, UK

- "Intra-operative cell salvage (ICS) is the accepted standard of care in vascular, orthopaedic and urological surgery, and is gaining popularity in obstetrics and gynaecology."

- "It is the final safety net in cases of heavy bleeding and an essential component of any patient blood management programme."

Background

The principle of saving blood lost during surgery or trauma was introduced nearly 200 years ago, when James Blundell washed blood-soaked swabs from obstetric haemorrhage in saline and reinfused the blood. Blood can be reinfused from ectopic pregnancy because it is defibrinogenated and remains liquid, but it was not until the principles of anticoagulation were established that simple canister-style devices were introduced for intra-operative 'autotransfusion'. Unwashed blood reinfusion was introduced in the 1970s, when techniques for minimising haemolysis were developed, but the most popular device, the Bentley ATS-100, was withdrawn after several deaths from air embolism.

Edwin J. Conn, in the 1950s, developed techniques for separating blood components using centrifugation, but his equipment was not reusable (Figure 1). Allen 'Jack' Latham was an engineer whose best

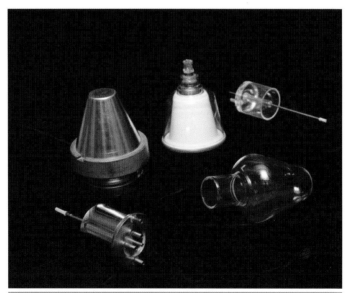

Figure 1. Conn's early glass and original 1952 aluminium cell separator with Latham's 1972 bowl.

friend, Abner Nichols, was critically injured in a chemical explosion at their workplace. Latham volunteered to help him with a direct transfusion, which sadly did not save his life. As a result, Latham developed a lifelong interest in blood transfusion and worked with Conn. The result of his painstaking research was the Latham bowl (Figure 1), whose unique plastic seal could withstand the 5000 rpm required to separate blood, without overheating.

Intra-operative use of the Latham bowl was initially patchy, but the huge transfusion demands of open heart surgery made it an attractive economic option. The equipment saw further development during the Vietnam conflict but the hepatitis scandals and HIV epidemic of the mid 1980s were the main drivers towards widespread use of ICS. Latterly, the provision of ICS has been written into quality standards worldwide, for example, the National Abdominal Aortic Aneurysm Screening Programme and associated quality improvement programme for aortic surgery [1].

The principle of cell washing is shared by several different machines (Figures 2 and 3; see also Appendix XI for a list of suppliers of intra-operative cell salvage machines). Blood is collected using a standard sucker and mixed with either citrate or heparin in the collection tubing. It enters the centrifuge where the cellular components are trapped at its circumference. Saline is then introduced, washing away supernatant contaminants and anticoagulant in a helical vortex. After washing, the red cells are resuspended in saline for reinfusion. The product has a high oxygen content, low viscosity, good-quality red cells (older cells are lysed by the process) but no coagulation factors or functional platelets.

In theory, non-washed blood should be inferior to washed as it contains fibrin degradation products, decreased levels of clotting factors, inactive platelets, activated white cells and elevated inflammatory mediators. This has been shown to lead to increased markers of fibrinolysis in recipients, but there have been no reports of clinical sequelae [2]. In practice, however, it is only possible to salvage non-washed blood from patients that are fully heparinised, which limits the technique to certain phases of vascular and cardiac surgery. For this practical reason, washed systems have taken over in clinical practice.

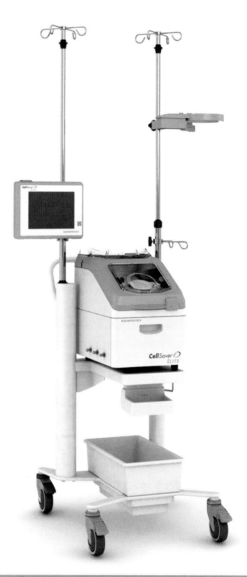

Figure 2. Cell Saver® Elite® autotransfusion system. *Reproduced with permission from Haemonetics Corporation. © Haemonetics Corporation, 2016.*

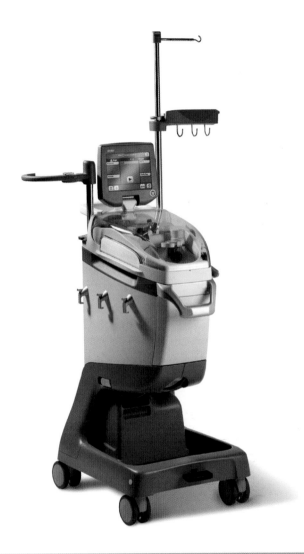

Figure 2. LivaNova XTRA™ autotransfusion system. *Reproduced with permission from LivaNova PLC. © LivaNova PLC, 2016.*

The incentive to use cell salvage rather than to rely on allogeneic transfusion is both clinical and economical. Avoiding transfusion reduces tumour recurrence, postoperative infection, myocardial infarction, lung injury, alloimmunization and even 5-year mortality. In cases of major blood loss, such as a ruptured aortic aneurysm, ICS becomes more effective. It is difficult to argue against the provision of an ICS service in a modern hospital [3].

Evidence

Despite the lack of good-quality randomised trials, the evidence from the literature is that cell salvage is highly effective at conserving blood. In many ways, events have overtaken science in much the same way as when laparoscopic cholecystectomy was adopted. The advantages were obvious to both clinicians and patients. Randomised trials are difficult to justify from an ethical point of view; good-quality 'real time' information regarding the efficacy of ICS is now available from sources such as the Vascular Society's National Vascular Registry.

The recent National Institute for Health and Care Excellence (NICE) guideline development group have painstakingly analysed the overall evidence for the use of ICS [4]. The final guidance acknowledged the relatively poor scientific quality of the large number of trials studied, but the overall treatment effect demonstrated a significant reduction in bank blood transfusion (RR 0.78: 0.78-0.94), reduced exposure to allogeneic transfusion (RR 0.74: 0.58-0.93) and a reduction in infectious complications (RR 0.4: 0.8-0.97) in patients deemed at high risk of blood loss.

Vascular surgery

Pooled data from five randomised controlled trials (RCTs) showed that ICS reduced allogeneic transfusion by 37% in elective aortic surgery [5]. This has been confirmed by two prospective and one retrospective review. One of the studies included ruptured aneurysms whose exposure to bank blood was reduced by three units. Our own experience of 247 ruptured

AAAs demonstrated no complications and an in-hospital mortality of 13% in patients receiving ICS compared to 26% in those having bank blood alone. Recovery of blood from washed swabs via ICS may increase the volume of blood saved but data are poor.

Cardiothoracic surgery

There is a great variation in transfusion rates between cardiac centres. Improved surgical techniques have largely eliminated the need for cross-matched blood in primary coronary artery bypass grafting (CABG) but there is a need for ICS in valve surgery and redo operations. A large meta-analysis of 31 trials showed a reduction in blood product exposure of 37% and red cell transfusion of 40%, with no increased morbidity or mortality [6]. Since the publication of this work there have been four randomised trials with relatively low numbers, one of which found no benefit for ICS, but the results are diluted by the use of ICS in first-time CABG and straightforward valve replacement. The conclusion is that ICS should be set up to 'collect only' as a safety precaution for valve replacement or redo cases and probably abandoned for straightforward primary CABG.

Cardiopulmonary bypass can be complicated by neurocognitive loss caused by microembolism to the brain. ICS with washing of the blood from cardiotomy suction, along with ultrafiltration, removes most of the microemboli responsible and halves the incidence of this unpleasant complication, as well as improving pulmonary function after cardiopulmonary bypass [7].

Orthopaedics

Orthopaedic surgeons are frankly more motivated by complications, especially infection, than blood transfusion. In a study of 308 patients, ICS significantly reduced the rate of infections in a series of patients having primary arthroplasty [8]. There are good studies involving revision hip and knee arthroplasty that support the use of ICS, but variable data in primary hip and scoliosis surgery. In addition to the clinical advantages there are significant cost savings associated with ICS in terms of bank blood and the high costs of revision surgery.

Obstetrics and gynaecology

Although peri- and post-partum haemorrhage are an important cause of maternal death it is generally not practical to salvage blood following vaginal delivery. However, high-risk Caesarean section, due to placenta accreta or praevia, is an ideal setting for ICS. Initial concerns regarding the danger of amniotic fluid embolus have been allayed by good-quality experimental studies followed by clinical use, with no complications associated with ICS combined with filtration to remove foetal squamous cells and lamellar bodies. The overall data are poor but enthusiasts are increasing their use of ICS, which is now fully supported by NICE, the Confidential Enquiry into Maternal and Child Health (CEMACH), the Association of Anaesthetists of Great Britain and Ireland (AAGBI), the Obstetric Anaesthetists' Association (OAA) and similar professional organizations worldwide such as the American Association of Blood Banks.

In gynaecology, ICS use is increasing with the identification of cases likely to bleed, such as larger myomectomies, hysterectomy and cancer surgery, with no influence on survival rates.

Urology

Concerns about the dissemination of cancer cells during ICS was a major concern in the 1980s, but these were offset by a reluctance to transfuse bank blood because of the known (and perceived) risks, as well as immune suppression. This led to the publication of several studies in prostate, bladder and renal surgery showing that ICS was safe, with and without filtration, that it significantly reduced bank blood transfusion and did not decrease survival. The NICE guideline IPG 258 endorsed the technique. Since then, however, there has been an explosion in the use of laparoscopic and robotic surgery which has largely overtaken the need for ICS.

Other areas

There is a small but generally encouraging literature advocating cell salvage in paediatric cardiac surgery, orthotopic liver transplantation, osteosarcoma resection and general surgery. In cases where the operative field may be contaminated, such as bowel trauma, studies have shown no correlation between bacteria cultured from the salvaged blood and postoperative infection. The consensus view is that wash volumes should be increased and broad-spectrum antibiotics administered; ICS is no longer contraindicated [9].

Patients who refuse blood transfusion on religious grounds are discussed in a separate chapter; in general, ICS is acceptable as long as there is a continuous circuit to keep the blood in contact with the patient.

Adverse events

The reporting of adverse events involving ICS has been included in the Serious Hazards of Transfusion (SHOT) programme for many years. The SHOT system records procedural problems including operator error, technical failures and the non-availability of an operator, as long as they impact on the care of the patient. Adverse events during the ICS process and reactions during reinfusion are also recorded. There are, however, no national data regarding the number of operations in which ICS is used; the denominator is very large.

In the latest SHOT report [10], there were 16 cases of minor adverse events, but no deaths or serious morbidity associated with ICS. Fifteen of these cases were reviewed by the appropriate hospital committee. There was one case of hypotension following reinfusion of blood through a leucocyte depletion filter, which was reversed when reinfusion was stopped. The need for a filter is increasingly being questioned as several large series have reported no adverse events without their use. Two cases involved delayed reinfusion >6h after salvage (studies have shown that this arbitrary time limit may be too strict), eight cases involved machine failure (6/8 from one institution) and one involved salvage from a contaminated area (which might be clinically justified in some circumstances). In conclusion, ICS is extremely safe.

ICS and tranexamic acid (TXA)

The NICE guidelines considered the use of ICS in combination with other interventions, namely postoperative cell salvage (POCS) and tranexamic acid. POCS is very effective but is seldom used outside cardiac surgery where mediastinal drain collection has been used effectively in the past. Postoperative drains were also used in joint replacement surgery in the past but this has become less popular.

The CRASH II (Clinical Randomisation of an Antifibrinolytic in Significant Haemorrhage) trial [11] and other data considered by NICE confirmed the efficacy of tranexamic acid in reducing blood loss and transfusion requirements, particularly in medium blood loss scenarios. Pragmatically, the recommendation is that TXA should be used in all such operations. ICS works in an entirely complementary way and is particularly effective in heavy bleeding which would overwhelm the effect of TXA's antifibrinolytic action. The recommendation is, therefore, that ICS should always be used in combination with TXA.

How to do it

Introducing an ICS service should be easy to justify to hospital managers. There are several cost efficiency studies reporting savings in terms of allogeneic blood, but the main financial benefit results from a reduction in complications such as infection and transfusion reactions (please refer to the detailed economic analysis in the NICE guidelines). Hospital stay and mortality are reduced in ICS cases [12]. Regular audit on an institutional level will identify cases where ICS is undoubtedly effective (e.g. ruptured AAA) or less so (e.g. primary hip replacement). Setting up the suction and collection reservoir alone saves money. The more expensive processing disposables are only opened if there is deemed to be sufficient blood to process. Processing small volumes of blood may prevent bank blood transfusion if the ICS blood is enough to exceed the agreed transfusion trigger.

Training staff is an essential component of an ICS service. A responsible clinician should be in charge of the service and be a part of the hospital transfusion team/committee. Guidelines and a toolkit for competency are freely available online, courtesy of the UK Cell Savage Action Group, which was set up to promulgate ICS (www.transfusionguidelines.org.uk). Extensive support and advice is also available from the Australian National Blood Authority (www.blood.gov.au/ics). Training can be delivered in-house or electronically, using the competency assessment workbook. It is useful to regularly rotate staff through theatres so that they can keep their knowledge and experience up to date using a suitable training register.

It is vital that key data from each case are recorded. The newer machines have the facility to store information for download, but as yet there are no agreed standards. ICS volumes, bank blood transfusion requirements, blood product transfusion, and the type of surgery are a minimum and are often part of the dataset required for registries.

Finally, regular quality control of the ICS process with regard to wash efficiency is essential. There are several markers which are used. Free plasma haemoglobin is the most important as it can lead to renal tubular damage, but assays are not commonly in use. Plasma albumin and calcium are more suitable and the latter can be measured in real time on a standard blood gas machine.

Conclusions

Cell salvage is an extremely safe quality improvement intervention that has been proven to reduce blood transfusion and improve clinical outcomes. It should be available for all operations where there is the potential for bleeding that may lead to anaemia requiring transfusion. No matter what other PBM interventions are available, ICS provides a safety net in cases of unexpected haemorrhage that might otherwise have rendered them ineffective. Institutions should identify candidate operations, train and certify operators, organize rotas and institute regular audit and quality control. ICS should be used alongside tranexamic acid in all cases unless there is a special risk of thromboembolism.

Checklist summary

✓ Engage a senior manager and rehearse the advantages of ICS, clinical and economic.

✓ Befriend your local anaesthetists.

✓ Involve an ICS 'champion' in theatre, such as the senior operating department practitioner or operating room technician.

✓ Identify, through audit and consultation with the transfusion laboratory, procedures that might be suitable for ICS.

✓ Hold presentations at the relevant departmental audit meetings.

✓ Invite one of the companies to become involved in training a small key group of operators, who will then 'buddy' train others. It is not practical to train large groups due to rota and staffing issues.

✓ Use the ICS workbook as core knowledge.

✓ Rotate staff to maintain experience.

✓ Keep accurate records of salvage volumes and quality assurance results.

✓ Involve and inform your patients.

✓ Enjoy the benefits of ICS.

References

1. http://www.vascularsociety.org.uk/wp-content/uploads/2012/11/National-AAA-QIP-Interim-Report.pdf.

2. Konig G, Waters JH. Washing and filtering of cell-salvaged blood - does it make autotransfusion safer? *Transfus Altern Transfus Med* 2012; 12(3-4): 78-87.

3. Ashworth A, Klein AA. Cell salvage as part of a blood conservation strategy in anaesthesia. *Br J Anaesth* 2010; 105: 401-16.

4. National Institute for Health and Care Excellence. Blood transfusion - assessment and management of blood transfusion, NG24. London, UK: NICE, 2015. http://www.nice.org.uk/guidance/ng24.

5. Takagi H, Seishiro S, Takayoshi K, *et al.* Intraoperative autotransfusion in abdominal aneurysm surgery: meta-analysis of randomized controlled trials. *Arch Surg* 2007; 142: 1098-101.

6.   Wang G, Bainbridge D, Martin J, Cheng D. Efficacy of an intraoperative cell saver during cardiac surgery: a meta-analysis of randomized trials. *Anesth Analg* 2009; 109: 320-30.

7.   Jonsson H. The rationale for intraoperative blood salvage in cardiac surgery. *J Cardiothorac Vasc Anesth* 2009; 23: 394-400.

8.   Innerhofer P, Klingler A, Klimmer C, *et al.* Risk of postoperative infection after transfusion of white blood cell-filtered allogenic or autologous blood components in orthopedic patients undergoing primary arthroplasty. *Transfusion* 2005; 45: 103-10.

9.   http://www.aagbi.org/publications/guidelines/docs/cell%20_salvage_2009_amended.pdf.

10.   http://www.shotuk.org/wp-content/uploads/SHOT-2014-Annual-Report_v11-Web-Edition.pdf.

11.   CRASH trial collaborators. Final results of MRC CRASH, a randomised placebo-controlled trial of intravenous corticosteroid in adults with head injury - outcomes at 6 months. *Lancet* 2005; 365(9475): 1957-9.

12.   Duffy G, Tolley K. Cost of autologous blood transfusion, using cell salvage, compared with allogeneic blood transfusion. *Transfus Med* 1997; 7: 189-96.

Chapter 15

Surgical methods to prevent blood loss

John Thompson MS FRCSEd FRCS
Consultant Surgeon, Royal Devon and Exeter Hospitals, University of Exeter Medical School, Exeter, UK

- "Will all Great Neptune's ocean wash the blood clean from my hand?"
  Macbeth

- "Knowledge depends on long practice, not from speculations."
  Marcello Malphigi 1698

- "Choose your surgeon with care!"

Background

There have been huge advances in surgery in the last 20 years, many of which have been driven by the parallel imperatives of blood conservation arising in the wake of the human immunodeficiency virus (HIV) crisis of the 1980s. The previous generation of surgeons worked quickly and boldly, relying on natural haemostasis, packing and ligatures applied to principal vessels alone. Today's surgeons have been trained differently. Although an individual surgeon's technique is the most important determinant of blood loss within an institution, there is clear evidence of huge variation between hospitals [1].

The shift towards blood conservation by promoting the appropriate use of blood is one of the most important drivers that has led to better surgical technique. The emergence of hospital transfusion/blood management committees enabled surgeons to be informed of their blood transfusion data (use and wastage) for specific operations. The data could then be presented in an anonymised fashion in audit meetings. Perceived (or real!) peer pressure led to surgeons examining ways in which their blood loss could be reduced [2]. More recently the publication of individual surgeon's results in the USA, similarly followed by several European nations, has been a great incentive to improve standards.

General approaches

The most important aspect of surgical bleeding is for the surgeon to adopt a philosophy of blood conservation. Trainees should imagine that the patient has no blood available for transfusion, which is of course a fact in many countries.

Dissection should be careful and all bleeding should be dealt with immediately by the use of cautery, ligature or suture. Meticulous technique is an important part of bloodless surgery that fits well with advances in orthopaedic, vascular and especially oncological surgery that promote dissection through avascular tissue planes such as mesorectal excision.

There are many other common sense techniques to reduce blood loss (Table 1).

Table 1. Basic surgical techniques to reduce blood loss.

Meticulous dissection:

- Dissect in avascular planes.
- Deal with bleeding immediately.
- Ensure adequate lighting exposure and assistance.

Reduce blood pressure:

- Patient position such as 'deck chair'.
- Proximal inflow control such as the Pringle manoeuvre.
- Tourniquets.

Normothermia:

- Warm fluids, gases, patient with 3M™ Bair Hugger™.
- Minimise heat loss (internal packing rather than evisceration).
- Warm irrigation solutions and use impermeable drapes.

In cases of major unexpected bleeding, it is vital for solo surgeons to immediately summon experienced help (it is astonishing to discover that this was not done in medicolegal cases with a bad outcome). The bleeding vessels should be packed until the following are present:

- Adequate lighting.
- Assistance.
- Suction.
- Cell salvage if possible.
- Blood (cross-matched if possible, group-specific if available or emergency O Rh neg).

Assistants should be trained to use finger or swab pressure if possible at all times rather than continuous suction. It is no good to have a dry field in an exsanguinating patient!

Reducing blood pressure

Volume blood flow in the vein draining an organ is roughly equal to the arterial input. As a result surgeons have a healthy respect for venous bleeding, which can be torrential and difficult to control. Positioning the patient can moderately reduce arterial pressure but it is particularly effective in reducing venous bleeding. Examples include the use of the head-down position for varicose vein surgery or the deck chair position for neurosurgery. For spinal surgery the patient is placed prone on a Montreal mattress enabling the abdomen to hang clear. This reduces diaphragmatic splinting and lowers the pressure in the vertebral venous plexus [3].

During surgery the arterial inflow to an organ may be temporarily interrupted such as by clamping the hepatic artery during liver resection. Permanent ligation can also be used, as with ligation of the internal iliac arteries in cases of major obstetric haemorrhage. Tourniquets provide a completely bloodless field and are invaluable in cases of trauma (Figure 1).

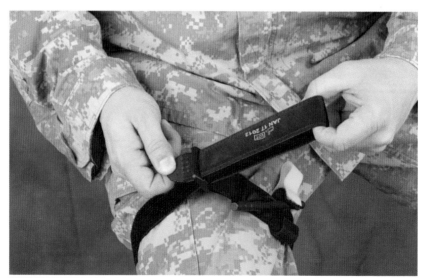

Figure 1. The C-A-Tourniquet® (http://combattourniquet.com). *Reproduced with permission from C-A-T Resources, LLC, Rock Hill, SC, USA. © Phil Durango, LLC.*

Elective orthopaedic, plastic and vascular surgery operations are facilitated by the use of tourniquets. In lower limb amputation the use of a tourniquet not only reduces transfusion but can also reduce revision rates [4].

Normothermia

Platelet function is severely impaired after a quite modest reduction in temperature — below 35°C [5]. The enzymes of the coagulation cascade are similarly affected, so prevention of heat loss along with active warming is an essential component of surgical haemostasis. The ambient temperature of the operating theatre can be raised in paediatric cases. All anaesthetic gases and fluids should be warmed and devices such as the Level 1® infuser (Smiths Medical, Dublin, OH, USA) enable rapid infusion of fluids and blood. Impermeable drapes, warm irrigation fluids and avoiding exenteration of bowel are also helpful.

Interventional radiology

Interventional radiology (IR) is an essential part of any trauma service and has replaced surgery in the management of several difficult scenarios (Figures 2-5). Catheter embolisation is the method of choice in cases of retroperitoneal haemorrhage especially from the kidney. Feeding arteries can be interrupted by means of coils, occlusion devices or synthetic copolymers such as Onyx® (Covidien). Bleeding vessels may be repaired by means of covered stent grafts and false aneurysms can be treated by percutaneous thrombin injection. Pre-operative embolisation can reduce the vascularity of tumours and selective devascularisation can be used for ischaemic pre-conditioning prior to liver resection or oesophagectomy.

Endovascular aneurysm repair (EVAR) has replaced open surgical repair for abdominal and thoracic aneurysms in approximately 70% of cases (nearly 100% in some centres). EVAR can be done percutaneously and even under local anaesthetic as a day case. Blood loss is minimal and emergency conversion to open surgery is a very rare event. For open surgery blood conservation techniques, especially cell salvage, mean that most elective AAA repairs can be done with a group and save alone.

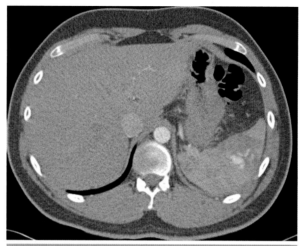

Figure 2. CT angiogram of a 28-year-old man whose motorcycle had hit a telegraph pole. He sustained multiple fractures and a ruptured spleen. Active bleeding can be seen in the upper pole.

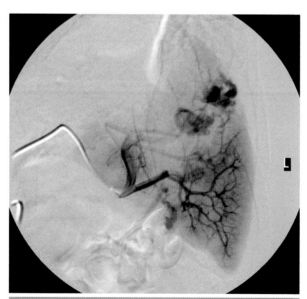

Figure 3. Transfemoral angiography demonstrates active extravasation of contrast from the upper pole splenic artery.

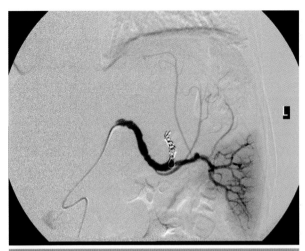

Figure 4. After coil embolisation bleeding from the spleen has been arrested. The patient left the hospital after 5 days.

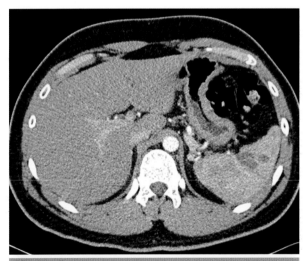

Figure 5. Follow-up CT at 6 weeks showing a well-perfused splenic remnant. No long-term antibiotic prophylaxis was required.

Minimally invasive surgery and robotics

In the era of open surgery there was a move towards smaller and smaller incisions; mini-incision cholecystectomy, for example. Laparoscopic surgery is minimally invasive in terms of the port sites, but the same procedure as an open operation is performed internally. High definition and, recently, 3-D monitors provide better visualisation than open surgery. Blood loss is immediately obvious and it is possible to maintain meticulous haemostasis from the outset. Surgical strategies such as the medial to lateral approach for laparoscopic colectomy enable the principal vessels to be ligated first. This improves oncological results as well as haemostasis. The increased use of laparoscopic surgery has been so successful that recruitment to studies of the use of intravenous iron in such procedures have been virtually impossible.

In cardiac surgery, off-pump techniques have been shown to improve platelet function and to decrease blood transfusion requirement.

Robotic surgery is now the clear technique of choice in several areas and, in particular, urology. Open cystectomy, radical prostatectomy and nephrectomy were once operations requiring major transfusion support. The 3-D platform of robotic surgery combined with the degrees of freedom of movement of the tiny instruments are ideal for careful haemostasis. Although it is hardly ever needed, cell salvage can be used via the suction port. In our institution, radical prostatectomy can now be performed as a day case with only two transfusions in over 300 procedures [6].

Cell salvage

Cell salvage is considered in the previous chapter, but it is worth emphasising that optimum use of the equipment can contribute to increased efficiency. The equipment should be available for all cases where bleeding might be sufficient to lead to transfusion. The 'suck and save' approach avoids breaking out the more expensive centrifuge until it is needed. At the end of the procedure a near-patient Hb estimation should be performed. If the patient is just below the agreed transfusion trigger, it may well be worth processing a small volume of salvaged blood to exceed the trigger and avoid transfusion. Washing blood-soaked swabs and processing the saline can increase cell salvage efficiency by 30% [7].

Surgical instruments

There are a wide variety of instruments available that are used to achieve haemostasis and as an adjunct or alternative to sharp dissection. All work on the principle of delivery of energy to generate heat (Table 2).

Table 2. Haemostatic surgical instruments.

	Mechanism	Disadvantages	Applications
Monopolar diathermy	Heat	Collateral damage Pacemakers Ignition of gases	Most surgery
Bipolar diathermy	Heat	Ignition of gases	Precise surgery Use near nerves Pacemakers
Argon beam	Heat	As monopolar	Hepatobiliary Pelvic
Laser	Heat	As monopolar Cost Special theatre	Laparoscopic surgery Gynaecology
Ultrasound dissector	Sonic and heat	Cost	Solid organs Large tumours, e.g. sarcoma
Water jet dissector	Mechanical	Cost	As above

Monopolar diathermy is the most widely used technique. High-frequency current passes through the patient via a large surface area adhesive electrode. High resistance at the diathermy tip generates heat which can be used to coagulate or dissect. Various combinations of wave form are available which can blend the cutting and sealing functions, or 'spray' the current over a broad area. The argon beam coagulator uses a stream of argon gas to enhance the delivery of heat and has the added advantage of dispersing tissue and fluid, making it especially useful for liver resection.

Bipolar diathermy involves the current passing between the tips of the forceps without the use of a remote earthing plate. This is useful in cases where surgery is in close proximity to delicate structures such as nerves or when the patient has a pacemaker *in situ*, although most modern pacemakers can be deactivated during surgery by the placement of a magnet over the control box. The LigaSure™ device (Medtronic) is a variant of bipolar diathermy where the tissue to be divided is placed in the jaws of the instrument, where it is heated, sealed and then mechanically cut (Figures 6 and 7). LigaSure™ is particularly useful for cancer surgery, splenectomy and thyroidectomy [8].

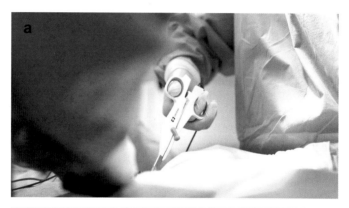

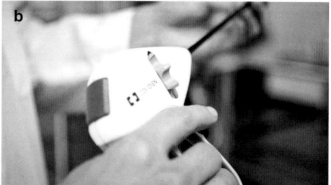

Figure 6. a) LigaSure™ small jaw instrument. b) LigaSure™ blunt tip laparoscopic instrument. *Reprinted with permission from Medtronic. All rights reserved.*

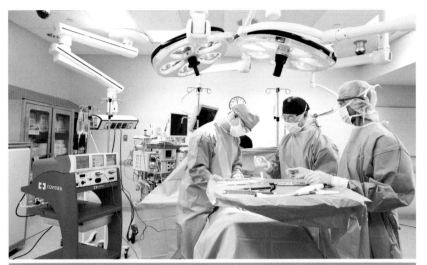

Figure 7. The ForceTriad™ energy platform which delivers monopolar, bipolar and LigaSure™ energy. *Reprinted with permission from Medtronic. All rights reserved.*

Lasers

There are a wide variety of lasers available for medical use [9]. All of them use thermal energy to achieve the desired effect but the characteristics of the laser energy emitted and the power influence the extent and depth of penetration. The use of laser mandates local rules, a responsible officer, training and certification of operators and a secure theatre with signage and secure doors.

Neodynium-yttrium-aluminium-garnet (Nd-YAG) lasers produce light at a wavelength of 1.06μm penetrating to a depth of 3-5mm. This destructive capacity is used to treat bleeding peptic ulcers endoscopically or to resect oesophageal tumours for palliation.

Carbon dioxide (CO_2) lasers operate at 10.6μm. At this wavelength the energy is rapidly dissipated and absorbed by water so these lasers are useful in dealing with superficial lesions such as skin and cervical malignancy.

Argon lasers emit light at the 0.49-0.51µm wavelength which is blue/green and is therefore absorbed by red pigments. Their main use is in dealing with retinal lesions.

Holmium-YAG lasers have a longer wavelength of 2.1µm which penetrates tissue up to 1mm in depth, making them most useful in endourology. Laser prostatectomy is a largely bloodless procedure and has been approved by the UK's National Institute for Health and Care Excellence (NICE). NICE has concluded that the procedure is equivalent in efficacy to standard transurethral prostatectomy and has the benefit of reduced blood loss.

Ultrasound and water jet dissectors

These instruments are invaluable for dissecting parenchyma in solid organs, especially the liver. The Harmonic Scalpel® (Ethicon, USA) delivers vibration energy to its shears at 55.5kHz which has the effect of disrupting cells but leaving collagen fibres intact. These are present in vessels, bile ducts and nerves which can then be ligated or divided under direct vision. The Harmonic Scalpel® produces modest temperatures of up to 100°C. A refinement of the technique is the Cavitational Ultrasonic Surgical Aspirator® (CUSA®, Integra, NJ, USA) which has an aspiration channel that removes debris and allows very clear views of the bile ducts and vessels. This is invaluable during segmental hepatectomy.

Water jet dissectors provide the same advantages of CUSA® using a high-pressure saline jet. Randomised trials support the use of water jet and ultrasonic dissectors but there have been negative results when compared to traditional techniques; this emphasises the importance of individual surgical technique.

Topical haemostatic agents

These are applied over a bleeding surface and act by encouraging the tissue factor or fibrin pathway to enhance haemostasis. In general, surgeons should only use these agents after all the traditional methods have been exhausted; they are particularly useful if there is a raw area or oozing due to dual antiplatelet therapy.

There are three main categories:

* Haemostatic swabs/patches/powders.
* Fibrin glue/sealants.
* Exothermic agents.

Haemostatic swabs, patches and powders

These use various preparations of oxidised cellulose, calcium alginate or collagen as a fabric, microfibres or powder, which provides a large surface area promoting extrinsic activation of coagulation and platelets. They are very effective and in wide use. Many surgeons, however, are not aware that with the earlier haemostatic products on the market that the instructions for use state that the material should not be left in place. For some newer products, however, these can be left in the body after surgery (see overleaf). This should be checked in advance before use. Material such as oxidised cellulose swells on activation so there is a potential risk of nerve compression in confined spaces [10]. Foreign body reactions have also been reported. Clinical judgement is therefore required.

The haemostat field is constantly evolving and new devices are being introduced into the surgical arena. One such example is Medtronic's Veriset™ haemostatic patch (Figure 8) which combines oxidised regenerated cellulose, polyethylene glycol (PEG) and trilysine, resulting in a fast-acting haemostat that works by lowering the blood pH, thus accelerating the natural coagulation cascade, and creating a PEG hydrogel barrier to exponentially increase the concentration of platelets at the bleeding site. All this occurs in less than 1 minute. The Veriset™ patch can be left inside the patient, dissolving after 1 month.

Figure 8. Veriset™ haemostatic patch. *Reproduced with permission from Medtronic Inc.*

A recent development is a fine polysaccharide powder (HaemoCer™ PLUS; BioCer Entwicklungs GmbH, Germany) which is derived from plant starch (Figure 9). The powder can be used off the shelf and results in rapid activation of coagulation factors and platelets. Residual starch is hydrolysed and metabolised and there is no risk of antigenicity or infection. There is no preparation time and the resultant gel is translucent. It is reabsorbed by the body within 48 hours. Data on the use of this product is awaited with interest.

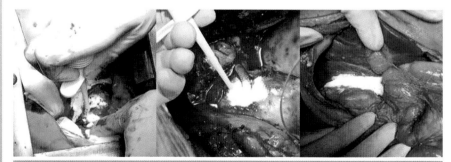

Figure 9. HaemoCer™ PLUS haemostatic powder. *Reproduced with permission from BioCer Entwicklungs GmbH.*

Fibrin glue and sealants

There is a wide range of products available which provide an exogenous supply of fibrin clot to boost local haemostasis. The source may be autologous (providing the patient's fibrinogen levels are sufficient) or exogenous. The essential component of all products consists of separate vials of thrombin and fibrinogen. An antifibrinolytic agent such as aprotinin, factor XIII to stabilise the clot and calcium chloride as an activator complete the recipe. Fibrin glue is useful in patients who have depleted coagulation factors.

The evidence surrounding the efficacy of fibrin sealants is poor. There are perennial problems with poor study design, heterogeneity, surrogate endpoints and very few data regarding transfusion. Despite this, most surgeons have experienced very positive results in difficult bleeding situations and operating theatres should keep a stock for emergency use. The general consensus is that fibrin sealants do have a role to play especially in cardiovascular surgery [11].

Exothermic materials

The most effective example of these is QuikClot® (Z-Medica, Wallingford, CT, USA), which was originally designed as a powder containing zeolite. The zeolite interacts with blood in a wound creating an exothermic reaction which can cause second-degree burns. QuikClot® has been used in Iraq and Afghanistan and is highly effective as can be seen in internet videos, but it is not used in civilian practice [12].

Conclusions

The most important contributor to patient blood management in surgery is for the whole surgical team and the surgeon in particular to develop a philosophy of bloodless surgery. This will be rewarded by improved outcomes as well as decreased reliance on blood. Simple methods such as warming, positioning and careful dissection should be the norm. More expensive adjuncts such as lasers and ultrasonic instruments should be reserved for special situations.

Checklist summary

✓ Surgical technique is the single most important factor in reducing intra-operative blood loss.

✓ Basic techniques such as positioning and approach can result in significant reduction in blood loss.

✓ Modern haemostatic instrumentation can contribute to bloodless dissection, particularly in cancer surgery.

✓ Topical haemostatic agents can be helpful when all other interventions have failed.

✓ The move towards endovascular, laparoscopic and robotic surgery has significantly reduced reliance on blood transfusion.

References

1.   Hébert PC, Wells G, Martin C, *et al.* Variation in red cell transfusion practice in the intensive care unit: a multicentre cohort study. *Crit Care* 1999; 3(2): 57-63.

2.   http://www.acssurgerynews.com/specialty-focus/traumacritical-care/single-article-page/peer-pressure-moves-dial-on-restricting-rbc-transfusions/87789ef87207a94b50f009dccb217649.html.

3.   Lee TC, Yang LC, Chen HJ. Effect of patient position and hypotensive anaesthesia on inferior vena cava pressure. *Spine* 1999; 23: 941-7.

4.   Wolthuis AM, Whitehead E, Ridler BM, *et al.* Use of a pneumatic tourniquet improves outcome following trans-tibial amputation. *Eur J Vasc Endovasc Surg* 2006; 31(6): 642-5.

5.   Van Poucke S, Stevens K, Marcus AE, Lancé M. Hypothermia: effects on platelet function and haemostasis. *Thromb J* 2014; 12: 31.

6.   http://lib.ajaums.ac.ir/booklist/1-s2.0-S156990561450190X-main.pdf.

7.   Haynes SL, Bennett TR, Torella F, McCollum CN. Does swab washing improve red cell recovery in aortic surgery? *Vox Sang* 2004; 87(S3): 50.

8.   Contin P, Gooßen K, Grummich K, *et al.* ENERgized vessel sealing systems versus CONventional hemostasis techniques in thyroid surgery - the ENERCON systematic review and network meta-analysis. *Lang Arch Surg* 2013; 398: 1039-56.

9.   http://www.uptodate.com/contents/basic-principles-of-medical-lasers.

10.   Brodbelt AR, Miles JB, Foy PM, Broome JC. Intraspinal oxidized cellulose (Surgicel) causing delayed paraplegia after thoracotomy - a report of three cases. *Ann Roy Coll Surg Eng* 2002; 84: 97-9.

11.   Rousou JA. Use of fibrin sealants in cardiovascular surgery: a systematic review. *J Card Surg* 2013; 28(3): 238-47.

12.   Grissom TE, Fang R. Topical hemostatic agents and dressings in the prehospital setting. *Curr Opin Anaesth* 2015; 28(2): 210-16.

Chapter 16

Anaesthetic methods to minimise blood loss

Richard Telford BSc (Hons) MBBS FRCA
Consultant Anaesthetist, Royal Devon and Exeter Hospital/Peninsula Medical School, Exeter, UK

Claire Todd BSc MBChB (Hons) MRCP FRCA
ST7 Anaesthetics, Royal Devon and Exeter Hospital/Peninsula Medical School, Exeter, UK

- **"Bleeding is due to cutting blood vessels."**
  A Synopsis of Anaesthesia, 9th ed, 1982

- **"Once the practice of anaesthesia became established, although the surgeon caused the bleeding, the anaesthetist took the blame."**
  Leigh JM. The history of controlled hypotension. *Br J Anaesth* 1975; 47: 745-9

- **"It was dry when I closed!"** Anon

- **"The amiable juice; a rich liquid asset, a priceless deposit which can neither be spent or accumulated."**
  Dr Jonathan Miller, *The Nation's Health*

Background

The training, care and technique of the surgeon performing the operative procedure are the most crucial factors in minimising bleeding. However, the anaesthetic technique plays an important role in minimising peri-operative blood loss. It was evident to Humphry Davy in 1800 when he wrote "... it (nitrous oxide) may probably be used with advantage during surgical operations in which no great effusion of blood takes place" [1]. Following the discovery that ether produced insensibility during surgical operations in 1846 [2], although the bleeding was frequently the result of surgical trauma the anaesthetist commonly took the blame. This had some justification since patients anaesthetised with volatile agents bled more than those conscious during the surgical procedure.

The conduct and technique of anaesthesia can influence the degree of intra-operative blood loss. The techniques to minimise this are discussed in this chapter.

How to do it

Patient positioning

One of the most simple and yet effective methods for reducing intra-operative blood loss is meticulous care and attention to the positioning of the patient to minimise venous pressure. The operative site should be raised to slightly above the level of the heart. For head and neck surgery a head-up posture should be used, and for lower limb, pelvic and lower abdominal procedures the head-down (Trendelenburg) position should be used. Caution should be exercised, however, if large veins are exposed during surgery because of the risk of air embolism.

Tourniquets

When operating on extremities blood loss can be reduced by the application of a limb tourniquet to create a bloodless field. Tourniquets are most commonly used during orthopaedic and plastic surgery procedures.

The limb is exsanguinated using elevation and/or an Esmarch bandage before the tourniquet is inflated. The tourniquet pressure should be 100-150mmHg above the systolic blood pressure of the patient. The tourniquet is frequently deflated close to the end of surgery to identify any bleeding points prior to closure of the surgical wound. Tourniquet time should be limited to 2 hours in order to minimise the risk of distal ischaemia. The use of a tourniquet is contraindicated in patients with sickle cell disease/trait (because of the risk of precipitating a sickle crisis) and where the blood supply to the limb is already tenuous (e.g. severe atherosclerosis). Disadvantages of tourniquets include compression, ischaemia, and also toxic metabolite release after tourniquet deflation which can lead to nerve, vascular and muscular injury, and cardiac dysfunction.

Vasoconstrictors

Vasoconstrictor drugs are used to limit the bleeding locally at the site of surgery. The most commonly used drug is adrenaline which may be used in isolation or in combination with a local anaesthetic such as lignocaine or bupivacaine. Combination of local anaesthetic with adrenaline has the advantage of contributing to postoperative analgesia. The total dose of adrenaline should not exceed 100µg in an adult, which is equivalent to 20ml of a 1 in 200,000 strength solution. Care must be taken not to exceed the recommended doses of local anaesthetics because of their potential side effects. This is a particular problem when the surgical field covers a large surface area of the body. In addition, care should be taken not to inject vasoconstrictors intravascularly. The use of vasoconstrictors is contraindicated in areas where there are end arteries, e.g. fingers and toes.

Surgical technique

This is probably the most crucial factor in reducing operative blood loss. Surgery causes bleeding directly through tissue and vascular damage.

Development of avascular planes, meticulous attention to haemostasis and the pre-emptive ligation of major feeding vessels are important. Laser and ultrasonic scalpels (Figure 1) and water jet dissectors are helpful in certain types of surgery. Topical haemostatic agents such as collagen and fibrin glue may be useful.

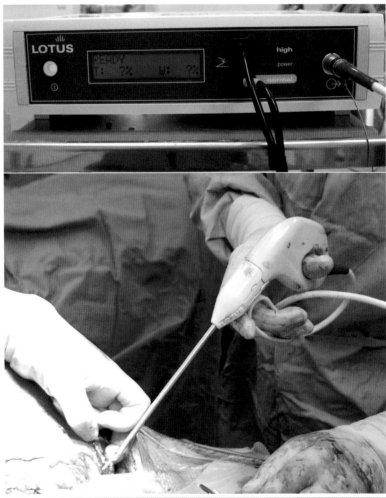

Figure 1. Lotus® ultrasonic scalpel.

Thermoregulation

Anaesthetised patients become hypothermic for a variety of reasons. Loss of behavioural responses to cold, impairment of thermoregulatory mechanisms, anaesthetic-induced peripheral vasodilatation and the use of unwarmed intravenous or irrigation fluids all contribute. Heat loss occurs via:

* Radiation (responsible for 40-50% of loss): this is transfer of heat to a cooler object from the body to the surroundings.
* Convection (30%): air next to the body is warmed by conduction and carried away in convection currents.
* Evaporation (20-25%): as moisture evaporates from the body it loses latent heat of evaporation, causing the body to cool. Evaporative heat losses are increased in open body cavity surgery and when inspired anaesthetic gases are not humidified.
* Conduction (5%)

Peri-operative hypothermia impairs coagulation and leads to an increase in intra-operative blood loss. Hypothermia causes platelet dysfunction, alteration of coagulation enzyme kinetics, enhanced fibrinolysis, an increased affinity of haemoglobin for oxygen, an increased release of red cell potassium and a decreased breakdown of lactate.

All surgical patients are at risk of developing intra-operative hypothermia but risk factors include:

* A combination of general and regional anaesthesia.
* Prolonged surgical time.
* A low body mass index.
* Open body cavity surgery.
* Extremes of age.

Core temperature should be regularly measured during the peri-operative period and steps should be taken to prevent hypothermia. These include the use of forced air warmers, warmed intravenous fluids and maintenance of high ambient theatre temperature.

Balanced anaesthesia

The triad of anaesthesia comprises analgesia, muscle relaxation and unconsciousness. Balancing these components plays an important role in minimising blood loss. Adequate levels of anaesthesia and analgesia should be maintained to minimise intra-operative hypertension and tachycardia which increase blood loss. Adequate control of ventilation avoids hypercarbia (higher than normal levels of carbon dioxide) which results in vasodilation and increased intra-operative blood loss. Finally, a balanced anaesthetic technique will avoid the patient coughing or straining which would increase venous pressure and increase blood loss.

The use of regional anaesthesia, particularly central neuraxial blockade (epidural/spinal) reduces intra-operative blood loss and the requirement for blood transfusion. The haemodynamic effects, which lower arterial blood pressure, venous blood pressure and central venous pressure explain the reduction in blood loss [3].

Permissive hypotension

This refers to the technique of inducing hypotension during a surgical procedure in order to reduce bleeding and the need for blood transfusion. It also has the advantage of reducing the amount of blood in the surgical field, therefore improving the surgeon's view. It is mostly commonly requested in maxillofacial surgery, middle ear surgery, major orthopaedic surgery (particularly joint replacements), cardiac surgery and open clipping of intracranial aneurysms.

There are several definitions of permissive hypotension including a reduction in mean arterial blood pressure (MAP) by 30% of the baseline reading, a MAP of 50-65mmHg or a systolic blood pressure of less than 90mmHg. It is not uncommon for surgeons to request the blood pressure to be increased to pre-operative levels near the end of the procedure to check for haemostasis.

The two most commonly used techniques to induce hypotension include regional anaesthesia (most commonly epidural anaesthesia) and a combination of an intravenous infusion of the potent opioid, remifentanil, with either propofol or an inhalational anaesthetic agent. Other pharmacological agents to induce hypotension can be used but this is relatively uncommon outside cardiac surgery. Examples include β-blockers (e.g. esmolol), sodium nitroprusside, glyceryl trinitrate (GTN) and centrally acting alpha-2 agonists (clonidine).

The main risk of permissive hypotension is decreased perfusion of vital organs with a potentially increased risk of stroke, myocardial infarction and renal failure. It is only appropriate in the hands of an experienced anaesthetist with access to comprehensive monitoring facilities. Patients must be carefully selected; permissive hypotension must be used cautiously in patients with cardiac or vascular disease because of the increased risk of end-organ damage.

Acute normovolaemic haemodilution

Acute normovolaemic haemodilution (ANH) was first introduced in the 1970s [4]. ANH involves the collection of whole blood from the patient with simultaneous infusion of crystalloid to maintain normovolaemia. Any surgical bleeding then entails a smaller loss of red cells. ANH can be performed immediately before or after the onset of anaesthesia. Blood is withdrawn into citrated blood bags (Figure 2), which can be stored at room temperature for 6 hours. This may be prolonged to 12 hours with appropriate cooling. ANH has several advantages over allogeneic blood donation. The blood procured by haemodilution requires no testing. The blood is fresh, containing functional platelets and clotting factors. The units are not removed from the operating theatre, so the possibility of an administrative error resulting in an ABO incompatible blood transfusion, is virtually eliminated. Bacterial contamination is less likely. The calculated volume of blood is withdrawn from a venous or arterial line connected to a three-way stopcock into citrated collection bags. Haemodilution kits that contain a Y-type Luer locking adapter simplify the process and improve sterility.

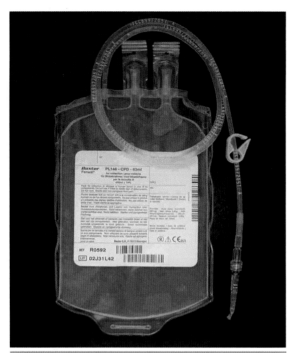

Figure 2. Blood bag which can be used for acute normovolaemic haemodilution (ANH).

Calculation of the volume of blood to be withdrawn is done using the simplified formula published by Goss [5]:

Volume of blood to be removed = EBV (70ml/kg) x $\dfrac{(H_i - H_f)}{H_{av}}$

where EBV = estimated blood volume; H_i = initial haematocrit; H_f = final haematocrit; H_{av} = average of H_i and H_f.

450-500ml of blood is withdrawn into each bag which is gently agitated during the collection process until the target haematocrit is reached. The bags containing the autologous (patient's own) blood are labelled, numbered sequentially and stored at room temperature (by the patient's side) to maintain platelet function. Euvolaemic (normal circulatory volume) patients maintain cardiac output and oxygen delivery to the tissues because of the improved rheology (blood flow) associated with a decreased haemoglobin concentration.

The blood is reinfused into the patient as needed, ideally once surgical blood loss has ceased, although it can be administered during the surgical procedure if clinically indicated. ANH can be used as a standalone blood conservation technique or in combination with intra-operative cell salvage. The collected units are normally returned to the patient in reverse order, thus the first unit collected (which has the highest number of platelets, coagulation factors and haematocrit) is returned last.

Intra-operative haemodilution should be considered for operations with an estimated blood loss >1000ml (or >20% of blood volume) and in patients with a high initial haematocrit. It is contraindicated in patients with cardiac disease, impaired renal function and anaemia. The amount of blood removed depends on the patient's blood volume, tolerance of the procedure and anticipated blood loss. Generally, clinicians aim for a pre-operative haemoglobin of 80-90g/L (haematocrit of 24-27%). The potential benefits and risks of intra-operative haemodilution have been debated [6]. The major benefit of intra-operative haemodilution is quoted as a decrease in exposure to allogeneic blood. It also has the benefit of increasing tissue perfusion as haemodilution decreases blood viscosity. The main disadvantages are that it is time consuming and requires trained and dedicated personnel. Mathematical modelling has suggested that severe haemodilution (peri-operative haematocrit less than 20%) accompanied by substantial blood loss would be required before the red cell volume saved becomes clinically important. Therefore, ANH, where appropriate, is employed alongside other blood conservation measures such as intra-operative cell salvage.

Conclusions

The anaesthetist can make a significant contribution to minimising peri-operative blood loss. Meticulous attention to the anaesthetic technique, careful patient positioning and maintenance of normothermia are pivotal. Permissive hypotension and acute normovolaemic haemodilution have a useful role in carefully selected fit patients free from cardiorespiratory disease.

Checklist summary

✓ Employ simple techniques such as patient positioning.

✓ Avoid peri-operative hypothermia.

✓ Consider using permissive hypotension in carefully selected patients but be aware of the risk of organ hypoperfusion and damage.

✓ Consider acute normovolaemic haemodilution if the potential operative blood loss is likely to exceed 20% of the patient's blood volume and the patient has no cardiorespiratory disease.

References

1.   Davy H. *Researches, Chemical and Philosophical Chiefly Concerning Nitrous Oxide.* London, UK: J. Johnson, 1800: 556.

2.   Bigelow HJ. Insensibilty during surgical operations produced by inhalation. *The Boston Medical and Surgical Journal* 1846; 35 (Nov 18th): 309-7.

3.   Modig J. Regional anaesthesia and blood loss. *Acta Anaesthesiology Scand Supplement* 1988; 89: 44-8.

4.   Mesmer K. Haemodilution. *Surg Clin North Am* 1975; 55: 659.

5.   Goss JB. Estimating allowable blood loss: corrected for dilution. *Anaesthesiology* 1983; 58: 277-80.

6.   Segel JB, Blasco-Colmenares E, Norris EJ, Guallar E. Preoperative acute normovolaemic haemodilution: a meta-analysis. *Transfusion* 2004; 44: 632-44.

Chapter 17

Pharmacological methods for minimising blood loss

Beverley J. Hunt FRCP FRCPath MD

Professor of Thrombosis & Haemostasis, King's College University; Consultant, Guy's & St Thomas' NHS Foundation Trust, London, UK

- "Tranexamic acid reduces bleeding in surgical patients by one third."

- "Tranexamic acid reduces bleeding deaths in trauma by one third."

- "Increasing the dose of tranexamic acid from 1-2g does not increase efficacy but does lead to neurological side effects."

Background

There has been an explosion of interest in the use of pharmacological agents to reduce bleeding in the last 30 years since the discovery in 1986 that aprotinin reduced bleeding in high-risk cardiac surgery. Unfortunately, aprotinin has fallen out of favour and since the Clinical Randomisation of an Antifibrinolytic in Significant Haemorrhage (CRASH-2) study was published in 2010, research efforts have concentrated on using tranexamic acid (TXA). Tranexamic acid has been shown to reduce mortality due to traumatic bleeding by a third, without apparent safety issues. It is now clearly established that intravenous TXA reduces blood loss in patients with surgical bleeding and the need for transfusion. It can also be used topically to reduce bleeding. Its use is being explored further in large pragmatic trials in traumatic head injury, postpartum haemorrhage and in upper gastrointestinal haemorrhage. There are few side effects from the use of TXA except when administered in a high dose where neurological events have been noted, possibly relating to TXA interfering with cerebral gamma-amino butyric acid (GABA) and glycine receptors. However, clinical studies suggest that there is no increased efficacy in using a higher dose, and that a dose of 1g intravenously in an adult patient has maximal efficacy, which is not increased by higher doses. The CRASH-2 trauma trial clearly showed no increase in thrombotic events after its use in trauma; indeed, there was a significant reduction in myocardial infarction. Trials of TXA in surgery have failed to adequately study its effects on the risk of postoperative venous and possible reduction in arterial thromboembolism, and this needs to be the subject of future research. We await the results of the WOMAN study, which will show whether TXA is efficacious in reducing death due to postpartum haemorrhage.

Introduction

In the last 30 years there has been a massive increase in interest in the utility of pharmacological agents to reduce bleeding, all prompted by the original study of a cardiothoracic team at the Hammersmith Hospital in the mid 80s[1]. They showed that the peri-operative use of aprotinin reduced bleeding significantly after cardiothoracic surgery. This was duplicated in numerous clinical trials and the effect attributed to its antifibrinolytic action. Unfortunately, the use of aprotinin was curtailed by the publication of the BART study [2]. This study showed that despite reducing bleeding, aprotinin was associated with a higher mortality when compared to two other antifibrinolytic agents: tranexamic acid (TXA) and ε-aminocaproic acid (EACA). A large pragmatic randomised controlled study called CRASH-2 was published in 2010 [3], the largest trauma trial ever conducted. It showed a reduction in mortality with the use of TXA. Since this study there have been many other clinical trials in surgery and interest in the role of fibrinolysis in bleeding. This chapter presents an overview of our current understanding as to where TXA may have clinical benefit, the appropriate dose and possible side effects.

Pharmacology of tranexamic acid (TXA)

Tranexamic acid (trans-4- [aminomethyl] cyclohexanecarboxylic acid) is a synthetic derivative of the amino acid lysine that competitively inhibits the activation of plasminogen to the serine protease, plasmin, via binding to kringle domains. Tranexamic acid is a competitive inhibitor of tissue plasminogen activator. It blocks the lysine-binding sites of plasminogen, resulting in inhibition of plasminogen activation and fibrin binding to plasminogen and therefore impairment of fibrinolysis [4].

Tranexamic acid is about ten times more potent *in vitro* than ε-aminocaproic acid, and binds more strongly than ε-aminocaproic acid to both the strong and weak receptor sites of the plasminogen molecule in a ratio corresponding to the difference in potency between the compounds. Tranexamic acid is distributed throughout all body tissues and the plasma half-life is 120 minutes.

The efficacy of tranexamic acid in reducing traumatic bleeding

The largest trial to date of antifibrinolytics, the CRASH-2 trial, assessed the effects of early administration of TXA in trauma patients with, or at risk of, substantial bleeding (Table 1) [3]. A total of 20,211 trauma patients from 40 countries were randomly assigned within 8 hours of injury to either TXA

(1g load, then 1g over 8h) or placebo. The primary outcome was in-hospital mortality within 4 weeks of injury. All-cause mortality was significantly reduced with TXA (14.5% vs. 16%; relative risk 0.91, 95% CI 0.85-0.97; p = 0.0035). The data from CRASH-2 showed that, following the second day, bleeding is not the main cause of mortality, and was ascribed to head injury, multi-organ failure and vaso-occlusive complications, all of which were reduced, although all except myocardial infarction were non-significantly reduced in those receiving TXA. However, the critical question was whether there was a reduction in bleeding deaths, and indeed, a significant reduction in death due to bleeding by one third was seen. The excitement about the application of the findings of CRASH-2 is that death due to traumatic bleeding is a global problem, and if TXA was given to all those with, or at risk of, traumatic bleeding, this would result in a worldwide reduction in the number of deaths of 120,000 per annum. The response in the UK has been positive, with NHS England ensuring that all ambulances and paramedics carry TXA; moreover, TXA needs to be administered in patients "receiving blood products within 3 hours of injury" under the Major Trauma Best Practice Tariff [5].

Despite the reduction in mortality due to bleeding, TXA did not reduce transfusion requirements. Why might this be? The management of blood loss during trauma is not fine-tuned to compensate for losses as it is in surgical practice; blood is given empirically and blood losses are not accurately measured. Also, investigators were asked to use their normal

Table 1. The efficacy of tranexamic acid in reducing traumatic bleeding — CRASH-2 trial.

- A total of 20,211 trauma patients from 40 countries were randomly assigned within 8 hours of injury to either TA (1g load, then 1g over 8h) or placebo.
- All-cause mortality was significantly reduced with TXA.
- A significant reduction in death due to bleeding by one third was seen.
- TXA did not reduce transfusion requirements.
- TXA treatment given in the first 3 hours reduced the risk of death due to bleeding.
- TXA treatment given after 3 hours seemed to increase death due to bleeding.

practice and the availability of blood components is variable between the 40 countries involved in the study — it is widely recognised that blood transfusion practice varies widely. We also hypothesised that a proportion of the reduction in deaths was not due to reduced bleeding but other mechanisms, perhaps due to the anti-inflammatory and/or anti-thrombotic effects of TXA [6].

The timing of TXA administration is important. Further analysis of CRASH-2 showed that treatment given in the first 3 hours reduced the risk of death due to bleeding, with relative risk (RR) reduction in the first hour of 0.68 (95% CI 0.57-0.82; p<0.0001) and 0.79 (95% CI 0.64-0.97; p = 0.03) between 1 and 3 hours. However, treatment given after 3 hours seemed to increase death due to bleeding, with a RR of 1.44 (95% CI 1.12-1.84; p = 0.004) [7]. Thus, TXA should be given as early as possible to bleeding trauma patients. For trauma patients admitted late after injury, TXA is less effective, and could be harmful.

Efficacy of tranexamic acid in reducing surgical bleeding

Since the withdrawal of aprotinin, TXA has been widely used to reduce bleeding in cardiac surgery, but it is now also used in other types of surgery (Table 2). In 2007, a systematic review of randomised trials assessing TXA in elective surgery identified 53 studies that included 3836 patients [8]. Tranexamic acid reduced the need for blood transfusion by a third (RR 0.61, 95% CI 0.54-0.70). A further systematic review in 2012 [9], reflecting the increased interest in TXA over the intervening years, identified 129 trials that included 10,488 patients, carried out between 1972 and 2011. In this meta-analysis, TXA reduced the probability of receiving a blood transfusion by a third (RR 0.62, 95% CI 0.58-0.65; p<0.001). This effect remained when the analysis was restricted to trials using adequate allocation concealment (RR 0.68, CI 0.62-0.74; p<0.001). Fewer deaths occurred in the TXA group (RR 0.61, CI 0.38-0.98; p = 0.04), although when the analysis was restricted to trials using adequate concealment there was considerable uncertainty (RR 0.67, 0.33 to 1.34; p = 0.25). The authors concluded that cumulative meta-analysis showed reliable evidence that TXA reduces the need for transfusion.

Table 2. The efficacy of tranexamic acid in reducing surgical bleeding.	
Henry *et al* [8]	• TXA reduced the need for blood transfusion by a third.
Ker *et al* [9]	• TXA reduced the probability of receiving a blood transfusion by a third. • Fewer deaths occurred in the TXA group.
Ker *et al* [10]	• The use of TXA was associated with an overall reduction in surgical bleeding by about a third. • There was no improved reduction in bleeding with doses of TXA >1g.

Another systematic review of 104 randomised trials examined whether the effect of TXA on blood loss varies with the extent of surgical bleeding. The results suggest that, despite variation in the magnitude of blood loss between procedures and the heterogeneity of the studies included, the use of TXA was associated with an overall reduction in surgical bleeding by about a third. This reduction in bleeding with TXA is almost identical to the reduction in the risk of receiving a blood transfusion with TXA suggesting, as expected in the closely monitored environment of an operating theatre, that unlike traumatic bleeding in CRASH-2, blood transfusion use was closely titrated to blood loss [10].

Efficacy of tranexamic acid in postpartum haemorrhage

A Cochrane review in 2010 [11] concluded that TXA decreased postpartum blood loss after vaginal delivery and Caesarean section, but since there were only two randomised controlled trials, which were small and of unclear quality, further studies were needed to establish efficacy and safety. In a subsequent study, Xu *et al* [12] conducted a randomised, double-blind, case-controlled study of TXA 10ml/kg^{-1} vs. placebo in 174 primiparous patients undergoing Caesarean section. Blood loss up to 2 hours postpartum was significantly lower (p <0.01) in the TXA group (mean [SD] 46.6 [42.7] ml) than in the control group (84.7 [80.2] ml), but the blood loss in the period from placental delivery to the end of the Caesarean section did not differ between the TXA and control groups (p = 0.17). No significant abnormal vital signs were observed after TXA administration. Ducloy *et al* [13] studied the use of high-dose TXA in a randomised, controlled, multicentre, open-label trial. Women with postpartum haemorrhage (PPH) >800ml following vaginal delivery were randomly assigned to receive TXA (loading dose 4g over 1 hour, then infusion of 1g/hr[-1] over 6 hours) or not. Blood loss between enrolment and 6 hours later was significantly lower in the TXA group (median [IQR] 173 [59-377] ml) than in controls (221 [105 to 564] ml); p = 0.041. In the TXA group, bleeding duration was shorter and progression to severe PPH was less frequent than in controls (p <0.03). Red cell transfusion was needed in 93% of women in the TXA group versus 79% of controls (p = 0.016). This study is the first to demonstrate that high-dose TXA can reduce blood loss and maternal morbidity in women with PPH (Table 3). However, this and previous studies were not adequately powered to address safety issues, notably the rate of venous thromboembolism (VTE) postpartum. Postpartum women are at high risk of VTE; it remains one of the major causes of maternal mortality, and there is concern that using an antifibrinolytic drug may increase this risk.

Table 3. The efficacy of tranexamic acid in postpartum haemorrhage.

Novikova *et al* [11]	• TXA decreased postpartum blood loss after vaginal delivery and Caesarean section.
Xu *et al* [12]	• Blood loss up to 2 hours postpartum was significantly lower in the TXA group than in the control group. • Blood loss in the period from placental delivery to the end of Caesarean section did not differ between the TXA and control groups.
Ducloy *et al* [13]	• Blood loss between enrolment and 6 hours later was significantly lower in the TXA group. • Bleeding duration was shorter and progression to severe PPH was less frequent than in controls.

The WOMAN study [14] is a large, pragmatic, randomised, double-blind, placebo-controlled trial designed to determine the effect of early administration of TXA on mortality, hysterectomy and other morbidities (surgical interventions, blood transfusion, risk of non-fatal vascular events) in women with clinically diagnosed PPH. The use of health services and safety, especially thromboembolic effect will be assessed. Treatment entails a dose of TXA (1g by intravenous injection) or placebo (sodium chloride 0.9%) given as soon as possible after randomisation. A second dose may be given after 30 minutes if bleeding continues, or if it stops and restarts within 24 hours after the first dose. The main analyses will be on an 'intention to treat' basis, irrespective of whether the allocated treatment was received or not. The study aims to recruit 20,000 women (and has recruited over 14,000 at the time of writing), and will have over 90% power to detect a 25% reduction from 4% to 3% in the primary endpoint of mortality or hysterectomy; it is due to report in 2016/7.

Topical use of tranexamic acid

There is reliable evidence that topical application of TXA reduces bleeding and blood transfusion in surgical patients; however, the effect on the risk of thromboembolic events is uncertain [15]. Further high-quality trials are warranted to resolve these uncertainties before topical TXA can be recommended for routine use.

Other areas where tranexamic acid is being trialled

There are inadequate studies to ascertain whether TXA will be beneficial in reducing gastrointestinal (GI) bleeding and mortality, and it is debatable whether the results of CRASH-2 should be extrapolated from trauma to GI bleeding. Thus, an ongoing trial is addressing this research question. The Haemorrhage Alleviation with TXA — Intestinal Symptoms (HALT-IT) is currently randomising 8000 patients with acute upper GI haemorrhage to TXA vs. placebo [16]. The CRASH-3 trial is an international, multicentre, pragmatic, randomised, double-blind, placebo-controlled trial to quantify the effects of the early administration of TXA on death and disability in patients with traumatic brain injury. Ten thousand adult patients will be randomised to receive TXA or placebo. Treatment will entail a 1g loading dose followed by a 1g maintenance dose over 8h [17].

Dose of tranexamic acid

The original studies by Horrow *et al* showed that, in cardiac surgery, a dose of TXA of 10mg/kg^{-1} followed by 1mg/kg^{-1}/hr^{-1} decreased bleeding during cardiac surgery and larger doses did not produce haemostatic benefit [18, 19]. CRASH-2 used this information to produce an empirical dose to provide adequate plasma levels to have an antiplasmin effect in adults. The meta-analysis by Ker *et al* [9] also suggested that a dose of 1g produced a reduction in bleeding that was not improved by giving higher doses. This study showed that a total dose of 1g was likely to be sufficient for most adults and there was no evidence to support higher doses.

Since 2010, there have been a number of articles describing seizures with high-dose TXA; using doses much greater than the original Horrow recommendations [19, 20]. In an elegant set of studies, Lecker *et al* [21] showed there is structural similarity between the TXA and inhibitory neurotransmitter-gated Cl$^-$ channel glycine receptors, and demonstrated that TXA inhibits glycine receptors and binds competitively to GABA type-A receptors. They proposed that the higher rate of TXA-related seizures seen in cardiac surgery might relate to disruption of the blood brain barrier by cerebral emboli. However, it may also be that cardiac surgery is one of the few areas where very high doses of TXA have been used. Anaesthetic agents with glycine receptor agonist properties such as isoflurane or propofol may be uniquely suited to prevent such seizures after surgery; although ultimately limiting the dose of TXA to the original dose as suggested by Horrow appears as safe and efficacious as a higher dose.

Thrombotic risk

CRASH-2 showed that TXA significantly reduced the risk of myocardial infarction, and had no effect on the rate of venous thromboembolism, reassuring physicians that it is safe to use in a trauma setting. Although there is strong evidence that TXA reduces blood transfusion in surgery,

Table 4. Thrombotic risk of tranexamic acid.

CRASH-2 [3, 7]	• In traumatic bleeding TXA significantly reduced the risk of myocardial infarction, and had no effect on the rate of venous thromboembolism.
Ker *et al* [9]	• In general surgery the effect of TXA on myocardial infarction, stroke, deep vein thrombosis and pulmonary embolism was uncertain.
Poeran *et al* [22]	• In hip and knee replacement the use of TXA has suggested that there is no increased risk of vascular occlusive events.

there is still uncertainty as to whether TXA may be associated with an increased risk of arterial and venous thromboembolism, and this uncertainty limits its widespread use (Table 4). In a large meta-analysis [9], the effect of TXA on myocardial infarction (0.68, CI 0.43-1.09; p = 0.11), stroke (1.14, CI 0.65-2.00; p = 0.65), deep vein thrombosis (0.86, CI 0.53-1.39; p = 0.54), and pulmonary embolism (0.61, CI 0.25-1.47; p = 0.27) was uncertain. A newly published analysis of the use of TXA in hip and knee replacement in the USA has suggested that there is no increased risk of vascular occlusive events in this group of patients [22].

The effect of TXA on thromboembolic events and mortality requires further attention. The ongoing Aspirin and Tranexamic Acid for Coronary Artery Surgery trial [23] should help resolve uncertainties around cardiac surgery, but there is still a need for a large pragmatic trial in other surgical patients. Furthermore, there is an exciting suggestion from CRASH-2 that the use of TXA could reduce death due to postoperative myocardial infarction [24], making TXA a highly cost-effective way of improving surgical safety. It is timely to resolve this uncertainty in an adequately powered randomised controlled trial.

Conclusions

The management of major bleeding is changing very fast due to good-quality evidence from randomised controlled trials. Tranexamic acid (TXA) has been shown to be efficacious in reducing bleeding and mortality in several areas with trials in other areas ongoing. By 2020 there will be a substantial body of evidence around the use of TXA in all types of major bleeding. Will we be using TXA in every bleeding situation?

Checklist summary

✓ Tranexamic acid reduces bleeding during and after surgery by about one third.

✓ Tranexamic acid in trauma reduces bleeding deaths by one third.

✓ So far there is no evidence of an increased thrombotic risk with using tranexamic acid.

✓ The ideal dose of tranexamic acid for an adult is 1g and higher doses do not reduce bleeding further but have side effects.

References

1. Royston D1, Bidstrup BP, Taylor KM, Sapsford RN. Effect of aprotinin on need for blood transfusion after repeat open-heart surgery. *Lancet* 1987; 2(8571): 1289-91.

2. Fergusson DA, Hébert PC, Mazer CD, *et al*; BART Investigators. A comparison of aprotinin and lysine analogues in high-risk cardiac surgery. *N Engl J Med* 2008; 358(22): 2319-31.

3. CRASH-2 trial collaborators. Effects of tranexamic acid on death, vascular occlusive events, and blood transfusion in trauma patients with significant haemorrhage (CRASH-2): a randomised, placebo-controlled trial. *Lancet* 2010; 376: 23-32.

4. Astedt B. Clinical pharmacology of tranexamic acid. *Scand J Gastroenterol* 1987; 22: 22-5.

5. Department of Health. Payment by results guidance 2013-4. London, UK: Department of Health. https://www.gov.uk/government/uploads/system/uploads/attachment_data/file/214902/PbR-Guidance-2013-14.pdf.

6.   Godier A, Roberts I, Hunt BJ. Tranexamic acid: less bleeding and less thrombosis? *Crit Care* 2012; 16: 135.

7.   CRASH-2 trial collaborators. The importance of early treatment with tranexamic acid in bleeding trauma patients: an exploratory analysis of the CRASH-2 randomised controlled trial. *Lancet* 2011; 377: 1096-101.

8.   Henry DA, Carless PA, Moxey AJ, *et al*. Anti-fibrinolytic use for minimising perioperative allogeneic blood transfusion. *Cochrane Database Syst Rev* 2007; 4: CD001886.

9.   Ker K, Edwards P, Perel P, *et al*. Effect of tranexamic acid on surgical bleeding: systematic review and cumulative meta-analysis. *Br Med J* 2012; 344: e3054.

10.   Ker K, Prieto-Merino D, Roberts I. Systematic review, meta-analysis and meta-regression of the effect of tranexamic acid on surgical blood loss. *Br J Surg* 2013; 100: 1271-9.

11.   Novikova N, Hofmeyr GJ. Tranexamic acid for preventing postpartum haemorrhage. *Cochrane Database Syst Rev* 2010; 7: CD007872.

12.   Xu J, Gao W, Ju Y. Tranexamic acid for the prevention of postpartum hemorrhage after Cesarean section: a double-blind randomization trial. *Arch Gynecol Obstet* 2013; 287: 463-8.

13.   Ducloy-Bouthors AS, Jude B, Duhamel A, *et al*; EXADELI Study Group. High-dose tranexamic acid reduces blood loss in postpartum haemorrhage. *Crit Care* 2011; 15: R117.

14.   Shakur H1, Elbourne D, Gülmezoglu M, *et al*. World Maternal Antifibrinolytic Trial: tranexamic acid for the treatment of postpartum haemorrhage: an international randomised, double blind placebo controlled trial. *Trials* 2010; 11: 40.

15.   Ker K, Beecher D, Roberts I. Topical application of tranexamic acid for the reduction of bleeding. *Cochrane Database Syst Rev* 2013; 7: CD010562.

16.   Haemorrhage Alleviation with Tranexamic Acid - Intestinal Symptoms (HALT-IT). http://www.clinicaltrials.gov/show/NCT01658124.

17.   Dewan Y, Komolafe EO, Mejía-Mantilla JH, *et al*; CRASH-3 Collaborators. CRASH-3 - tranexamic acid for the treatment of significant traumatic brain injury: study protocol for an international randomized, double-blind, placebo-controlled trial. *Trials* 2012; 13: 87.

18.   Horrow JC, Hlavacek J, Strong MD, *et al*. Prophylactic tranexamic acid decreases bleeding after cardiac operations. *J Thorac Cardiovasc Surg* 1990; 99: 70-4.

19.   Horrow JC, Van Riper DF, Strong MD, *et al*. The dose-response relationship of tranexamic acid. *Anesthesiology* 1995; 82: 383-92.

20.   Murkin JM, Falter F, Granton J, *et al*. High-dose tranexamic acid is associated with nonischemic clinical seizures in cardiac surgical patients. *Anesth Analg* 2010; 110: 350-3.

21.	Lecker I, Wang DS, Romaschin AD, *et al.* Tranexamic acid concentrations associated with human seizures inhibit glycine receptors. *J Clin Invest* 2012; 122: 4654-66.

22.	Poeran J, Rasul R, Suzuki S, *et al.* Tranexamic acid use and postoperative outcomes in patients undergoing total hip or knee arthroplasty in the United States: retrospective analysis of effectiveness and safety. *Br Med J* 2014; 349: g4829.

23.	Aspirin and Tranexamic Acid for Coronary Artery Surgery: a randomised controlled trial. http://www.atacas.org.au.

24.	Ker K, Roberts I. Tranexamic acid for surgical bleeding. *Br Med J* 2014; 349: g4934.

Chapter 18

Postoperative blood salvage

Manuel Muñoz MD PhD
Professor, Peri-operative Transfusion Medicine, School of Medicine, University of Málaga, Málaga, Spain
Fernando Canilllas del Rey MD PhD
Department of Orthopaedic Surgery, Hospital "Cruz Roja", Madrid, Spain

- "The end of the surgical procedure does not signify the end of blood loss. Postoperative blood loss can take place through wound drains, third spacing into traumatized tissue, or aggressive phlebotomy during the postoperative period."

- "Postoperative cell salvage techniques are effective at reducing transfusion requirements where there is a predictable blood loss, and where that blood is relatively 'clean'."

- "Reinfusion of unwashed, salvaged blood reverses post-traumatic immunodepression, and it is attributed to immune stimulants generated during salvaged blood collection."

Background

Postoperative blood salvage (PBS) a well-recognised and common practice after surgical procedures, where significant amounts (≥400ml) of relatively clean blood can be collected within the first 6 postoperative hours, and returned to patients [1]. In this technique, the blood collected from a postoperative drain or chest tube is returned after micro-aggregate filtering alone or after washing and concentration. Although it is controversial, in orthopaedic procedures, the most common practice is to reinfuse the collected blood with simple micro-aggregate filtering and no washing, whereas in cardiac procedures, shed blood processing is highly recommended [2-5].

This chapter discusses the role for postoperative blood salvage within a patient blood management (PBM) program aimed to avoid unnecessary exposure to allogeneic blood transfusion (ABT) and improve clinical outcomes. It includes an analysis of devices, indications, efficacy, safety and cost of PBS, with a special focus on orthopaedic procedures.

Evidence

Efficacy of postoperative cell salvage

Orthopaedic surgery

The use of closed-suction drainage systems after major orthopaedic surgery (knee, hip, spine) is common practice, but not universally accepted. However, it can be postulated that if postoperative drains are to be used, low-vacuum salvage/reinfusion drains (i.e. an unprocessed blood device [UBD]) might be beneficial to the patient in the event of significant postoperative blood loss, especially when used in combination with a defined ABT protocol [6].

For total knee arthroplasty (TKA), salvaged and reinfusion of shed blood (378-564ml) reduced by 60% the relative risk of ABT when compared with a control group (11% vs. 30%, respectively; p<0.001), independently on whether washed (relative risk reduction: 63%) or unwashed shed blood (relative risk reduction: 62%) was reinfused (Grade 1B) [3]. Patients with a pre-operative haemoglobin (Hb) between 12 and 15g/dL would benefit most from this blood conservation technique. It would not be necessary in those with Hb >15g/dL and should be associated with other blood-saving techniques (e.g. iron, epoetin) if Hb <12g/dL [7].

Similarly, in primary total hip arthroplasty (THA), reinfusion of unwashed shed blood (203-441ml) reduced by 40% the relative risk of receiving ABT compared with the control (18% vs. 30%, respectively; p<0.001). On the other hand, reinfusion of washed peri-operatively salvaged (intra-operative and postoperative) blood has also been shown to be effective in reducing the ABT rate in primary and revision THA. Therefore, postoperative blood salvage is recommended in THA (Grade 1B) [3]. In most hip fractures not enough blood was collected for reinfusion in most patients [8].

In spinal surgery, the effectiveness of peri-operative cell salvage is controversial and its use is only recommended for selected operations with high peri-operative blood loss. It might be of use to complement intra-operative cell salvage at reducing ABT requirements, especially in patients undergoing extensive instrumented spine fusion (e.g. scoliosis correction) where postoperative blood loss is substantial (Grade 1C) [3].

Cardiac surgery

For cardiac surgery, postoperative mediastinal drainage can be much more significant with respect to the volume of blood lost. In cardiac procedures with extracorporeal circulation, peri-operative blood recovery, including the processing of blood from the cardiotomy reservoir, reduces the percentage of patients exposed to allogeneic blood (32% vs. 46%), but not the number of units per transfused patient (Grade 1B) [3-5].

This efficacy is increased when used in combination with antifibrinolytic agents. In a recent randomised study of 1047 cardiac surgery patients, who received intravenous tranexamic acid (TXA), the use of intra-operative and postoperative blood salvage with the Haemonetics cardioPAT® system (a processed blood device [PBD]) resulted in a significant reduction in patient exposure to allogeneic blood transfusion when compared with traditional intra-operative blood salvage followed by chest drain insertion (1.2 vs. 2.1 units per patient; p = 0.02). In addition, postoperative complications (e.g. deep venous thrombosis, atrial fibrillation) were slightly less frequent in the cardioPAT® group [9]. However, reinfusion of unwashed postoperative mediastinal drainage is not recomended and will not be discussed further [3-5].

Safety of unwashed blood

Safety concerns are related to the use of UBDs yielding blood with free haemoglobin, inflammatory mediators, fibrin split products, complement fractions, and fat particles at concentrations several-fold higher than circulating levels (see reference 6 for an update review) (Table 1). However, in orthopaedic surgery, the accumulated experience with the use of unwashed blood retransfusion (e.g. over 1,350,000 Bellovac ABT® devices have been sold in Europe since 2000) does not support the statements against its efficacy and safety (shivers, febrile reactions, and hypotension are the most commonly reported complications following unwashed, postoperative shed blood) [6]. A prospective audit was performed in 1819 consecutive patients (995 THA; 824 TKA) from 38 Dutch hospitals who received postoperative shed blood reinfusion using a low-suction UBD (average 460ml) within 6 hours postoperatively. The frequency of serious adverse events was 0.1%, whereas febrile reactions (fever, shivering) were observed in 3.1% of patients during retransfusion (5.8% in TKA and 1.5% in THA) [10]. A retrospective series of 1093 TKA reported no serious adverse events attributable to UBD use [7]. Based on the low incidence of side effects, postoperative cell salvage with such an UBD is considered safe [6].

In orthopaedic surgery, venous thromboembolism is of particular concern when an unwashed, shed blood product is reinfused. However, in a recent randomised comparison of 1759 THA or TKA procedures, postoperative cell salvage with UBD or PBD did not influence the rate of thromboembolic complications when compared with no reinfusion (15/1,061 [1.3%] vs. 8/698 [1.1%]; p = NS) [11]. Nevertheless, if one is to detect changes in the incidence of these low-incidence complications, samples of a much larger size than those in currently published reports are needed.

There is also concern regarding readministration of significant amounts of free Hb through UBDs might lead to renal dysfunction. However, if reinfusion is limited to 1000-1500ml, there seems to be enough haptoglobin in a patient's circulation to bound free Hb, thus avoiding the risk of renal impairment [6]. In two studies of THA patients receving intra-operatively and postoperatively salvaged unwashed blood (Sangvia™, Wellspect; n = 158) or no reinfusion (control, n = 164), only one case of transient acute renal dysfunction was observed in the reinfusion group [12]. Moreover, in TKA surgery, it has been recently shown that the amount of free Hb reinfused with the washed salvaged product was identical to that of the unwashed system [13]. In addition, the mechanical fragility index was significantly greater in the washed group, which indicates that in the recovery and processing by the washed device, significantly more damage was inflicted on the washed red cells [13]. Based on this work, the assumption of using the washing device, to provide a product that is expected to contain fewer contaminants, needs to be further evaluated.

Another point of controversy regarding the reinfusion of unwashed shed blood is the content of fat particles which may produce acute lung injury, but may also result in a postoperative neurological deficit, after orthopaedic and cardiac surgery. Common haematological cytometers allow the detection of fat particles in unwashed salvaged blood and verification of their elimination (as well as that of bacteria and tumour cells) by leukocyte filters, thereby avoiding these potential side effects. However, it must be borne in mind that the use of leukocyte-reducing filters in the retransfusion line will reduce the blood Hb content and may increase the risk of hypotensive episodes [6].

Data from several reports suggest a positive effect of unwashed shed blood reinfusion on a patient's immune function, which was attributed to immune stimulants, generated during salvaged blood collection, and might hasten a patient's recovery [14]. In a large observational study of patients undergoing TKA, reinfusion of postoperative unwashed shed blood significantly reduced the transfusion rate and length of hospital stay (with a trend to lower postoperative infection rate), and was cost-saving for most pre-operative Hb strata [7].

Postoperative blood salvage and local infiltration analgesia (LIA) are two important techniques in patient management after major orthopaedic surgery. In a review of six studies where the LIA technique was used (doses up to 490mg) and where analysis of ropivacaine concentration in patients and/or in the drain were performed, no patient had symptoms of systemic toxicity due to the local anaesthetic [15]. Therefore, the available data show that postoperative cell salvage with filtered blood can be combined safely with the use of LIA, performing a slow reinfusion during 30-60 minutes or more.

How to perform postoperative blood salvage

Devices

On the basis of function, there are two types of devices for postoperative blood salvage: those that reinfuse the shed blood without washing (unprocessed blood devices [UBDs]) and those that wash and concentrate the blood (processed blood devices [PBDs]).

Unprocessed blood devices

These include products such as the Hemovac® (Zimmer Corporate), SureTrans™ (Davol Inc), Bellovac ABT® (Wellspect Healthcare), ConstaVac™ CBCII (Stryker Corp.), or DONOR™ Autologous Blood Reinfusion System (Van Straten Medical) (Figure 1). General components of an UBD are depicted in Figure 2. This class dominates the market in orthopaedic surgery primarily because of simplicity, cost, and ease of use. Anticoagulant is not generally used here because most wound blood is already defibrinated, eliminating clot formation (if used, citrate is the anticoagulant of choice), and suction level should be kept <100mmHg to minimise haemolysis. Typical costs associated with UBDs total around ∈75 to ∈150, and economical evaluation indicates that their use is cost-effective when compared with PBD or allogeneic blood [7, 16].

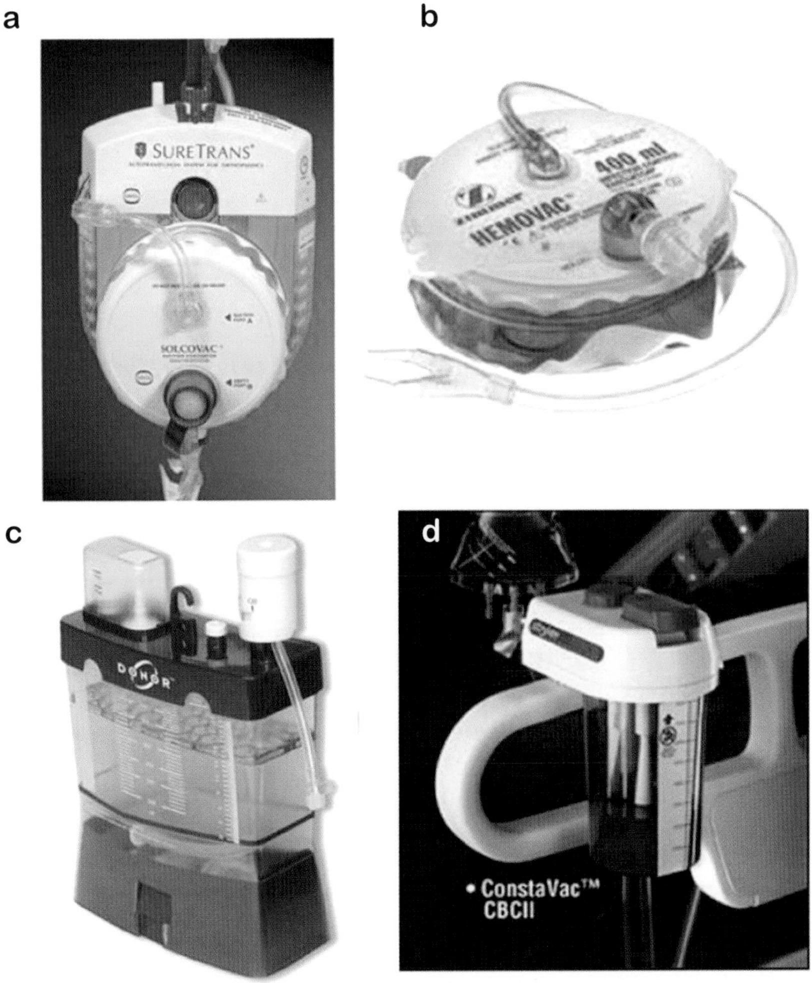

Figure 1. Some unprocessed blood recovery devices: a) SureTrans™ (Davol Inc.); b) Hemovac® (Zimmer Corp.); c) DONOR™ Autologous Blood Reinfusion System (Van Straten Medical); d) ConstaVac™ CBCII (Stryker Corp.).

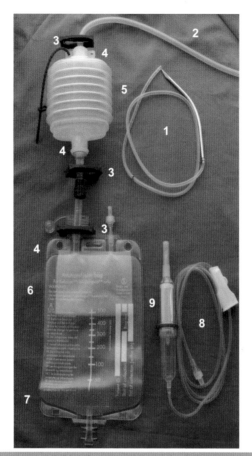

Figure 2. Unprocessed blood recovery device characteristics. Bellovac ABT® (Wellspect Healthcare): 1. Wound drain catheter with trocar; 2. Inlet tubing with connection port for drain catheter; 3. Inlet/oulet clamps; 4. Non-return valves; 5. Vacuum bellows (200ml; max. suction pressure — 90mmHg); 6. 200µm macro-filter; 7. Blood collection bag (500ml); 8. Blood giving set with drip chamber and roller clamp; 9. 80µm and 40µm micro-filters.

Processed blood devices

In PBDs, the blood is collected in a fashion similar to an UBD except that the blood is subsequently washed and concentrated before readministration, either in a discontinuous or continuous fashion. Among discontinuous PBDs, the OrthoPAT® and the CardioPAT® (Haemonetics Corp) incorporate a 'dynamic disk' (Figure 3) for effectively washing the shed blood [4]. Typical cost for the disposable used in these PBDs ranges from ∈ 300 to ∈ 400, although their use may be still cost-effective when compared with allogeneic blood [16].

a   b   c

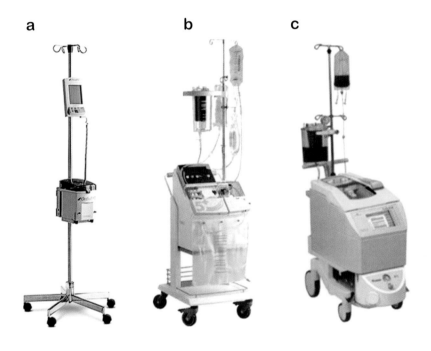

Figure 3. Some processed blood recovery devices: a) OrthoPAT® (Haemonetics Corp.); b) Cell Saver 5® (Haemonetics Corp.); c) CATS® Continuous Auto Transfusion System (Fresenius HemoCare).

Most commonly used discontinuous (Sorin/COBE BRAT II®, Bridgepoint Gambro Inc.; Medtronic autoLog™, Medtronic; Haemonetics CS5+®, Haemonetics Corp.) and continuous (CATS® Continuous Auto Transfusion System, Fresenius HemoCare) PBDs offer unique methods that provide effective concentration and washing (Figure 3). CATS® is more efficient in eliminating fat particles, whereas discontinuous systems eliminate more white blood cells, tumoral cells and platelets, and both systems efficiently eliminate proteins and anticoagulant [17]. Therefore, although all cell-saving devices use the same theory of centrifugation, the actual quality of the washed RBC product differs widely from one device to another. As opposed to CardioPAT® and OrthoPAT®, these devices have a large footprint and its use in the post-anaesthesia or intensive care unit environment can be cumbersome. Typical cost for the disposable used with one of these devices is around € 150 to € 300, though the collecting and the processing disposables can be purchased and used separately (except for CATS®).

Device selection

The three most common reasons for selecting a particular device are ease of use, cost, and product quality. UBD devices require the least amount of preparation, management, and cost. PBDs require additional training and are more costly, but they yield a processed end product with reduced undesirable wound contaminants. In this regard, it is worth noting that the use of a colloid-based sedimentation method reduces chemical and cellular contaminant of salvaged blood collected with an UBD after TKA. After colloid treatment, 90% of RBCs were recovered, and mean haemoglobin (Hb) was similar to that of standard leuko-reduced RBCs [18]. This method may provide a low-cost alternative to PBDs, although its clinical implications need to be further evaluated.

Contraindications and precautions

Contraindications to the use of postoperative, unwashed shed blood are determined by the particular conditions of the patient and the characteristics of salvaged blood. Contraindications include: kidney failure, impaired liver function, coagulation disorders, patients with erythrocyte abnormalities (e.g. sickle cell disease), the use of local haemostatic agents, patients with HIV, Hepatitis B or C, a patient's refusal to accept the technique, a lack of experience of the surgeon, anaesthesiologist or nurse in the use of the technique, infection or cancer at the surgical site [6]. The intra-operative use of betadine, chlorhexidine, hydrogen peroxide, local antibiotics or other agents not for parenteral administration is not a contraindication for postoperative cell salvage providing adequate lavage of the wound using saline is performed prior to closure [1]. On the other hand, given the haematological and biochemical characteristics of unwashed salvaged blood (Table 1), it is not recommended to reinfuse a volume of more than 1000-1500ml [6].

Table 1. Haematological and biochemical parameters of unprocessed postoperative shed blood (USB), colloid processed USB, OrthoPAT® processed blood, and banked allogeneic blood (leukodepleted red blood cell concentrates [LD-RBC]).

| | USB (n=40) | Colloid processed USB (n = 40) | | OrthoPAT® processed blood (n = 5)** | LD-RBC (n = 25) |
		Concentration	Total content reduction (%)*		
Haemoglobin (g/dL)	10.9 ± 1.5	18.9 ± 2.8	10	22.3 ± 1.9	19.6 ± 1.5
Haematocrit (%)	33 ± 5	57 ± 8	-	68 ± 5	59 ± 4
Leucocytes (x10³/µl)	3.5 ± 1.5	2.7 ± 1.3	60	2.3 ± 0.3	0.04 ± 0.04
Platelets (x10³/µl)	43 ± 19	51 ± 4	48	30 ± 3	2 ± 1
PFHB (g/dL)	0.50 ± 0.32	0.87 ± 0.49	53	0.24 ± 0.23	0.25 ± 0.14
GOT (U/ml)	110 ± 50	110 ± 50	70	23 ± 23	19 ± 9
CK (U/ml)	2194 ± 2352	1279 ± 1218	78	-	64 ± 27
LDH (U/ml)	939 ± 302	1101 ± 501	65	679 ± 356	164 ± 83
Haptoglobin (mg/dL)	74 ± 38	55 ± 36	80	-	6 ± 7
Total protein (g/dL)	4.3 ± 0.8	4.3 ± 0.9	75	0.7 ± 0.5	0.9 ± 0.5

PFHB = plasma-free haemoglobin; GOT = glutamate-oxalacetate transaminase, CK = creatine kinase; LDH = lactate dehydrogenase.
* The removal of the different blood and chemical contaminants in terms of a percentage value was calculated according to changes in volume and haematocrit of colloid processed USB with respect to unprocessed USB [7].
** Using diluted whole donor blood stored for <15 days as a model for postoperative blood salvage (650mL, haematocrit 24%) [20].

Actions to be taken

The vast majority of postoperative salvage is performed with little focus on quality. This lack of observation and auditing may account for limited safety data being published on this topic. Therefore, there are a number of actions to be taken:

- Postoperative blood salvage should only be targeted to the right procedure (indications) and the right patient (no contraindications).
- The patient should be involved through a process of informed consent.
- Surgeons, anaesthesiologists and nurses must be provided with adequate training in operating the different blood salvage devices and reinfusing the salvaged blood.
- Each case involving postoperative blood recovery should be recorded prospectively to comply with traceability regarding disposables and/or the machine used.
- The efficacy of this blood-saving strategy at reducing ABT requirements should be audited periodically, especially if changes in surgical techniques have been introduced.
- Quality control samples should be sent to the blood bank at regular intervals.
- Any adverse event should be reported to the National Haemovigilance Reporting System via the hospital transfusion committee or the blood bank responsible [1, 2].

Implications for everyday clinical practice

From this point of view, it could be said that the postoperative salvage and reinfusion of filtered blood offers the following benefits:

- It does not interfere with the standard surgical procedure.
- It does not require complex equipment, software, power supplies or a vacuum source; the UBD pack usually contains everything you need for the collection and reinfusion of drained blood.
- It is easy to use by the surgeon and nurses, with minimum training needs for its management.
- Most patients accept it (including Jehovah's Witnesses, just adding a line of continuity between the drain and the patient).
- It provides compatible blood immediately and almost the same amount that is collected from drains (approximately 1 unit/patient).

- It has an Hb concentration similar to that of the patient, but unlike stored blood, it has an optimal oxygenation capacity.
- It is clinically safe, saves allogeneic units and seems to be cost-effective.
- Its use is compatible with almost any other blood-saving strategy.

Recipe for success

The effectiveness of this transfusion therapy may be increased if it is associated with other blood-saving strategies within an individualized PBM program [19]. However, though the benefits of a PBM program for both the patient and the healthcare system are undisputable, its implementation is not so straightforward and there are several barriers to overcome:

- A PBM program takes a great deal of multidisciplinary planning and forethought, as it is simply too easy to order a unit of blood.
- To run a PBM program, strong leadership is required. The coordinator has to interact with medical and nursing staff for its planning, implementation and audit (efficacy and safety).
- The coordinator will need the direct or indirect support from the hospital managers (organisation), health authorities (funds and regulations), and medical societies (guidelines).
- Continuing medical education should be offered to health professionals to refresh and update their knowledge on PBM, thus facilitating their commitment with the program.

Conclusions

Postoperative blood salvage, using processed or unprocessed blood devices, may be useful when targeted to the right procedure (indications) and the right patient (no contraindications).

In orthopaedic procedures of the knee, hip and spine, postoperatively recovered, filtered blood appears to be an excellent source of viable red cells, with optimal functionality, without many of the risks associated with ABT and, possibly, some immune stimulatory effects. It was proved to reduce ABT requirements and costs, without relevant clinical complications (Grade 1B). Reinfusion of postoperatively recovered, washed blood seems to be equally effective (Grade 1B). Postoperative blood salvage after hip fracture repair is not efficacious and, therefore, not recommended [3].

In cardiac procedures, peri-operative salvaged and reinfusion of washed blood reduces the percentage of patients exposed to ABT (Grade 1B). Reinfusion of unwashed shed blood is not recommended in this clinical setting [3].

Checklist summary

✓ Postoperative blood loss after certain major procedures may be significant.

✓ Postoperative blood salvage has few contraindications and may be accomplished using processed or unprocessed blood devices.

✓ The reinfusion of both washed and unwashed postoperative shed blood has been proved to reduce transfusion requirements after orthopaedic surgery.

✓ The reinfusion of unwashed shed blood (up to 1000-1500ml) after orthopaedic procedures seems to be safe. However, it is not recommended after cardiac surgery.

✓ In cardiac procedures, peri-operative blood recovery, including the processing of blood from the cardiotomy reservoir, reduces allogeneic blood transfusion rates.

✓ The effectiveness of postoperative blood salvage may be increased when used within a patient blood management program.

✓ When using this technique, adequate training for using devices, quality control of salvaged blood, periodical auditing of efficacy and an adverse event reporting system should be implemented.

References

1.   Hamer A. Postoperative blood salvage. In: Thomas D, Thompson J, Ridler B, Eds. *A manual for blood conservation*. Shrewsbury, UK: tfm publishing Ltd, 2005: 123-32.

2.   Shander A, Rijhwani T, Dyga R, Waters JH. Postoperative blood management strategies. In: *Blood Management: Options for Better Patient Care*. Waters JH, Ed. Bethesda, DN: AABB Press, 2008.

3.   Leal-Noval SR, Muñoz M, Asuero M, *et al*. Spanish Consensus Statement on alternatives to allogeneic blood transfusion: the 2013 update of the "Seville Document". *Blood Transfus* 2013; 11: 585-610.

4.   Kozek-Langenecker SA, Afshari A, Albaladejo P, *et al*. Management of severe perioperative bleeding: guidelines from the European Society of Anaesthesiology. *Eur J Anaesthesiol* 2013; 30: 270-382.

5.   Society of Thoracic Surgeons Blood Conservation Guideline Task Force; Society of Cardiovascular Anesthesiologists Special Task Force on Blood Transfusion. 2011 update to the Society of Thoracic Surgeons and the Society of Cardiovascular Anesthesiologists blood conservation clinical practice guidelines. *Ann Thorac Surg* 2011; 91: 944-82.

6.   Muñoz M, Slappendel R, Thomas D. Laboratory characteristics and clinical utility of post-operative cell salvage: washed or unwashed blood transfusion? *Blood Transfus* 2010; 9: 248-61.

7.   Muñoz M, Ariza D, Campos A, *et al*. The cost of post-operative shed blood salvage after total knee arthroplasty: an analysis of 1093 consecutive procedures. *Blood Transfus* 2013; 11: 260-71.

8.   Muñoz M, Iglesias D, Garcia-Erce JA, *et al*. Utility and cost of low-vacuum reinfusion drains in patients undergoing surgery for subcapital hip fracture repair. A before and after cohort study. *Vox Sang* 2014; 106: 83-91.

9.   Weltert L, Nardella S, Rondinelli MB, *et al*. Reduction of allogeneic red blood cell usage during cardiac surgery by an integrated intra- and postoperative blood salvage strategy: results of a randomized comparison. *Transfusion* 2013; 53: 790-7.

10.   Horstmann WG, Slappendel R, Van Hellemondt GG, *et al*. Safety of retransfusion of filtered shed blood in 1819 patients after total hip or knee arthroplasty. *Tranfus Altern Tranfus Med* 2010; 11: 57-64.

11.   So-Osman C, Nelissen RG, Koopman-van Gemert AW, *et al*. Patient blood management in elective total hip- and knee-replacement surgery (part 2): a randomized controlled trial on blood salvage as transfusion alternative using a restrictive transfusion policy in patients with a preoperative hemoglobin above 13g/dL. *Anesthesiology* 2014; 120: 852-60.

12.   Horstmann WG. Perioperative blood saving measurements in total hip and knee arthroplasty. PhD Thesis. Amsterdam 2011: 127-56 (ISBN: 978-90-393-5624-1).

13.   Ley JT, Yazer MH, Waters JH. Hemolysis and red blood cell mechanical fragility in shed blood after total knee arthroplasty. *Transfusion* 2012; 52: 34-8.

14.   Islam N, Whitehouse M, Mehendale S, *et al.* Post-traumatic immunosuppression is reversed by anti-coagulated salvaged blood transfusion; deductions from studying immune status after knee arthroplasty. *Clin Exp Immunol* 2014; 177: 509-20.

15.   Jansson J-R, Slappendel R. Local infiltration analgesia (LIA) and postoperative blood salvage can be safely combined in major orthopedic surgery [Poster]. 30th Annual ESRA Congress, Dresden (Germany), September 2011. http://www.multiwebcast.com/eposter.esra/2011/30th/12427/

16.   Rao VK, Dyga R, Bartels C, Waters JH. A cost study of postoperative cell salvage in the setting of elective primary hip and knee arthroplasty. *Transfusion* 2012; 52: 1750-60.

17.   Dai B, Wang L, Djaiani G, Mazer CD. Continuous and discontinuous cell-washing autotransfusion systems. *J Cardiothorac Vasc Anesth* 2004; 18: 210-7.

18.   Muñoz M, García-Segovia S, Ariza D, *et al.* A sedimentation method for improving and standardizing the quality of postoperatively salvaged unwashed shed blood in orthopaedic surgery. *Br J Anaesth* 2010; 105: 457-65.

19.   Muñoz M, García-Erce JA, Villar I, Thomas D. Blood conservation strategies in major orthopaedic surgery: efficacy, safety and European regulations. *Vox Sang* 2009; 96: 1-13.

20.   Muñoz Gómez M, Ariza Villanueva D, Romero Ruiz A, *et al.* Evaluation of the OrthoPAT autologous transfusion system by experimental models simulating intra- and postoperative blood salvage. *Rev Esp Anestesiol Reanim* 2005; 52: 321-7.

Chapter 19

Haemostasis and sealing — the continuum concept

Arunesh Sil MS (ENT) MRCS DOHNS
Medical Advisor, Baxter Healthcare, Newbury, UK

- "Post-surgical bleeding complications can create a significant economic impact." [1]

- "No widely accepted guidelines exist to aid the process of patient blood management (PBM) implementation." [2]

- "Patient blood management (PBM) involves the use of multidisciplinary, multimodal, individualized strategies." [2]

- "Haemostasis and sealing are basic concepts that are relevant in every surgical procedure."

- "Where blood conservation is concerned, simple interventions matter."

Background

Surgical practice is fraught with several challenges, and can generate a significant risk to the operator and the patient. Bleeding from the operative site is no doubt a significant challenge during surgery. Management of such situations with difficult surgical bleeds costs time and money, and has an impact on the quality of life not only for the patient, but also for the treating physician.

A French study [1] has estimated an increase of approximately 20% in terms of additional hospital costs for length of stay, which is increased in patients having complications related to bleeding during surgery. In the current financial climate, this can be of material consideration in individual hospitals and treatment centres.

Along with bleeding, operative leaks and postoperative adhesion formation also present significant challenges in terms of patient management. Finding the solutions to the clinical needs of haemostasis, tissue repair and anti-adhesion are of paramount importance to achieve an optimal intra-operative and postoperative outcome.

The terms 'haemostasis' and 'sealing' are often used interchangeably in the surgical environment and it is important to differentiate between the two concepts. While 'haemostasis' simply refers to the process of stopping bleeding, 'sealing' refers to the process of achieving a seal, over a point of leak in the operative area. Both processes can occur simultaneously but the clinical needs served are different — while haemostats provide a solution for bleeding, sealants provide a solution for intra-operative or postoperative leaks. There are obviously situations where there is a need for both and in those situations it is useful to use an agent which has properties of haemostasis as well as sealing.

Therefore, based on the needs of the clinical scenario, haemostasis and sealing are continuum concepts where on one end of the spectrum haemostats stop the bleeding, while on the other end sealants provide a seal for an operative leak (Figure 1). Within the range of this spectrum several agents can provide a biphasic solution and can act as a haemostat and also as a sealant.

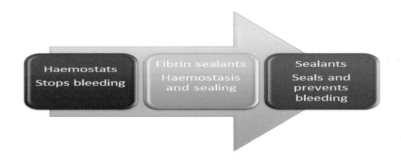

Figure 1. Haemostasis and sealing are continuum concepts in surgical practice with many interventions doing both at varying levels and degrees.

Relevance to blood conservation

Blood conservation is a multimodal strategy requiring the input of many experts, modalities and interventions. Three important strategic activities have been described in a few studies [2] as follows:

* Optimisation of haematopoiesis.
* The reduction of bleeding and minimisation of blood loss.
* Achievement of satisfactory postoperative outcome by adequate management of anaemia and optimising the tolerance to anaemia.

In the wider scheme of patient blood management, adequate levels of haemostasis and sealing therefore fall in the second strategic step, where the primary focus is to reduce bleeding and minimise blood loss. Within this strategy, the intra-operative management of bleeding has a vital role to play. As studies have shown [2, 3], overall blood management programs can significantly improve patient outcomes. Intra-operative blood loss has been identified to be a key risk factor that can affect postoperative bleeding and the postoperative transfusion rates [4].

Besides clinical benefit, the financial aspect of cost saving has also been studied in detail. As mentioned before, Ye et al [1] have reported a potential cost saving of approximately 19.9% with the ideal scenario of avoiding complications due to excess bleeding. A good proportion of this can be recognised by interventions such as the use of haemostats and sealants.

Based on a national comparative audit of blood use in the UK in 2006-7, studies have estimated a potential saving of ~£35 million to the National Health Service (NHS) based on data collected on total hip replacements and other major surgery [2]. Although further research is due in these areas, the scope of potential clinical and health economic benefit is very clear.

The annual cost of blood transfusions in the UK has been studied at the beginning of this millennium. Varney et al have estimated an increase by more than double from £252 million in 1994/95 to £898 million in 2000-2001. However, the number of whole blood donations only increased by 2% to 2.8 million and the number of apheresis donations decreased by 52% [5]. As a result, the financial penalty on the NHS for an adult transfusion is fairly high. The same study estimated the NHS cost for an adult transfusion at £635 for one unit of red blood cells [5].

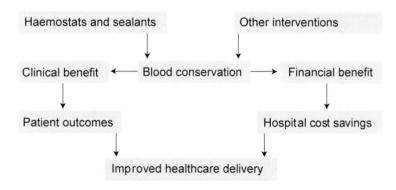

Figure 2. Cost/benefit interplay in blood conservation.

Since blood conservation is a multimodal strategy with various interrelated interventions, it is difficult to attribute clinical benefit to a single strategy like haemostasis (Figure 2). Nevertheless, in a health economic study in 2009, the potential for decreased length of stay as a result of avoiding bleeding was clearly demonstrated [1]. This illustrates the role that haemostats and sealants have to play in the overall scheme of clinical activities.

Haemostats — an introduction

A haemostat by definition is any agent that stops bleeding. Invariably, this is interlinked closely to either a direct or indirect interaction with the coagulation cascade.

Haemostasis has undergone a systematic evolution along with general progress made in surgery and surgical techniques. Traditionally, tamponade, ligation and diathermy have been the main cornerstones of stemming blood loss and stopping mild to severe bleeds. The importance of good surgical technique and skill cannot of course be underestimated.

However, this contemporary period has seen the advent of several topical haemostatic agents which range from synthetic to biological to human derived agents. Over the recent years these have played a significant role in surgical haemostasis, and the importance has also warranted a significant interest in cost assessment and consideration of regulatory parameters surrounding the use of these materials [6]. Five key performance categories with respect to the use of haemostats have been identified by the authors as safety, efficacy, usability, cost and approvability [6].

The coagulation cascade is crucial to the understanding of the mechanism of action of haemostats. Physiologically, there are two pathways (intrinsic and extrinsic) that stem from the site and cause of bleeding, but then converge to a single important step involving a reaction between fibrinogen and thrombin (Figure 3).

Types of haemostats in clinical practice

Haemostats have been described functionally as active or passive [7], or categorically as a mechanical, active, flowable and fibrin sealant [6].

It is generally preferable to use a functional terminology as the categories of haemostats continue to evolve with more advances in clinical and surgical research. Functionally, passive haemostats are materials or processes that accelerate a step in the coagulation cascade as shown below (Figure 3).

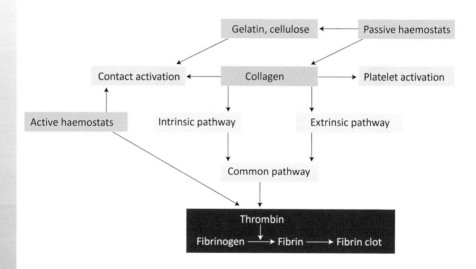

Figure 3. Coagulation cascade. This diagram shows the different levels of interaction of active and passive haemostats with the coagulation cascade.

Examples of passive haemostats include gelatin, collagen and cellulose, and such agents usually act by contact activation. Collagen not only acts by platelet activation but also facilitates platelet aggregation [7].

Passive haemostats provide a three-dimensional lattice structure where a 'clot matrix' can form and this enables and facilitates clot formation [7]. Even swabs and gauze pieces can act as a scaffold for the clot formation to occur. In addition, gelatin can provide a tamponade effect as it can swell on contact with the operative site [7]. Macroscopically, passive haemostats can take various forms including powders, paste, gel, patches and sheets.

Active haemostats (also called biophysical haemostats) in contrast are thrombin-containing agents. The presence of thrombin facilitates the interaction with fibrinogen at the end of the coagulation cascade and this augments the clot formation and achievement of haemostasis. Thrombin may be used either as an agent on its own [8] or as a combination with gelatin [9]. When used in combination with gelatin, the added advantage of a passive haemostat causes the combination to interact with the coagulation cascade at two points and, therefore, accelerates the time to haemostasis [10]. It is very important to remember that topical haemostats are an adjunct to haemostasis and are not a primary method of controlling bleeding, and are not a substitute for mechanical fixation. Therefore, while topical haemostats can certainly improve or stop bleeding, they will not replace the efficacy of mechanical fixation provided by a suture or a clip.

An important difference between the active and passive haemostats is related to the process of anticoagulation. This can have a significant effect on passive haemostats, since they only interact with a single step in the coagulation cascade. In contrast, active haemostats contain thrombin which also interact and influence the final step of the coagulation cascade, and therefore, are less susceptible to decreased efficacy in coagulopathies and during periods of anticoagulation [7] as is required quite often in long and complex surgeries.

The importance of haemostats and blood transfusion

Blood transfusion is commonplace in surgical practice and in some specialties like cardiac surgery has been shown to be strongly associated with infection, ischaemic postoperative morbidity, length of stay in hospital, mortality and hospital costs [11].

Studies have illustrated benefits both in terms of clinical outcome and economic outcome that can be achieved by prevention of transfusions either of whole blood or its components. This, therefore, is an important element of blood conservation strategy [2].

It has been shown that transfusions can be associated with increased morbidity, increased ICU (intensive care unit)/HDU (high dependency unit) dependence and increased cost of admission and length of stay [11]. The same study concluded that avoiding transfusion would have prevented 50% of all infections and ischaemic events following cardiac surgery and would have reduced the non-operative costs of an admission by nearly 40% [11]. They have also shown a significant association with mortality. Following transfusion, the risk of death was shown to be six times higher in the first 30 days in the cohort of patients who were transfused compared to the non-transfused patients. This increase in risk also continued through the first postoperative year [11]. It is important to bear in mind that the cohort of transfused patients are generally expected to be sicker and have more baseline morbidities compared to the non-transfused cohort and this is an important covariate; nevertheless, the high hazard ratio certainly attributes some causation to transfusion.

Fibrin sealants — an introduction

Fibrin sealants have both haemostatic and sealant properties and, therefore, fall in the middle of the continuum from haemostats to sealants.

Essentially, these are biocompatible and biodegradable combination agents that contain fibrinogen and thrombin. They may be plasma-derived [12] or recombinant (artificially synthesized molecules through genetic engineering). The fibrinogen combines with thrombin to form a clot and, therefore, this mimics the final step of the coagulation cascade (Figure 4). The result is a pearly-white opalescent clot which obviously does not have the red colour due to the absence of red blood cells. Such clots can form rapidly and can be stronger in terms of tensile strength than physiological blood clots [13].

Fibrin sealants can be manufactured with an added aprotinin [14] or without aprotinin [15]. The addition of aprotinin acts as a clot stabilizer. Normally, once

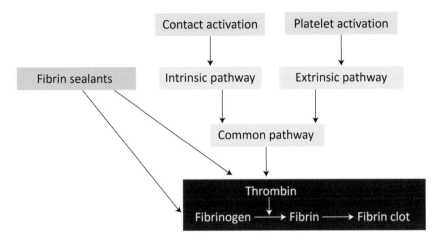

Figure 4. Coagulation cascade. This diagram shows how fibrin sealants augment the action of the coagulation cascade by providing fibrinogen and thrombin independent of the clotting cascade.

a fibrin clot is formed, the clot is then subject to rapid degradation by plasmin, which can happen in a matter of hours [13]. Aprotinin is an inhibitor of plasmin, and is therefore added to inhibit the activity of plasmin, thus serving to preserve the clot from degradation for 9-10 days [13]. When fibrin sealants are manufactured without aprotinin, chromatographic filtering techniques are used to reduce the amounts of plasminogen [6].

Fibrin sealants have been in the clinical environment for many years and are often referred to as 'fibrin glue' due to their adhesive properties. However, when used as a haemostat, it is important to remember that the haemostatic function is due to the thrombin that reacts with fibrinogen. In general, they are used for diffuse oozing types of bleeding rather than more severe bleeding. As previously mentioned, fibrin sealants are used as an adjunct to improve haemostasis rather than use as a primary measure.

In addition to commercial combinations of fibrinogen and thrombin, there are other methods of making fibrin sealants from the patient's own plasma. These involved specialised devices but have the advantage of being an autologous infusion as there is no transmission of foreign substances.

Fibrin sealants — applicability to clinical practice

There are plenty of indications for fibrin sealants and new studies concerning them are emerging continuously. While most applications relate to the haemostatic efficacy, some applications relate to the sealant function. It is important to note that the regulatory approval for these products being used can vary considerably from one product to another. Some products have site-specific sealing indications and these should be taken into consideration while using these products in the clinical environment, otherwise the application of the product can be off-licence. The fibrinogen component can vary and so can the thrombin content from product to product.

Some products like TISSEEL® (fibrin sealant) can be used for sealing function in gastrointestinal anastomosis, for mesh fixation in hernia repair and in neurosurgery for sealing the dura [14]. Some other products like EVICEL® sealant can be used for vascular surgery [15]. Yet another fibrin sealant, ARTISS® (fibrin sealant), can be used for plastic and reconstructive surgery.

In modern healthcare delivery, the three most important drivers of any modality of treatment are safety, efficacy and cost benefit/health economic outcomes.

Safety

Safety is a key factor that should be considered when fibrin sealants are being used. These products are usually delivered in the form of an aerosol with a spray device and, therefore, there is a potential risk of gas/air embolism. Therefore, education and training for surgeons with regard to the optimal pressure and distance of spraying is important to avoid risk to the patient. It is also important to ensure that surgeons do not use a thick layer of fibrin sealant which can interfere with wound healing [14]. Finally, as these products are human-derived, the risk of allergic reactions and viral transmission, although very rare, should be recognised [14].

Efficacy

Efficacy of the products and their use depends on the constitution, and this can vary considerably. In addition to the traditional fibrin sealants, a slow-setting fibrin sealant such as ARTISS® sealant indicated for plastic surgery contains a lower amount of thrombin (4IU) and this extends the polymerisation time of fibrin [16]. This is an important factor since it allows additional time which is crucial in repositioning of grafts following reconstructive surgery.

Health economic outcomes

Health economic models and conclusions are crucial in driving clinical practice and the adoption of change in practice. Such models usually revolve around the need to conserve blood and improve patient outcome, and fibrin sealants have an important role to play in both aspects.

Synthetic sealants — introduction and types

Sealants are products that provide a mechanical seal. Synthetic sealants do not have a biological origin and, therefore, do not interact with the coagulation cascade. The mechanical property of the sealing effect depends on the ability of the product to form covalent bonds with the underlying tissue of the patient.

Such covalent bonds are readily formed by a chemical called polyethylene glycol (PEG). These molecules are utilised for manufacture of sealants. Two commercially available products utilising this function of PEG are COSEAL® surgical sealant and DURASEAL® sealant. It is important to remember that there is a difference in the approved indications. While COSEAL® surgical sealant is indicated for sealing in vascular surgery, lung and cardiac procedures [17], DURASEAL® sealant is indicated for sealing the dura [18]. As for other topical products, these are used as adjuncts to primary surgical repair.

One of the important consequences for using PEG as sealants is swelling. PEG molecules form covalent bonds with the tissues and with themselves, and form a hydrogel which can absorb water and can swell. COSEAL® sealant can swell up to 400% [17] and DURASEAL® sealant can swell up to 50% [18].

Anti-adhesion

Postoperative adhesions are a significant challenge for surgeons. Adhesion formation, especially after abdominal surgery, can have an adverse effect on clinical outcome and can have a significant impact on hospital costs due to increased length of stay and prolonged hospitalisation. It has been shown that after colon cancer surgery, adhesions were associated with longer surgeries, longer hospital stays, and a delayed return to bowel function [19]. All of these have a significant impact on economic outcomes and can be reduced by the use of sealants as anti-adhesives. The surgeon should however bear in mind that the licensed use of sealants as anti-adhesives are restricted by regulatory approval and surgeons should carefully read the instructions for use before applying such products. COSEAL® sealant, for example, is approved for use as a site-specific anti-adhesive, namely in laparoscopic or abdominopelvic surgery and also in cardiac surgery.

Sealants in blood conservation

The prevention of bleeding by providing a mechanical seal can in fact result in improved outcomes related to blood conservation even though sealants are not haemostats. One study has shown that when used in vascular surgery, with sealants such as COSEAL® sealant, the median time to inhibit bleeding was 16.5 seconds compared to 189 seconds with GELFOAM® haemostat (gelatin sponge). There was also a significant difference in the immediate repair of anastomotic leak between the two [20].

Portfolio approach to surgical challenges

The surgical toolbox is full of new, interesting and evolving materials and methods in order to deal with surgical challenges.

In modern surgical scenarios, surgeons are presented with a range of measures and interventions. There is no substitute for good surgical judgement based on experience when the use of haemostats and sealants are concerned in order to achieve the optimum clinical outcome for the patient. Every challenging situation in the surgical arena is unique in many ways and, therefore, the importance of using the right product at the right place at the right time cannot be underestimated. This is facilitated by a portfolio approach where the surgeon needs to understand the entire range of haemostats and sealants in a continuum as opposed to looking at haemostats and sealants in isolation since the properties of these products and consequently their applications can be interrelated in many ways (Figure 5).

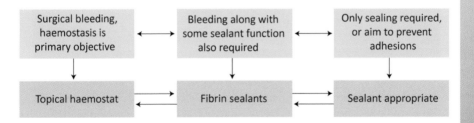

Figure 5. Illustration of the portfolio approach to surgical challenges. Note that the green boxes depict the surgical challenge, and the orange ones indicate potential solutions, but there is a considerable overlap and interchangeability between the needs and solutions. For example, a fibrin sealant in the appropriate situation can be used as a pure haemostat.

The astute surgeon has the ability to recognise the strengths and limitations of each product in this continuum in order to achieve the objectives of blood conservation and an optimised patient outcome.

Conclusions

Blood conservation is increasingly gaining ground as a crucial concept in surgical practice especially with the growing emphasis on patient outcomes. This interest is matched by a host of activities being undertaken at a hospital, regional and national level. What is needed in the future is a concerted and sustained effort by all stakeholders that looks at potential changes to our basic surgical and clinical practice at an operational level, and supported by development of robust evidence and guidelines at a strategic level regionally and nationally.

Checklist summary

✓ Haemostasis and sealing are continuum concepts when related to clinical practice.

✓ Both haemostats and sealants have a vital role to play in the blood conservation strategy in order to achieve optimum patient outcome.

✓ Haemostats stop bleeding by interacting with the coagulation cascade and depending on their level of interaction can be active or passive.

✓ Fibrin sealants result in a fibrin clot and provide a combination of haemostasis and sealing.

✓ Sealants are agents that provide a mechanical seal and are used for sealing, and for anti-adhesion.

✓ Sealants play a significant role in blood conservation by preventing bleeding through a 'tamponade effect' caused by the seal.

✓ Safety, efficacy and health economic benefits are key drivers to the adoption of haemostats and sealants in clinical practice.

✓ Good surgical practice results from a portfolio approach to surgical challenges.

References

1. Ye X, Lafuma A, Torreton E, Arnaud A. Incidence and costs of bleeding-related complications in French hospitals following surgery for various diagnoses. *BMC Health Serv Res* 2013; 13: 186.

2. Shander A, Van Aken H, Colomina MJ, *et al*. Patient blood management in Europe. *Br J Anaesth* 2012; 109(1): 55-68.

3. Ferraris VA, Brown JR, Despotis GJ, *et al*. 2011 update to the Society of Thoracic Surgeons and the Society of Cardiovascular Anesthesiologists blood conservation clinical practice guidelines. *Ann Thorac Surg* 2011; 91(3): 944-82.

4. Liu B, Belboul A, Larsson S, Roberts D. Factors influencing haemostasis and blood transfusion in cardiac surgery. *Perfusion* 1996; 11(2): 131-43.

5. Varney SJ, Guest JF. The annual cost of blood transfusions in the UK. *Transfus Med* 2003; 13(4): 205-18.

6. Spotnitz WD, Burks S. Hemostats, sealants, and adhesives: components of the surgical toolbox. *Transfusion* 2008; 48(7): 1502-16.

7. Samudrala S. Topical hemostatic agents in surgery: a surgeon's perspective. *AORN J* 2008; 88(3): S2-11.

8. Evithrom Product Information; www.ethicon360.com.

9. Floseal. Instructions for use. Baxter Healthcare Ltd., May 2012. www.baxterhealthcare.com.

10. Oz MC, Cosgrove DM 3rd, Badduke BR, *et al*. Controlled clinical trial of a novel hemostatic agent in cardiac surgery. *Ann Thorac Surg* 2000; 69(5): 1376-82.

11. Murphy GJ, Reeves BC, Rogers CA, *et al*. Increased mortality, postoperative morbidity, and cost after red blood cell transfusion in patients having cardiac surgery. *Circulation* 2007; 116(22): 2544-52.

12. Jackson MR. Fibrin sealants in surgical practice: an overview. *Am J Surg* 2001; 182(2 Suppl): 1S-7S.

13. Seelich TJ. Tissucol (Immuno, Vienna) biochemistry and method of application. *Head & Neck Pathol* 1982; 3: 65-60.

14. Tisseel. Summary of product characteristics. Baxter Healthcare Ltd., March 2013; 1-16.

15. Evicel solutions for sealant. Abbreviated prescribing information. Omrix Biopharmaceuticals Ltd., August 2013.

16. Artiss solutions for sealant. Summary of product characteristics. Baxter Healthcare Ltd., August 2010; 1-16.

17. Coseal surgical sealant. Instructions for use. Baxter Healthcare Ltd., January 2009; 1-3.

18.   Duraseal Dural Sealant System. Instructions for use. www.covidien.com.

19.   Amri R, den Boon HC, Bordeianou LG, *et al*. The impact of adhesions on operations and postoperative recovery in colon cancer surgery. *Am J Surg* 2013; 206(2): 166-71.

20.   Glickman M1, Gheissari A, Money S, *et al*. A polymeric sealant inhibits anastomotic suture hole bleeding more rapidly than gelfoam/thrombin: results of a randomized controlled trial. *Arch Surg* 2002; 137(3): 326-31; discussion 332.

Baxter, Artiss, Coseal and Tisseel are registered trademarks of Baxter International Inc.

Duraseal is a registered trademark of Confluent Surgical, Inc.

Evicel is a registered trademark of Johnson & Johnson Corporation.

Gelfoam is a registered trademark of Pharmacia & Upjohn Company LLC.

Chapter 20

Transfusion triggers for blood and blood products: the evidence

Akshay Shah BMedSci (Hons) BM BS MSc MRCP
NIHR Academic Clinical Fellow and Specialty Registrar, Anaesthesia & Intensive Care, Nuffield Division of Anaesthetics, John Radcliffe Hospital, Oxford, UK

Stuart McKechnie MBChB BSc (Hons) FRCA FFICM DICM PhD
Consultant in Anaesthesia & Intensive Care, Nuffield Division of Anaesthetics, John Radcliffe Hospital, Oxford, UK

Simon Stanworth MD DPhil
Consultant Haematologist and Senior Lecturer, NIHR Oxford Biomedical Research Centre, Oxford University Hospitals NHS Foundation Trust and The University of Oxford, UK

- "Contaminated blood inquiry begins."
  BBC News, 18th April 2007

- "Like all medical treatments, a blood transfusion should only be given if it is essential. Your doctor will balance the risk of you having a blood transfusion against the risk of not having one."
  NHS Blood & Transplant Patient Information leaflet

- "Analysis of incidents highlights need for a redesign of the transfusion process."
  SHOT Report, 2013

Background

Allogeneic red cell transfusion is a commonly used treatment to correct anaemia and improve the oxygen-carrying capacity of blood. Approximately 85 million red cell units are transfused worldwide annually [1], with around two million issued across the UK in 2011 [2]. Surgical patients receive approximately 40% of transfused allogeneic blood [3].

The last few years have seen a marked fall in the overall usage of red cells for transfusion. The reasons for this are multifactorial, and include national and local educational initiatives (now often covered by the term "patient blood management") aimed at increasing awareness of the risks of transfusion, improved surgical techniques, and the need to consider alternatives, supported by a striking lack of evidence to support maintaining higher haemoglobin concentrations by transfusion.

Aerobic metabolism is dependent upon adequate tissue oxygen delivery (DO_2), which in turn is dependent upon cardiac output (CO) and arterial oxygen content (CaO_2).

$$DO_2 = CO \times CaO_2$$
$$= CO \times (1.39 \times [Hb] \times SaO_2 + PaO_2 \times 0.003)$$

Under normal conditions, the vast majority of oxygen is carried by haemoglobin (Hb). The haemoglobin concentration is therefore critical in determining arterial oxygen content, with a fall in haemoglobin resulting in reduced arterial oxygen content and, unless compensated, a fall in DO_2.

Case reports [4] highlight survival with Hb as low as 20g/L and experimental studies have shown that young healthy adults can compensate for Hb as low as 40g/L without significant deleterious effects if the circulating blood volume is maintained with fluids [5]. However, acutely unwell and elderly patients, especially those with comorbidities, are less likely to tolerate such low levels.

In the context of inadequate oxygen delivery, a clinician must decide between increasing the cardiac output (fluids and/or inotropes), or increasing the arterial oxygen content (correction of hypoxaemia and/or red cell transfusion). Global markers of inadequate oxygen delivery, such as low central, or mixed, venous saturations and lactic acidosis, may be useful but lack specificity. Haemoglobin concentration, in the absence of other specific clinical and laboratory tests, remains the most widely used trigger for blood transfusion in clinical practice.

Evidence

Allogeneic red blood cell transfusion

Observational studies suggest that patients who receive allogeneic red blood cell (RBC) transfusion are at increased risk of mortality, ischaemic complications, delayed wound healing, and increased length of stay [6-8]. However, it is not clear whether this link is causal or associative, as the findings of most observational studies are confounded by the fact that sicker patients, with associated worse clinical outcomes, generally receive more blood.

A number of randomised studies have provided evidence regarding the risk-benefit ratio of red cell transfusion. These trials have typically randomly allocated patients to a restrictive or liberal transfusion strategy. A Cochrane systematic review [9], identifying 19 such randomised studies involving 6264 patients across a variety of clinical settings, concluded that a Hb threshold (or transfusion trigger) of 70 or 80g/L is associated with fewer red cell transfusions without adverse association with regard to mortality, cardiac morbidity, functional recovery or hospital length of stay. The authors do comment on the significant heterogeneity between studies. A more recent meta-analysis consisting of 31 trials and 9813 patients, which also included medical patients and children, also concluded that restrictive transfusion practices are safe, associated with lower healthcare costs and further highlighted the lack of benefit from liberal transfusion policies [10]. The evidence base for blood transfusion in different clinical settings is described below.

Peri-operative anaemia and blood transfusion

The World Health Organization (WHO) defines anaemia as a haemoglobin (Hb) concentration of <130g/L in men, <120g/L in non-pregnant women and <110g/L in pregnant women [11]. Approximately 1.26 billion people worldwide are anaemic [11].

The prevalence of pre-operative anaemia varies widely — from 5% to 76% [12], and has been linked to increased postoperative mortality, morbidity, length of stay, and decreased quality of life [12-14]. Certain subgroups, for example, those with colorectal cancer, have a higher prevalence of pre-operative anaemia ranging from 39% (Dukes A) to 76% (Dukes D) [15].

The Clinical Use of Blood handbook by the WHO states that "there is rarely a justification for the use of pre-operative blood transfusion simply to facilitate elective surgery" [16]. The British Committee for Standards in Haematology (BCSH) guidelines state that "there is no case for transfusion back to a normal haemoglobin level either before or after surgery, and to avoid transfusion when the Hb is above 10g/L" [17].

Intra-operative goal-directed fluid therapy, to optimise stroke volume and cardiac output, has become established practice in major elective surgery. However, most algorithms for intra-operative goal-directed fluid therapy are based on crystalloid and/or colloid administration. The role of red cell transfusion in intra-operative goal-directed therapy has not been extensively studied. A recent study investigating the effect of a peri-operative cardiac output-guided haemodynamic algorithm on outcomes in patients undergoing major gastrointestinal surgery (OPTIMISE) [18], included maintaining a Hb of >80g/L as part of the algorithm. Use of the algorithm did not improve a composite outcome of complications and 30-day mortality compared to usual care in this study, but inclusion of the OPTIMISE results in a meta-analysis did suggest a significant reduction in complications with the intervention [18].

Orthopaedic surgery

Orthopaedic surgery is a major consumer of red cells and two studies in the UK showed that approximately 20-30% patients undergoing primary/revision hip or knee arthroplasty were transfused [19, 20]. The FOCUS trial [21] showed that a restrictive transfusion strategy (symptoms of anaemia or at physician discretion for an Hb <80g/L) was safe, even in patients with a history of, or risk factors for, cardiovascular disease, in patients undergoing surgery for a fractured neck of the femur. These findings have been confirmed in two more recent, albeit smaller trials [22, 23]. Overall, a restrictive transfusion strategy appears to be safe for the majority of patients undergoing orthopaedic lower limb surgery.

Cardiac surgery and acute myocardial infarction

Cardiac surgery is a major consumer of red cells. TiTRE2 [24] was a large multicentre trial that randomised approximately 2000 postoperative cardiac surgical patients to a restrictive (<75g/L) or liberal (<90g/L) transfusion threshold and found no difference in morbidity (serious infection, ischaemic event) or healthcare costs between groups. However, this study did find an increase in mortality, a secondary outcome, in the restrictive group.

Two small trials in patients with acute myocardial infarction, consisting of a total of 154 patients, showed an increasing trend in mortality in the restrictive group compared to the liberal group [25, 26]. However, these results were not statistically significant and larger trials in this group of patients are needed. At present, it may be prudent to maintain the Hb >80-100g/L in patients with active myocardial ischaemia whilst larger trials are awaited.

Critically ill patients

The landmark TRICC trial [27] showed that a restrictive transfusion trigger of Hb 70g/L was as safe as a liberal strategy, except perhaps in patients with ischaemic heart disease. Subsequent trials have also shown no benefit of liberal transfusion strategies [28, 29]. Current UK guidelines recommend that a transfusion threshold of 70g/L or below, with a target Hb range of 70-90g/L, should be the default unless specific comorbidities or acute illness-related factors modify decision-making [30].

Sepsis

Early goal-directed therapy (EGDT) in severe sepsis and septic shock has traditionally included targeting a haematocrit of >30% (Hb 100g/L) as part of a package of protocol-driven care within the first 6 hours of presentation [30]. However, these recommendations are largely drawn from one single-centre study [31, 32].

The use of protocol-driven goal-directed therapy in sepsis in a wider context has recently been tested in three large multicentre trials in North America (ProCESS) [33], the UK (ProMISE) [34] and Australia (ARISE) [35], where the transfusion trigger was an Hct <30% or Hb <100g/L in the protocol-based EGDT group compared to a transfusion trigger of Hb <75g/L in the protocol-based standard therapy group. Meta-analysis of the three trials has shown no difference in 90-day mortality between groups and increased use of vasopressors, blood transfusion and ICU resources in the EGDT group.

Acute blood loss

In patients with acute upper gastrointestinal (GI) haemorrhage, Villanueva *et al* in 2013 [36] showed that clinical outcomes, including all-cause mortality, were significantly improved in a restrictive group (transfusion trigger <70g/L) when compared to a liberal group (transfusion trigger <90g/L). A large and more recent feasibility trial [37] in patients with acute upper GI haemorrhage also showed that a restrictive transfusion policy (Hb <80g/L) is safe, associated with fewer red cell transfusions (although this was not statistically significant) and with non-inferior clinical outcomes when compared to a liberal policy (Hb <100g/L).

Fresh frozen plasma, platelets, cryoprecipitate and fibrinogen concentrate

Fresh frozen plasma

Fresh frozen plasma (FFP) is human donor plasma, frozen within 8 hours of collection. After thawing, FFP contains almost normal levels of plasma coagulation factors, acute phase reactants, immunoglobulins and albumin [38]. Current UK and European Union guidelines require that only factor VIII levels need to be quality controlled [39]. The recommended dose of FFP is 12-15ml/kg.

FFP use can be divided into prophylactic (to prevent bleeding) or therapeutic (to stop bleeding). Recent UK national audits have shown a gradual reduction in the use of FFP over the past few years. Approximately 266,000 units were used in 2013 compared to approximately 300,000 units in 2009 [40]. This could be attributed to the lack of high-quality evidence supporting the efficacy of FFP. A systematic review [41] in 2012 and recent trials [42] have found no evidence of benefit for prophylactic or therapeutic FFP use across a wide range of clinical settings – prior to invasive procedures, liver disease, cardiac surgery, warfarin anticoagulation reversal, burns, shock and head injury.

FFP use is recommended in patients with disseminated intravascular coagulation (DIC) with evidence of bleeding to maintain a prothrombin time (PT) and activated partial thromboplastin time (APTT) of less than 1.5 times the normal control time [43]. In the setting of major haemorrhage in trauma, haemostatic management involves giving red cells, FFP (and platelets) in fixed ratios with limited use of crystalloid or colloid solution. The optimal ratio of red cells to FFP is subject to ongoing debate. The recent PROPPR trial [44] attempted to answer the question of the optimal ratio, randomising patients with trauma and severe bleeding to one of two plasma: platelet: red cell ratios – 1:1:1 or 1:1:2. The authors found no difference in 24-hour or 30-day mortality between the groups. However, a 1:1:1 ratio did result in a signification reduction in mortality from exsanguination within the first 24 hours (9.2% vs. 14.6%, p = 0.03) with similar complication rates to the 1:1:2 ratio group. Table 1 summarises the current recommendations for the use of FFP.

Table 1. Suggested indications for the transfusion of fresh frozen plasma. *Reproduced with permission from John Wiley & Sons* [56].

Indication	Recommendation
Disseminated intravascular coagulopathy (DIC)	Consider transfusion with FFP, platelets and cryoprecipitate if there is clinical evidence of bleeding. There is no supporting evidence for prophylactic transfusion in the absence of bleeding despite abnormal coagulation tests.
Reversal of warfarin effect	FFP should only be used for the reversal of warfarin anticoagulation in the presence of *major* bleeding if prothrombin complex concentrate is not available. In the absence of bleeding, over-anticoagulation should be managed by withholding warfarin therapy and initiating oral/intravenous vitamin K.
Peri-operative transfusions	The majority of FFP use in this setting is in cardiac surgery. Meta-analysis does not suggest a reduction in peri-operative blood loss with prophylactic FFP use.
Before invasive procedures	Regional/neuraxial blockade: For elective surgery, relevant anticoagulants and antiplatelets should be stopped according to local/national guidelines. With regards to warfarin reversal: • Urgent procedures — consider 2.5-5mg of oral/intravenous vitamin K. • Immediate reversal — consider FFP, although no high-level evidence exists to support this. Intensive care: Minor derangements in PT/INR are common in ICU patients and are often due to vitamin K deficiency. Trials have not shown any clear benefit of prophylactic FFP use to reduce bleeding related to planned procedures.

Platelets

In the UK, platelets are produced from centrifugation of whole blood or by apheresis [45]. Both methods generate the same number of platelets and are considered therapeutically equivalent. A unit of platelets also contains plasma (or platelet-additive solutions) to maintain platelet function during storage. Pooled platelet concentrates can be stored in a closed system at 22°C with continuous gentle agitation for up to 5 days. One unit of apheresis platelets would be expected to increase the platelet count in an average adult by 20-40 x 10^9/L [46]. Indications for platelet transfusion can be broadly classified into:

- Prophylactic:
  - routine use in non-bleeding patients with thrombocytopenia;
  - presence of risk factors for bleeding, e.g. sepsis;
  - pre-procedure to prevent bleeding following invasive procedures/ surgery.
- Therapeutic:
  - treatment of active bleeding.

Clinical guidelines typically use platelet number to guide platelet transfusion, but less regard is given to assessment of platelet function. Much of the evidence for prophylactic transfusion in non-bleeding patients has come from haematology patients with chemotherapy-associated thrombocytopenia. Randomised controlled trials in this cohort [46] have shown that a transfusion trigger of 10 x 10^9/L confers no increased bleeding risk when compared to a trigger of 20 x 10^9/L.

There is a lack of evidence to guide platelet transfusions to cover invasive/surgical procedures, with guidelines based mainly on expert opinion. There does not appear to be a role for the prophylactic transfusion of platelets in patients on cardiopulmonary bypass, with transfusion reserved for bleeding patients who have had a surgical cause excluded [46].

The use of prophylactic platelet transfusion is not recommended in patients with heparin-induced thrombocytopenia or idiopathic thrombocytopenic purpura and is contraindicated in patients with thrombotic thrombocytopenic purpura [46]. Table 2 summarises the current recommendations for platelet transfusion.

Table 2. Suggested indications for the use of platelet transfusions. *Reproduced with permission from John Wiley & Sons* [56].

Indication	Transfusion trigger
Routine prophylactic use to reduce bleeding risk.	10×10^9/L
Prophylactic use in patients with additional risk factors, e.g. sepsis.	$10\text{-}20 \times 10^9$/L
Prophylactic use pre-procedure:	
• Surgery involving critical sites — brain, eye.	100×10^9/L
• Non-critical site surgery (e.g. laparotomy) or invasive procedure.	50×10^9/L
• Neuraxial blockade.	75×10^9/L is normal risk

Cryoprecipitate and fibrinogen concentrate

Cryoprecipitate is an allogeneic blood product prepared from human plasma. Cryoprecipitate is derived from controlled thawing of FFP at 1° to 6°C to precipitate higher molecular-weight proteins such as factor VIII, von Willebrand factor, fibronectin, factor XIII and fibrinogen [47].

Amazingly and despite almost 50 years of use, evidence of the efficacy of cryoprecipitate is limited. A Cochrane review evaluating the effectiveness of fibrinogen concentrate for bleeding patients found six small trials in elective surgery, all of which were low quality and underpowered for mortality but demonstrating a clear reduction in the incidence of allogeneic transfusions [48]. Cryoprecipitate/fibrinogen concentrates should be reserved for use in patients with documented dysfibrinogenaemia or hypofibrinogenaemia secondary to major haemorrhage, massive transfusion, or DIC. Guidelines recommend transfusion of cryoprecipitate if the fibrinogen level is <1.5g/L with clinical evidence of bleeding, although there is no high-level evidence to support this [49].

Risks associated with blood and blood products

The risks of allogeneic red cell transfusion include those common to all blood components, such as transfusion transmitted infection and errors in the processing and administration, and those specific to red cells, such as the storage lesion. The annual Serious Hazards of Transfusion (SHOT) reports provide insight into the risks of transfusions in UK practice. More than half of the cases reported were due to preventable mistakes, with the leading error being incorrect blood component transfusion. Acute transfusion reactions were the commonest cause of pathological and unpredictable incidents [50]. These risks are summarised in Table 3.

Table 3. Early and late hazards of allogeneic red cell transfusion. *Reproduced with permission from John Wiley & Sons* [56].

Early:

- Haemolytic reactions — immediate or delayed.
- Non-haemolytic febrile reactions.
- Transfusion-associated circulatory overload (TACO).
- Transfusion-associated acute lung injury (TRALI).
- Citrate toxicity.
- Electrolyte disturbances — hyperkalaemia.
- Hypothermia.
- Post-transfusion purpura.

Late:

- Infection:
  - viral — hepatitis A, B, C, E, HIV;
  - bacterial;
  - parasites.
- Graft vs. host disease.
- Transfusion-related iron overload.
- Immunomodulation.

Risks commonly associated with FFP include transfusion-related acute lung injury (TRALI), transfusion-associated circulatory overload (TACO) and allergic/anaphylactic reactions. Less common risks include infection transmission, haemolytic and febrile non-haemolytic transfusion reactions and red cell alloimmunization [51].

The potential benefits of platelet transfusion must be balanced against the risks. Non-haemolytic febrile reactions and mild allergic reactions are common with an estimated incidence of 2% and 4%, respectively. Anaphylaxis occurs rarely (1:20,000 to 1:50,000 of transfusions), but accounts for approximately 40% of the serious adverse events. Platelets are more commonly implicated in TRALI than red cells [50]. As with all blood components, there is a potential risk of transfusion transmitted infection. The rate of viral transmission — human immunodeficiency virus, hepatitis B, and hepatitis C — appears extremely low. Transfusion transmitted bacterial infection has an estimated incidence of 1:10,000 platelet transfusions, because, unlike other blood components, platelets are processed and stored at room temperature. Bacterial screening has been introduced to reduce the risk of transfusion transmitted bacterial infection.

How to do it

What is the clinical setting?

Although the evidence base for red cell transfusion practice is incomplete, as highlighted above, randomised studies consistently support the restrictive use of red cells in most settings, with little evidence of benefit for maintaining patients at higher haemoglobin thresholds (liberal strategy).

The degree to which the optimal Hb or transfusion trigger should be modified for patients with additional specific risk factors, especially ischaemic heart disease, remains less clear. It seems sensible to modify the decision to transfuse in the presence of symptoms such as chest pain, heart failure, or tachycardia unresponsive to fluid resuscitation. Guidelines suggest there is no evidence to transfuse when the Hb is >100g/L.

Is there a need to transfuse?

Increasing arterial oxygen content by increasing Hb does not necessarily increase tissue oxygen delivery or uptake. Transfused cells have altered rheological properties and increasing Hb increases the haematocrit (Hct) and blood viscosity which can reduce blood flow through the microcirculation.

Red cell transfusions rarely increase oxygen uptake (VO_2) except in extreme situations where oxygen uptake is directly dependent upon oxygen delivery such as severe circulatory shock [52, 53]. Blood loss of up to 30% can be adequately treated with crystalloids or colloids [3].

Old blood or new blood?

Current UK practice allows for the storage of red cells to a maximum of 35 days. It is well recognised that adverse biochemical and physiological changes occur in stored red cells but the clinical consequences of red cell storage lesions remains unclear.

The ABLE trialists [54] randomised critically ill patients to 'new' blood (less than 8 days) or 'old' blood (oldest compatible units available in the blood bank) and found no difference in the primary outcome (90-day mortality) or secondary outcomes (duration of organ support, length of stay and transfusion reactions) between groups. Other randomised trials aiming to answer the same question are ongoing [55].

What about blood products?

FFP should not be used prophylactically to correct minor derangements in coagulation markers in the absence of bleeding. Therapeutic indications include major haemorrhage and DIC. Guidelines for the prophylactic administration of platelets are largely based on platelet number (rather than function) and are drawn from studies in haematological malignancy patients and expert opinion. There is an urgent need for studies to determine the optimal use of both FFP and platelets in non-bleeding patients.

As for platelets, cryoprecipitate transfusion is largely based on a fibrinogen level trigger of <1.5g/dL with no high-level evidence to support this. Fibrinogen concentrate appears to reduce transfusion requirements, but there is also an urgent need for higher-quality studies to define indications for its use.

Practicalities

Local protocols should be followed when transfusing blood and blood products. This includes the management of samples and inclusion of the patient in the transfusion decision-making process, through consent for transfusion (or information in retrospect) that a transfusion was necessary.

Conclusions

A restrictive transfusion strategy using thresholds of 70-80g/L appears to be clinically safe in a wide range of clinical settings with subsequent reduction in red cell usage and patient exposure to the risks of transfusion. Larger, well-designed clinical trials are needed in high-risk patients such as those with acute coronary syndrome. No high-quality evidence supports the use of blood products such as FFP, platelets, and cryoprecipitate/ fibrinogen concentrate in the absence of bleeding.

Checklist summary

✓ Where possible, always involve the patient in the decision-making process for blood and/or blood product transfusion.

✓ Educate staff on patient blood management strategies to minimise transfusion.

✓ Adopt a restrictive transfusion policy for patients who need allogeneic red blood cell transfusion in the absence of major haemorrhage and acute coronary syndrome.

✓ Where possible, avoid prophylactic blood component administration in the absence of bleeding.

References

1. Takei T, Amin NA, Schmid G, *et al.* Progress in global blood safety for HIV. *J Acquir Immune Defic Syndr* 2009; 52: S127-31.
2. Bolton-Maggs PHB (Ed), Cohen H, on behalf of the Serious Hazards of Transfusion (SHOT) Steering Group. The 2011 Annual SHOT Report, 2012. http://www.shotuk.org/shot-reports/shot-annual-report-summary-2011/.
3. Association of Anaesthetists of Great Britain and Ireland (AAGBI). Blood transfusion and the anaesthetist. Red cell transfusion 2. London, UK: AAGBI, 2008.
4. Kulvatonyou N, Heard SO. Care of the injured Jehovah's Witness patient: case report and review of the literature. *J Clin Anesthesiol* 2004; 16: 548-53.
5. Weiskopf RB, Viele MK, Feiner J, *et al.* Human cardiovascular and metabolic response to acute, severe, isovolemic anemia. *JAMA* 1998; 279: 217-21.
6. Spahn DR, Theusinger OM, Hofmann A. Patient blood management is a win-win: a wake up call. *Br J Anaesth* 2012; 108: 889-92.
7. Murphy GJ, Reeves BC, Rogers CA, *et al.* Increased mortality, postoperative morbidity, and cost after red blood cell transfusion in patients having cardiac surgery. *Circ* 2007; 116: 2544-52.
8. Isbister JP, Shander A, Spahn DR, *et al.* Adverse blood transfusion outcomes: establishing causation. *Trans Med Rev* 2011; 25: 89-101.
9. Carson JL, Carless PA, Herbert PC. Transfusion thresholds and other strategies for guiding allogeneic red blood cell transfusion. *Cochrane Database Syst Rev* 2012; 4: CD002042.
10. Holst LB, Petersen MW, Haase N, *et al.* Restrictive versus liberal transfusion strategy for red blood cell transfusion: systematic review of randomised trials with meta-analysis and trial sequential analysis. *Br Med J* 2015; 350: 1354.
11. de Benoist B, McLean E, Egli I, *et al*, Eds. Worldwide prevalence of anaemia 1993-2005. Geneva, Switzerland: World Health Organisation, 2008.
12. Shander A, Knight K, Thurer R, *et al.* Prevalence and outcomes of anaemia in surgery: a systematic review of the literature. *Am J Med* 2004; 116: 58S-69S.
13. Shander A, Javidroozi M, Ozawa S, *et al.* What is really dangerous? Anaemia or transfusion? *Br J Anaesth* 2011; 107 (S1); i41-9.
14. Musallam KM, Tamim HM, Richards T, *et al.* Pre-operative anaemia and post-operative outcomes in non-cardiac surgery. *Lancet* 2011; 378: 1396-407.
15. Cappell MS, Goldberg ES. The relationship between the clinical presentation and spread of colon cancer in 315 consecutive patients: a significant trend of earlier cancer detection from 1982 through 1988 at a university hospital. *J Clin Gastroenterol* 1992; 14: 227-35.

16.   World Health Organization Blood Transfusion Safety. *The Clinical Use of Blood Handbook*. Geneva, Switzerland: World Health Organization, 2001.

17.   British Committee for Standards in Haematology. Guidelines for the clinical use of red cell transfusions. *Br J Haematol* 2001; 113: 24-31.

18.   Pearse RM, Harrison DA, MacDonald N, *et al*. Effect of a perioperative, cardiac output-guided hemodynamic therapy algorithm on outcomes following major gastrointestinal surgery. *JAMA* 2014; 311: 2181-90.

19.   Kotze A, Carter LA, Scally AJ. Effect of a patient blood management programme on preoperative anaemia, transfusion rate, and outcome after primary hip or knee arthroplasty: a quality improvement cycle. *Br J Anaesth* 2012; 108: 943-52.

20.   Saleh E, McClelland DB, Hay A, *et al*. Prevalence of anaemia before major joint arthroplasty and the potential impact of preoperative investigation and correction on perioperative blood transfusions. *Br J Anaesth* 2007; 99: 801-8.

21.   Carson JL, Terrin ML, Noveck H, *et al*. Liberal or restrictive transfusion in high-risk patients after hip surgery. *N Engl J Med* 2011; 365: 2453-62.

22.   Parker MJ. Randomised trial of blood transfusion versus a restrictive transfusion policy after hip fracture surgery. *Injury* 2013; 44: 1916-8.

23.   Gregerson M, Borris LC, Damsgaard EM. Postoperative blood transfusion strategy in frail, anaemic elderly patients with hip fracture. *Acta Orthopaedica* 2015; 86: 1-10.

24.   Murphy GJ, Pike K, Rogers CA, *et al*. Liberal or restrictive transfusion after cardiac surgery. *N Engl J Med* 2015; 372: 997-1008.

25.   Cooper HA, Rao SV, Greenberg MD, *et al*. Conservative versus liberal red cell transfusion in acute myocardial infarction. *Am J Cardiol* 2011; 108: 1108-11.

26.   Carson JL, Brooks MM, Abbott JD, *et al*. Liberal versus restrictive transfusion thresholds for patients with symptomatic coronary artery disease. *Am Heart J* 2013; 165: 964-71.

27.   Herbert PC, Wells G, Blajchman MA, *et al*. A multicenter randomised controlled trial of transfusion requirements in critical care. *N Engl J Med* 1999; 340: 409-17.

28.   Walsh T, Boyd J, Watson D, *et al*. Restrictive versus liberal transfusion strategies in older mechanically ventilated critically ill patients. *Crit Care Med* 2013; 41: 2354-63.

29.   Holst LB, Haase N, Wetterslev J, *et al*. Lower versus higher haemoglobin threshold for transfusion in septic shock. *N Engl J Med* 2014; 371: 1381-91.

30.   Retter A, Wyncoll D, Pearse R, *et al*. Guidelines on the management of anaemia and red cell transfusion in adult critically ill patients. *Br J Haem* 2013; 160: 445-64.

31.   Rivers E, Nguyen B, Havstad S, *et al*. Early goal-directed therapy in the treatment of severe sepsis and septic shock. *N Engl J Med* 2001; 345: 1368-77.

32.   Dellinger RP, Levy MM, Rhodes A, *et al*. Surviving Sepsis Campaign: international guidelines for management of severe sepsis and septic shock, 2012. *Intensive Care Med* 2013; 39: 165-228.

33.   The ProCESS Investigators. A randomised trial of protocol-based care for early septic shock. *N Engl J Med* 2014; 370: 1683-93.

34.   Mouncey PR, Osborn TM, Power GS *et al*. Trial of early goal-directed resuscitation for septic shock. *N Engl J Med* 2015; 372: 1301-11.

35.   The ARISE Investigators and the ANZICS Clinical Trials Group. Goal-directed resuscitation for patients with early septic shock. *N Engl J Med* 2014; 371: 1496-506.

36.   Villanueva C, Colomo A, Bosch A, *et al*. Transfusion strategies for acute upper gastrointestinal bleeding. *N Engl J Med* 2013; 368: 11-21.

37.   Jairath V, Kahan BC, Gray A, *et al*. Restrictive versus liberal blood transfusion for acute upper gastrointestinal bleeding (TRIGGER): a pragmatic, open-label, cluster randomised feasibility trial. *Lancet* 2015: 386; 137-44.

38.   Stanworth SJ. The evidence-based use of FFP and cryoprecipitate for abnormalities of coagulation tests and clinical coagulopathy. *Haematol* 2007; 179-86.

39.   BCSH Guidelines for the use of fresh frozen plasma. *Br J Haem* 2004: 126: 11-28.

40.   Serious Hazards of Transfusion Annual Report 2013. http://www.shotuk.org/wp-content/uploads/74280-SHOT-2014-Annual-Report-V12-WEB.pdf.

41.   Yang L, Stanworth S, Hopewell S, *et al*. Is fresh-frozen plasma clinically effective? An update of a systematic review of randomized controlled trials. *Transfusion* 2012; 52: 1673-86.

42.   Muller MC, Sesmu Arbous M, Spoelstra-de Man AM, *et al*. Transfusion of fresh-frozen plasma in critically ill patients with a coagulopathy before invasive procedures: a randomized clinical trial. *Transfusion* 2015; 55: 26-35.

43.   Levi M, Toh CH, Thachil J, *et al*. Guidelines for the diagnosis and management of disseminated intravascular coagulation. *Br J Haematol* 2009; 145: 24-33.

44.   Holcomb JB, Tilley BC, Baraniuk S, *et al*. Transfusion of plasma, platelets and red blood cells in a 1:1:1 vs. a 1:1:2 ratio and mortality in patients with severe trauma. *JAMA* 2015; 313: 471-82.

45.   British Committee for Standards in Haematology, Blood Transfusion Task Force. Guidelines for the use of platelet transfusions. *Br J Haematol* 2003; 122(1): 10-23.

46.   Stanworth SJ, Estcourt LJ, Powter G, *et al*. The effect of a no-prophylactic versus prophylactic platelet transfusion strategy on bleeding in patients with hematological malignancies and severe thrombocytopenia (TOPPS trial). A randomized controlled, non-inferiority trial. *N Engl J Med* 2013; 368: 1771-80.

47.   Stanworth SJ. The evidence-based use of FFP and cryoprecipitate for abnormalities of coagulation tests and clinical coagulopathy. *Haematol* 2007; 179-86.

48.   Wikkelso A, Lunde J, Johansen M, *et al*. Fibrinogen concentrate in bleeding patients. *Cochrane Database Syst Rev* 2013; 8: CD008864.

49.   Thomas D, Wee M, Clyburn P, *et al*. Blood transfusion and the anaesthetist: management of massive haemorrhage. *Anaesthesia* 2010; 65: 1153-61.

50.   Bolton-Maggs PHB (Ed), Cohen H, on behalf of the Serious Hazards of Transfusion (SHOT) Steering Group. The 2011 Annual SHOT Report, 2012. http://www.shotuk.org/shot-reports/shot-annual-report-summary-2011/.

51.   Pandey S, Vyas GN. Adverse effects of plasma transfusion. *Transfusion* 2012; 52 (Suppl 1): 65S-79S.

52.   Bakker J, Vincent JL. The oxygen supply dependency phenomenon is associated with increased blood lactate levels. *J Crit Care* 1991; 6: 152-9.

53.   Gilbert EM, Haupt MT, Mandanas RY, *et al*. The effect of fluid loading, blood transfusion and catecholamine infusion on oxygen delivery and consumption in patients with sepsis. *Am Rev Resp Dis* 1986; 134: 873-8.

54.   Lacroix J, Hebert PC, Fergusson DA, *et al*. Age of transfused blood in critically ill adults. *N Engl J Med* 2015; 372: 1410-8.

55.   Kaukonen KM, Bailey M, Ady B, *et al*. A randomised controlled trial of standard transfusion versus fresher red blood cell use in intensive care (TRANSFUSE): protocol and statistical analysis plan. *Crit Care Resusc* 2014; 16: 255-61.

56.   Shah A, Stanworth SJ, McKechnie S. Evidence and triggers for transfusion of blood and blood products. *Anaesthesia* 2015; 70: 10-e3.

Chapter 21

Trauma-induced coagulopathy

Lewis Gall BMSc (Hons) MRCS
Trauma Clinical Research Fellow, Centre for Trauma Sciences, Queen Mary University of London, UK
Karim Brohi BSc FRCA FRCS
Professor of Trauma Sciences, Centre for Trauma Sciences, Queen Mary University of London, UK

- "A greater understanding of the mechanisms underpinning trauma-induced coagulopathy is key to reducing the number of preventable deaths from haemorrhage."

- "Timely targeted intervention for haemorrhage control will result in better patient outcomes and reduced demand for blood products."
  Gruen RL, Brohi K, Schreiber M, *et al*.
  Haemorrhage control in severely injured patients.
  Lancet 2012; 380: 1099-108.

Background

Traumatic injuries account for the death of almost 6 million people worldwide each year with this number projected to have risen by 40% by the year 2030 [1]. Haemorrhage is responsible for 30-40% of deaths following trauma and is the most common cause of early in-hospital mortality within the first few hours following major trauma [2]. Of those patients with potentially survivable injuries, who subsequently die, the majority do so because of haemorrhage [3]. A greater understanding of the mechanisms underpinning trauma-induced coagulopathy (TIC) is key to reducing the number of preventable deaths from haemorrhage.

Coagulopathy following injury is not a new concept having first been reported during the Korean War in the early 1950s [4]. However, it was not until the identification of an early, endogenous acute traumatic coagulopathy (ATC) in 2003 that significant knowledge gains were made. ATC is present in nearly 25% of patients presenting to the emergency department following major trauma [5]. ATC is characterised by systemic anticoagulation and hyperfibrinolysis [6]. ATC is associated with a significantly increased requirement for blood product transfusion, greater incidence of multiple organ failure, longer intensive care and hospital lengths of stay and an overall mortality approaching 50% [7].

Trauma represents a significant and growing public health burden with the treatment of the injured, bleeding and coagulopathic patient placing huge demands on all clinical services including those of blood transfusion. In an effort to reduce the early mortality from haemorrhage it is therefore important that care providers working in the fields of both trauma and transfusion medicine have an understanding of TIC. This chapter outlines the current understanding of the pathophysiology of TIC. The availability of diagnostic tests for the identification of TIC and their current limitations are also discussed.

Revision of the classical description of coagulopathy

Coagulation requires a delicate balance between the creation of an impermeable platelet and fibrin clot at the site of injury whilst at the same time maintaining blood vessel patency to allow distal blood flow and localisation of the procoagulant process to the site of injury. The classical description of coagulation views it as a cascade of clotting factors which begins with two discrete pathways — the intrinsic and the extrinsic pathways. This coagulation cascade concept has been revised and haemostasis is now considered a cell-based model in which coagulation occurs on specific cell surfaces [8]. Haemostasis is therefore dependent upon complex interactions between tissue factor bearing cells, platelets and the vascular endothelium.

Drivers of trauma-induced coagulopathy (Figure 1)

Coagulopathy following major trauma was previously attributed to loss through bleeding, consumption, dilution and dysfunction of clotting factors. In addition, coagulopathy was considered a relatively late event that occurred as part of the 'lethal triad' along with acidosis and hypothermia. Contemporary understanding recognises that in the immediate post-injury phase, these factors alone do not result in TIC. Instead, early coagulopathy occurs as a consequence of endogenous ATC.

The primary drivers of ATC are the combination of tissue injury and shock with systemic hypoperfusion. In the presence of injury, as tissue hypoperfusion measured by base deficit (BD) increases, patients display

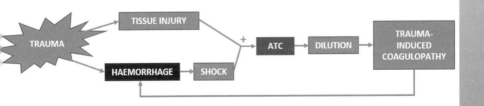

Figure 1. Drivers of trauma-induced coagulopathy.

a prolongation of their prothrombin time (PT) and activated partial thromboplastin time (APTT). Injured patients without hypoperfusion do not develop ATC. Similarly, shocked but non-injured patients do not develop ATC, highlighting that it is the combination of both injury and shock together which drives early coagulopathy [9].

Haemodilution exacerbates ATC. Dilution of remaining coagulation factors occurs during resuscitation, by the transfusion of hypocoagulable fluids such as crystalloids or packed red blood cells. The combination of haemodilution, along with ongoing blood loss, hypothermia, severe acidosis and consumption of clotting factors exacerbates ATC and contributes collectively to the establishment of a global TIC. Therefore, TIC is due in part to both endogenous ATC and iatrogenic factors.

Mechanisms of acute traumatic coagulopathy

ATC results from the activation of anticoagulant and fibrinolytic pathways. Activation of the protein C pathway is implicated in both of these processes. Fibrinogen depletion, vascular endothelial activation and platelet dysfunction also contribute to ATC.

Systemic anticoagulation via protein C activation

In the cell-based model of normal haemostasis, activated protein C functions as an anticoagulant and is believed to be one of the methods by which the body restricts clot formation to the area of vascular injury [8]. Following trauma, activation of this anticoagulant pathway appears to be one of the key mechanisms of ATC.

As BD increases, plasma levels of soluble thrombomodulin (TM) and activated protein C increase. It is proposed that following injury and in the presence of tissue hypoperfusion, TM is expressed on the vascular endothelium and thrombin binds to it. The thrombin-TM complex activates protein C, which in turn inactivates coagulation factors Va and VIIIa. The net effect is that less thrombin is available to cleave fibrinogen and systemic anticoagulation ensues [9]. Thrombin is essentially converted from a procoagulant to an anticoagulant.

Hyperfibrinolysis

Fibrinolysis or clot breakdown is physiologically required to prevent extension of the clot beyond the site of injury and to break down clots once tissue healing has had time to occur. Fibrinolysis is increased following trauma as identified by raised D-dimer levels [9]. However, in ATC, a major mechanistic component is excess clot degradation or hyperfibrinolysis [6].

The exact mechanism by which hyperfibrinolysis is activated in major trauma remains unclear. However, hypoperfusion activation of the protein C pathway has again been implicated. Tissue plasminogen activator (tPA) is released by the vascular endothelium following injury and shock. tPA cleaves plasminogen, forming plasmin which initiates fibrinolysis. In ATC, excess activated protein C will consume plasminogen activator inhibitor-1 (PAI-1), thus leading to 'de-repression' of tPA and reduced clot stability as a consequence of hyperfibrinolysis [7].

Fibrinolysis in ATC has likely been underestimated due to difficulties in its detection. Using rotational thromboelastometry (ROTEM®) alone, the reported incidence ranges from 5% to 20% [10, 11]. However, ROTEM® is an insensitive measure of fibrinolytic activity in trauma. Plasmin-antiplasmin complex (PAP) levels which correspond to the current activity level of the fibrinolytic system have also been used. Measurement of PAP levels suggests that almost 60% of trauma patients have evidence of fibrinolytic activity. Patients with 'moderate' or 'severe' fibrinolytic activity have a worse clinical outcome with a higher mortality, higher packed red blood cell and fresh frozen plasma transfusion requirements and will require longer hospital stays [10]. A greater understanding of the fibrinolysis pathways involved in ATC and better methods of detecting hyperfibrinolysis could lead to novel targeted therapies which could subsequently improve clinical outcomes.

Fibrinogen depletion

Fibrinogen is a vital substrate for blood clot formation and it has been demonstrated that fibrinogen depletion is a hallmark of ATC. On admission, the proportion of patients with a fibrinogen level below 1.5g/L,

1.0g/L and 0.8g/L has been found to be 14%, 5% and 3%, respectively. Specifically, fibrinogen levels on admission are reduced by one third in coagulopathic patients [12]. The mechanism by which fibrinogen depletion occurs remains unclear; however, fibrinogen consumption and fibrinogenolysis have been proposed as potential explanations. Low fibrinogen levels are associated with increased mortality. Supplementation of fibrinogen (with cryoprecipitate) during damage control resuscitation has been found to maintain fibrinogen levels and be associated with a lower mortality rate. In patients with ATC, by the *ex vivo* addition of fibrinogen concentrate or cryoprecipitate to their admission blood samples, it is possible to reverse ATC as measured by ROTEM® [12]. These findings highlight the importance of fibrinogen in the pathophysiology of ATC and although further clinical studies are required, if reproducible *in vivo*, early fibrinogen supplementation has the potential to completely reverse ATC and improve patient outcomes.

Endothelial activation

On the innermost aspect of each blood vessel wall is the single cell layer of the vascular endothelium which is then covered by the endothelial glycocalyx. The role of the vascular endothelium in the activation of protein C and its mechanistic contribution to ATC development has already been discussed. Research exploring the impact of trauma and shock on the vascular endothelium and glycocalyx has highlighted that both are active participants in the pathophysiology of ATC; however, the specific mechanisms by which the endothelium contributes to ATC remain unclear. Initial studies have demonstrated that following major trauma, endothelial glycocalyx degradation (represented by high levels of syndecan-1) occurs and is associated with increased sympatho-adrenal activity and increased mortality. It is postulated that following trauma, systemic hypoperfusion and sympatho-adrenal activation, with a rapid rise in catecholamine levels, may contribute to glycocalyx degradation. Endothelial glycocalyx degradation is associated with increased inflammation, lower protein C levels (inferring activation of protein C), increased hyperfibrinolysis and increased coagulopathy [13]. These findings are significant because glycocalyx degradation itself can trigger local thrombin formation, activation of protein C and hyperfibrinolysis. Although further research is required, glycocalyx degradation and endothelial activation have the potential to be an important mechanism of ATC.

Platelet dysfunction

Platelets are an essential component of haemostasis although our understanding of the role they play in the pathophysiology of TIC is somewhat limited. Platelet counts are generally maintained within the normal range following trauma, with only 5% of trauma patients presenting with a count <150 x 10^9/L[14]. Although yet to be fully characterised, platelet dysfunction rather than insufficient number of platelets is believed to contribute to TIC. A small but significant reduction in platelet function, as measured by multiple electrode impedance aggregometry (MEA), has been identified between survivors and non-survivors of trauma [15]. MEA relies upon the presence of a normal fibrinogen level. Therefore, in ATC which is characterised by fibrinogen depletion, the true cause of any identified platelet dysfunction by MEA is difficult to interpret.

Platelet dysfunction has also been detected using thromboelastography (TEG®) platelet functional analysis assays when comparing trauma patients to healthy volunteers. Shock, tissue injury and blood transfusion requirements were independently associated with the degree of platelet dysfunction on admission to hospital [16]. Further research is required to advance our knowledge of platelet dysfunction in trauma and to investigate the potential benefits of early platelet transfusion in the management of TIC.

Early diagnosis of trauma-induced coagulopathy

There is no universally available or definitive method to rapidly identify patients with TIC. Currently available diagnostics and definitions of TIC are highlighted along with mention of each of their main strengths and limitations. It should be emphasised that the haemostatic competence of a bleeding trauma patient can change rapidly and therefore repeated timely reassessment of coagulation function by whichever means available is advisable.

Laboratory coagulation screens

The initial studies into TIC used laboratory coagulation screens including PT, APTT and the International Normalised Ratio (INR) to define coagulopathy. A variety of different cut-off values or definitions of coagulopathy have previously been used [5]. A suggested clinically relevant definition of ATC using laboratory coagulation screens is a prothrombin time ratio (PTr) >1.2 [17]. A prolonged PTr beyond this level is associated with increased mortality and increased transfusion requirements.

Laboratory coagulation tests in clinical practice are slow, usually taking over 60 minutes for the result to be available [18]. In the context of the exsanguinating patient following major trauma, with massive haemorrhage and TIC, laboratory coagulation tests are essentially 'out-of-date' by the time the results become available and are of limited use in guiding transfusion management. These tests are measured using platelet-poor plasma. In light of our recent understanding of the cell-based model of haemostasis, the meaning of these lab coagulation tests is questionable. Additionally, PT and APTT measure the first 20 and 60 seconds, respectively, of clot formation only and are unable to quantify overall clot strength or clot propagation versus fibrinolysis [7].

Point-of-care devices which measure PT are faster and more convenient than their laboratory equivalent, but are inaccurate in the diagnosis of ATC as they rely upon a normal haematocrit [18]. Overall, therefore, both laboratory coagulation screens and currently available point-of-care devices are inadequate in the diagnosis of TIC.

Fibrinogen measurement

Fibrinogen appears integral to TIC development yet it is inconsistently measured as part of major trauma care. Patients with TIC have a low fibrinogen level on admission and are likely to benefit from fibrinogen supplementation. A laboratory fibrinogen level should be requested on all bleeding trauma patients on admission. Additionally, ROTEM® clot amplitude at 5 minutes can be used as an early surrogate measure of fibrinogen concentration and help to guide fibrinogen supplementation during 'damage control resuscitation'. A FIBTEM CA5 <9.5mm can discriminate patients with a fibrinogen level below 1.5g/L with a sensitivity of 78% and specificity of 70% [12].

Point of care — viscoelastic haemostatic assays

Increasingly in both research and clinical settings, viscoelastic haemostatic assay devices, such as TEG® and ROTEM®, are being used to characterise coagulation and to diagnose TIC. TEG® and ROTEM® are point-of-care devices which measure the viscoelastic properties of whole blood under low shear conditions and display the dynamics of clot formation, clot lysis and the influence of fibrinogen and platelets on their real-time display screens. It is possible to rapidly diagnose TIC using ROTEM®. A clot amplitude at 5 minutes (EXTEM CA5, which represents clot firmness at 5 minutes) of ≤35mm can successfully diagnose TIC and is more accurate than the PTr at predicting the need for massive blood transfusion (detection rate of 71% versus 43%, respectively) [18]. Of the currently available diagnostics for TIC, ROTEM® and TEG® have the greatest potential for obtaining an early diagnosis, predicting the need for massive transfusion and in their ability to visualise clot dynamics including fibrinolysis. However, their uptake and widespread use in trauma management worldwide has been limited due to their cost and the requirement to train personnel to perform the test competently and then interpret the results appropriately.

Clinical scoring systems

Clinical scoring systems can be used in the absence of TEG® or ROTEM® as an alternate method to identify patients with TIC and predict massive blood transfusion requirements. The Coagulopathy of Severe Trauma (COAST) score is the only score that has been developed to predict TIC. It uses five variables based upon pre-hospital observations and results in a score out of 7. It can be performed early in a patient's clinical course, with a score of ≥3 able to predict TIC with a specificity of 96.4% and a sensitivity of 60% [19]. Although specific for diagnosing TIC, the sensitivity of the COAST score is less than ROTEM® (CA5 ≤35mm) which by comparison has a specificity of 87% and sensitivity of 77% [18].

There have been several different scoring systems developed to predict the need for massive transfusion following traumatic injury. The Trauma-Associated Severe Haemorrhage (TASH) score, the Assessment of Blood Consumption (ABC) score and the McLaughlin score are three examples of scoring systems which use a variety of clinical and laboratory variables in addition to injury characteristics to predict the probability of massive transfusion.

Scoring systems for diagnosing TIC and predicting massive transfusion are not widely used in clinical practice. The poor sensitivity of the COAST score compared to ROTEM® limits its usefulness in the diagnosis of TIC. Incorporating scoring systems into major haemorrhage protocols remains difficult. An inherent limitation is that scoring systems are restricted by their static nature. They use one-off values and are therefore limited in their ability to guide trauma care which by contrast is often a dynamic rapidly evolving clinical situation.

Surrogate markers of TIC

Hypoperfusion is closely linked to TIC. An arterial blood gas (ABG) is typically the first blood result available in the management of trauma patients. ATC is driven by systemic hypoperfusion which can be identified by an elevated BD or lactate. In the absence of all other diagnostic tools, clinicians should anticipate TIC in those with major injuries and evidence of shock. An ABG could be used alone or in combination with the COAST score to increase the likelihood of diagnosing TIC.

Conclusions

TIC results from a combination of early endogenous ATC, compounded by haemodilution, loss of coagulation factors through bleeding, hypothermia and acidosis. ATC is driven by tissue injury in combination with systemic hypoperfusion. Activation of the protein C pathway is a key mechanism in the pathophysiology with resultant systemic anticoagulation and hyperfibrinolysis. The mechanism of fibrinogen depletion and the role of the endothelium in ATC have yet to be fully explored.

TIC has a mortality approaching 50% and is highly predictive of massive blood transfusion. Early diagnosis of coagulopathy could improve the accuracy of detecting those patients who are bleeding and require haemostatic resuscitation. Better means of detecting TIC could allow for targeted individualised resuscitation which may improve patient outcomes and avoid unnecessary and costly waste of blood products. In an attempt to achieve these improvements and reduce the number of preventable deaths from uncontrolled haemorrhage, ongoing research within this field is essential in order to advance our understanding of the mechanisms underpinning TIC.

Checklist summary

✓ Trauma-induced coagulopathy (TIC) is associated with increased blood product transfusion requirements and a significantly increased mortality.

✓ TIC is a combination of early endogenous acute traumatic coagulopathy (ATC) compounded by iatrogenic dilution, hypothermia and acidosis.

✓ ATC is driven by systemic hypoperfusion and major tissue injury.

✓ The key mechanism of ATC is protein C activation leading to systemic anticoagulation and hyperfibrinolysis.

✓ Fibrinogen depletion is a hallmark of TIC.

✓ ROTEM® and TEG® are superior to laboratory coagulation tests in diagnosing TIC in a clinically relevant timeframe.

References

1. Mathers CD, Loncar D. Projections of global mortality and burden of disease from 2002 to 2030. *PLoS Med* 2006; 3: e442.

2. Kauvar DS, Lefering R, Wade CE. Impact of hemorrhage on trauma outcome: an overview of epidemiology, clinical presentations, and therapeutic considerations. *J Trauma* 2006; 60(6 Suppl): S3-11.

3. Davis JS, Satahoo SS, Butler FK, *et al*. An analysis of prehospital deaths: who can we save? *J Trauma Acute Care Surg* 2014; 77: 213-8.

4. Scott R, Crosby WH. Changes in the coagulation mechanism following wounding and resuscitation with stored blood; a study of battle casualties in Korea. *Blood* 1954; 9: 609-21.

5. Brohi K, Singh J, Heron M, *et al*. Acute traumatic coagulopathy. *J Trauma* 2003; 54: 1127-30.

6. Brohi K, Cohen M, Ganter M, *et al*. Acute coagulopathy of trauma: hypoperfusion induces systemic anticoagulation and hyperfibrinolysis. *J Trauma* 2008; 64: 1211-7.

7. Brohi K, Cohen M, Davenport R. Acute coagulopathy of trauma: mechanism, identification and effect. *Curr Opin Crit Care* 2007; 13: 680-5.

8. Hoffman M, Monroe DM 3rd. A cell-based model of hemostasis. *Thromb Haemost* 2001; 85: 958-65.

9. Brohi K, Cohen M, Ganter M, *et al*. Acute traumatic coagulopathy: initiated by hypoperfusion: modulated through the protein C pathway? *Ann Surg* 2007; 245: 812-8.

10. Raza I, Davenport R, Rourke C, *et al*. The incidence and magnitude of fibrinolytic activation in trauma patients. *J Thromb Haemost* 2013; 11: 307-14.

11. Kutcher ME, Cripps MW, McCreery RC, *et al*. Criteria for empiric treatment of hyperfibrinolysis after trauma. *J Trauma Acute Care Surg* 2012; 73: 87-93.

12. Rourke C, Curry N, Khan S, *et al*. Fibrinogen levels during trauma hemorrhage, response to replacement therapy, and association with patient outcomes. *J Thromb Haemost* 2012; 10: 1342-51.

13. Johansson PI, Stensballe J, Rasmussen LS, *et al*. A high admission syndecan-1 level, a marker of endothelial glycocalyx degradation, is associated with inflammation, protein C depletion, fibrinolysis, and increased mortality in trauma patients. *Ann Surg* 2011; 254: 194-200.

14. Hess JR, Lindell AL, Stansbury LG, *et al*. The prevalence of abnormal results of conventional coagulation tests on admission to a trauma center. *Transfusion* 2009; 49: 34-9.

15. Solomon C, Traintinger S, Ziegler B, *et al.* Platelet function following trauma. A multiple electrode aggregometry study. *Thromb Haemost* 2011; 106: 322-30.

16. Wohlauer MV, Moore EE, Thomas S, *et al.* Early platelet dysfunction: an unrecognized role in the acute coagulopathy of trauma. *J Am Coll Surg* 2012; 214: 739-46.

17. Frith D, Goslings JC, Gaarder C, *et al.* Definition and drivers of acute traumatic coagulopathy: clinical and experimental investigations. *J Thromb Haemost* 2010; 8: 1919-25.

18. Davenport R, Manson J, De Ath H, *et al.* Functional definition and characterization of acute traumatic coagulopathy. *Crit Care Med* 2011; 39: 2652-8.

19. Mitra B, Cameron PA, Mori A, *et al.* Early prediction of acute traumatic coagulopathy. *Resuscitation* 2011; 82: 1208-13.

Chapter 22

Massive haemorrhage

Jane Graham MBChB MRCP FRCPath PGCMedEd
Haematology Specialty Trainee Doctor (ST7), NHS Blood and Transplant/Central Manchester University Hospitals NHS Foundation Trust, Manchester, UK
Kate Pendry MBChB FRCP FRCPath
Consultant Haematologist, NHS Blood and Transplant/Central Manchester University Hospitals NHS Foundation Trust, Manchester, UK

- "Efficient communication is paramount for effective management and good outcomes."[1]

- "Hospitals must have a major haemorrhage protocol in place and this should include clinical, laboratory and logistic responses."[2]

- "Tranexamic acid safely reduces the risk of death in bleeding trauma patients."[3]

- "Local protocols should... enable the issue of blood and blood components without the approval of a haematologist, as this may result in delays in its provision."[1]

Background

The past 10 years have seen significant changes to the way we manage massive blood loss, with a move towards pre-emptive treatment rather than reliance on laboratory parameters. Analysis of the UK's haemovigilance system (Serious Hazards of Transfusion [SHOT]) and National Reporting and Learning System have identified cases where delays in provision of blood/blood components have negatively impacted on patient outcome. These problems may have arisen as a result of poor knowledge, experience, judgement and especially poor communication [1]. The latter is a particular problem in massive haemorrhage due to difficulties in diagnosis, particularly when bleeding is occult or difficult to quantify. Definitions of massive haemorrhage vary across the literature but are generally agreed to be transfusion of 1 blood volume (70ml/kg) within 24 hours or 50% within 3 hours, transfusion of 10 units of packed red cells over 24 hours or acute blood loss of 150ml/minute. Pragmatically in the clinical setting, massive haemorrhage can be clinically diagnosed as bleeding which results in a systolic blood pressure of <90mmHg or a pulse rate >110bpm.

Retrospective studies of the management of massive haemorrhage, mainly in the trauma setting, have identified the importance of early plasma use [4]. There is a move towards 1:1 red-cell:plasma ratios to better mirror the natural constituents of blood and the concept of massive haemorrhage packs or 'shock packs' reflect this change in practice, particularly in the management of trauma haemorrhage. With coagulopathy an increasingly recognised problem, the importance of tranexamic acid administration in the trauma setting is now firmly established [3]. Point-of-care testing of the coagulation system to provide real-time laboratory data is being increasingly used in the setting of massive haemorrhage, although the evidence for this, and the use of coagulation factor concentrates rather than blood components, are awaited.

Successful management of massive haemorrhage requires a protocol-driven multidisciplinary approach to patient care and blood component support [1]. Implementing a massive haemorrhage toolkit enables healthcare providers to put evidence into practice when managing patients with massive bleeding. The evidence-based algorithms reflect the international guidelines available [2, 5, 6] and are designed to be tailored to local requirements and clinical situations. Providing an algorithm-driven approach to massive haemorrhage management ensures the rapid delivery of blood components to the patient without over-reliance on laboratory testing or repeated communication. It provides clear lines of communication with the laboratory and key specialties, e.g. surgery, endoscopy.

The use of a massive haemorrhage protocol (MHP) may, however, be associated with increased blood component wastage, especially when the protocol is triggered inappropriately. The recommendations are based on limited evidence (levels III and IV), so the protocol results in increased exposure to blood components with the associated risks of acute transfusion reactions and may result in depletion of platelet and plasma stocks. The balance between the pros and cons of this approach to the management of massive haemorrhage means that ongoing review of the management, and emerging evidence, are both integral to successful implementation of this toolkit into clinical practice.

Evidence

The management of massive haemorrhage can be divided into three distinct areas: recognition, assessment and resuscitation; control of bleeding; and haemostatic/transfusion support. This chapter focuses on the latter; however, a holistic multidisciplinary approach to massive haemorrhage is required for successful management.

Red cell transfusion

The transfusion of packed red cells restores the oxygen-carrying capacity of the blood and enhances functioning of the coagulation system. During massive haemorrhage, however, the haemoglobin concentration (Hb) and haemocrit are unreliable. A pragmatic approach to red cell transfusion must therefore be taken to reflect the degree of blood loss, tissue oxygenation and haemodynamic instability. Transfusion rates may be rapid (<10 minutes), although transfusions should be given through a blood warmer to prevent hypothermia and acquired coagulopathy. In patients with acute but not massive upper gastrointestinal bleeding, a more restrictive approach should be taken to reduce the risk of rebleeding [7]. Once the patient has stabilised and blood loss is under control, there is increasing evidence that a restrictive policy for transfusion is best, aiming for a Hb of 70-80g/L [8].

If the urgency of the situation is such that there is no time to wait for the result of blood grouping and antibody screening, emergency Group O RhD negative blood should be given to all females under 50 years of age; this should also be Kell negative. To conserve blood stocks, group O RhD positive blood may be given to adult males and women beyond child-bearing age. Blood should be administered only after a cross-match sample has been taken and it is essential to ensure that minimum patient identifiers are adhered to even in the emergency setting. Group-specific blood should be made available as early as possible to conserve group O blood stocks, remembering that two separate samples are often required by the laboratory to confirm a patient's blood group [9]. It is important for the laboratory to specify the time required to supply group-specific and cross-matched blood, to aid the team leader in deciding how many group O units are required.

Cell salvage is a recognised method to minimise allogeneic transfusion in massive haemorrhage, particularly in trauma, cardiac, vascular and obstetric surgery [2]. One allogeneic red cell unit is equivalent to 250ml washed salvaged red cells.

Coagulopathy

Massive haemorrhage is commonly associated with coagulopathy. This occurs due to consumption of clotting factors, endothelial damage, fibrinolysis, and the dilutional effects of IV fluids; 25% of patients presenting with traumatic haemorrhage will be coagulopathic on presentation [10]. Fibrinogen levels typically fall first, reaching sub-haemostatic levels (<1.5g/L) after the replacement of 1-1.5 blood volumes. Coagulopathy is worsened by hypothermia, acidosis and hypocalcaemia — which should all be monitored for and actively prevented/treated. Those patients with massive haemorrhage receiving anticoagulant or antiplatelet drugs must be established early, so specific action, e.g. administration of reversal agents, can be taken as appropriate.

Laboratory assessment of the coagulation system is performed by the prothrombin time (PT) and activated partial thromboplastin time (APTT), which assess the extrinsic, intrinsic and common pathways of the coagulation system *in vitro*. Assessment of fibrinogen levels should be through Clauss fibrinogen assays, as PT-derived fibrinogen levels may be falsely elevated, e.g. in liver and renal disease, disseminated intravascular coagulation (DIC) and those receiving anticoagulants [11]. These coagulation tests have a relatively long turnaround time so are less useful in the setting of acute massive haemorrhage, with reliance on these tests historically leading to delays in the administration of blood components. The tests are, however, useful to guide haemostatic blood component usage once management has been initiated and should be repeated every 30-60 minutes depending on the clinical situation.

Assessment of clotting time, clot strength and fibrinolysis is possible using viscoelastometric assays, e.g. thromboelastography® (TEG®) and rotational thromboelastometry (ROTEM®). This technology is becoming increasingly commonplace as it has the benefit of providing 'real-time' data; however, limited evidence shows its use may reduce blood component usage but does not improve morbidity or mortality [12]. Outside cardiac surgery there is currently little evidence to support its use in either monitoring or managing haemostasis apart from in the context of clinical trials[13].

Haemostatic blood component transfusion

There has been a move towards the administration of fresh frozen plasma (FFP) upfront in massive haemorrhage to prevent the onset of coagulopathy and improve outcome. The concept of a 1:1 red cell:plasma ratio stems from military research [4], although the influence of survival bias and differing patient populations has brought into question the applicability of this approach to civilian practice, particularly beyond trauma. Whilst the PROPPR trial (NCT01545232) in North America is addressing the issue in civilian trauma, current recommendations in massive haemorrhage are to take baseline clotting tests and administer FFP 12-15ml/kg (4-6 units for an adult), before clotting test results are known. Further FFP administration should be guided by the clinical picture and laboratory tests, to keep PT/APTT ratios >1.5. Where fibrinogen levels are known to be low, alternative fibrinogen sources of replacement should take priority over FFP. There is no evidence to support prothrombin complex concentrate (PCC) usage in massive haemorrhage unless as part of a clinical trial or the patient is receiving a vitamin K antagonist.

Within the UK, cryoprecipitate has historically been used as a source of fibrinogen in bleeding associated with hypofibrinogenaemia. Cryoprecipitate is made by thawing UK donor FFP at 4°C to produce a cryoglobulin rich in fibrinogen, factor VIII and von Willebrand factor, with two pools of 5 units typically raising the fibrinogen level by 1g/L. There is, however, an increasing interest in the use of fibrinogen concentrate to replace cryoprecipitate usage, although at present this therapy is only licensed for UK use in congenital hypofibrinogenaemia. The potential benefits of fibrinogen concentrate over cryoprecipitate are: a shorter duration to obtain the product (15 minutes vs. 40 minutes), a shorter administration time and exact known fibrinogen content. In comparison to cryoprecipitate, fibrinogen concentrate is also virally inactivated although it must be noted that donor exposure with fibrinogen concentrate is 1000+ rather than 10, which may prove to be a problem if new emergent pathogens are resistant to the viral inactivation process [14]. Clinical trials assessing the effectiveness of fibrinogen concentrate and correct dosing in massive haemorrhage are required.

The role for platelet transfusions is established where there is a known platelet defect, e.g. those patients receiving antiplatelet drugs or following cardiopulmonary bypass surgery. One adult therapeutic dose (ATD) of platelets is expected to raise the platelet count by 20-40 x 10^9/L. Within massive haemorrhage, the role of platelet transfusions is to maintain a platelet count above 50 x 10^9/L and a fall to this level can be expected when 1.5-2.5 blood volumes have been replaced. It is therefore recommended that 1 ATD of platelets be administered when the platelet count has fallen <75 x 10^9/L, to achieve the target of >50 x 10^9/L. Time delays in the acquisition of platelets in some hospitals may mean that platelets should be ordered early within the MHP.

Pharmacological treatments

The role of the antifibrinolytic drug, tranexamic acid, is firmly established in massive haemorrhage associated with trauma. Results of the international randomised placebo-controlled CRASH-2 trial demonstrated it safely reduced all-cause mortality and death due to bleeding in trauma patients with, or at risk of, bleeding when administered within 8 hours (ideally 3 hours) of injury [3]. Tranexamic acid should therefore be administered to all trauma patients as soon as possible after injury at a dose of 1g intravenously over 10 minutes followed by 1g intravenously over 8 hours. It should be considered in non-traumatic causes of massive haemorrhage as evidence suggests it is most probably beneficial, although patients with gastrointestinal bleeding should only be given tranexamic acid in the context of a trial (HALT-IT). Tranexamic acid should be used with caution in patients with active thromboembolic disease and/or a history of convulsions. The antifibrinolytic, aprotinin, is not recommended due to safety concerns [15].

Recombinant activated factor VIIa (rFVIIa) has historically been used as a 'last-ditch' therapy in cases of massive haemorrhage. Increasingly, the evidence shows that the drug is associated with harm and no real benefit. There is a significant increase in arterial thrombosis associated with use of rFVIIa, especially with increasing age [16]. There is no role for this drug outside of its licensed indications, which include the management of acquired haemophilia and congenital haemophilia with inhibitors.

After treatment of massive haemorrhage and haemostasis has been achieved, it is important to ensure appropriate thromboprophylaxis is prescribed and given. Trauma, surgery and bleeding per se are all associated with an increased venous thromboembolism (VTE) risk.

Specific considerations

Obstetrics

Within obstetric practice there is a major role for uterotonic drugs and obstetric intervention in the case of massive haemorrhage associated with postpartum haemorrhage (PPH). Advanced pregnancy is associated with increased fibrinogen and clotting factor levels, and normal values for viscoelastometric assays in pregnancy have now been established which reflect this physiological difference. With the exception of placental abruption, most cases of PPH are associated with normal coagulation despite significant blood loss and a Clauss fibrinogen level <3g/L taken in the early stages of PPH, reflects the risk of progressing to severe PPH, especially when <2g/L [17]. This measurement, and most probably the results of viscoelastometric assays, is helpful in guiding fibrinogen replacement therapy during PPH, although results from ongoing randomised studies exploring the role of viscoelastometric assays and fibrinogen concentrate usage are awaited. There is preliminary evidence for the use of tranexamic acid in PPH [18], although more definitive evidence will come from the double-blind randomised study of tranexamic acid versus placebo in this context (the WOMAN study).

Paediatrics

Definitions of massive haemorrhage can be summarised as 40ml/kg blood loss in 3 hours or 2-3ml/kg/min, which reflects the increased blood volume of children. A specific policy should be in place which takes into account appropriate age-specific reference ranges for laboratory tests, blood volumes for transfusion and special requirements, e.g. non-UK sourced, methylene blue/solvent detergent treated FFP/cryoprecipitate in those born after 1996.

Haematology

Those patients with known congenital bleeding disorders who present with massive haemorrhage should be discussed with a tertiary haematology provider. Hospital protocols should be in place for the reversal of anticoagulants in those patients presenting with bleeding. Cases should be discussed with a clinical haematologist where necessary.

Research

The strength of recommendations will change with the outcome of current and future research into the field of massive haemorrhage management. In particular, they include the optimal ratios of red-cells:plasma, use of tranexamic acid in non-trauma settings, the role of fibrinogen concentrate and impact of near-patient viscoelastometric testing.

How to do it

Make it work for you

The massive haemorrhage protocol (MHP) or toolkit is designed to be adapted to meet the clinical situation and local environment. Example MHP templates are provided in Figures 1 and 2. Separate MHPs are required for trauma, obstetrics, paediatrics, surgery (consider general/vascular and cardiac) and medicine (which most commonly presents as gastrointestinal bleeding). Ensure you formulate which team members are required for each clinical situation where massive haemorrhage may arise and provide contact details on the appropriate MHP. Implementation of a MHP requires buy-in from all those involved. It is vital to get laboratory staff, clinicians and other relevant parties, e.g. porters, involved in its implementation from the outset to ensure it works for all.

The MHP provides guidance on the best transfusion practice in addition to providing reference to appropriate resuscitation measures and methods to stop the bleeding. It is essential to ensure that the appropriate support services and resources are available to ensure this is possible, e.g. surgery, endoscopy and interventional radiology. The role of near-patient testing is likely to become increasingly popular in certain situations, e.g. obstetrics, trauma, cardiac surgery. The MHP should specify the availability of any near-patient testing in each clinical setting. The interpretation and actions to be taken when using near-patient testing need to be clearly outlined and should be evidence-based.

Transfusion management of massive haemorrhage in adults

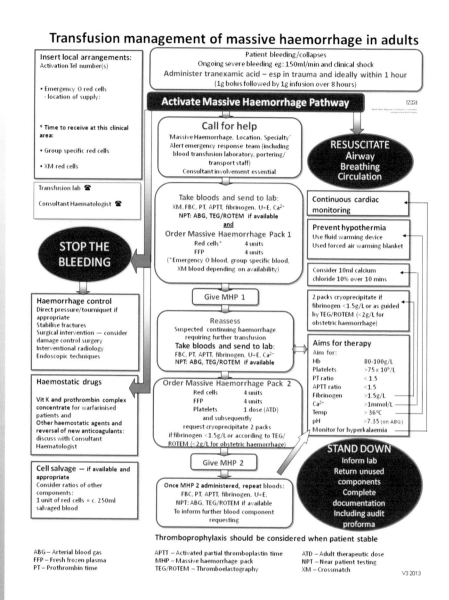

Figure 1. Flow chart outlining the management of massive haemorrhage in adults taken from the North West Regional Transfusion Committee (RTC) [19]. *Reproduced with permission from the North West Regional Transfusion Committee.*

Massive haemorrhage recognition and protocol activation

Failure to activate the MHP is a common problem and may result in suboptimal patient care and increased mortality. Inappropriate activation of the MHP may result in component wastage and potentially unnecessary exposure to additional blood components. It is therefore essential to provide clear guidance on how to recognise massive haemorrhage and trigger the MHP. These skills should be taught and assessed on a regular basis in all clinical areas and should involve the use of simulation training.

Clinical audit should be a routine part of the MHP each time it is triggered. Audit should also take place each time the MHP should have been triggered but was not. A robust system to identify these situations, e.g. through laboratory records or clinical incident reporting, should be specified in each pathway. Regular audit provides evidence to hospital transfusion committees and clinical users on the effectiveness and appropriateness of the MHP strategy and enables evidence-based modifications to be adopted to improve effectiveness and efficiency.

Effective communication

On activation of the MHP there should be rapid allocation of the four key team roles to ensure effective application of the pathway: the 'team leader', 'communication lead', 'runner' and 'scribe'. The team leader is often the most senior member of staff and is responsible for coordinating clinical care at the patient's bedside. They are responsible for deciding on the use of emergency group O red cells for immediate use and the subsequent use of group-specific or cross-matched blood. It is therefore necessary for the MHP to indicate the location of the nearest emergency group O red cells. The team leader is responsible for deciding on the use of additional blood components and haemostatic medications. They should allocate the other MHP roles to designated individuals.

The communication lead is the named individual solely responsible for liaising between the team leader/clinical setting and the laboratory and

Recognise blood loss and trigger major blood loss protocol

↓

Take baseline blood samples before transfusion for:
- Full blood count, group and save, clotting screen including Clauss fibrinogen
- Near-patient haemostasis testing if available

↓

If trauma and <3h from injury, give tranexamic acid 1 g bolus over 10 minutes followed by IV infusion of 1 g over 8h (consider tranexamic acid 1 g bolus in non-traumatic)

↓

Team leader to coordinate management and nominate a member of team to liaise with transfusion laboratory
- State patient unique identifier and location when requesting components
- To limit use of Group O NEG: until patient group known, use O NEG units in females and consider O POS in males
- Use group-specific blood as soon as available
- Request agreed ratio of blood components (e.g. 6 units RBS and 4 units FFP). Send porter to lab to collect urgently

↓

If bleeding continues

Until lab results are available:
- Give further FFP 1L (4 units) per 6 units red cells
- Consider cryoprecipitate (2 pools)
- Consider platelets (1 adult therapeutic dose (ATD))

If lab results are available:

IF	GIVE
Falling Hb	Red cells
PT ratio >1.5	FFP 15–20 mL/kg
Fibrinogen <1.5 g/L	Cryoprecipitate (2 pools)
Platelets <75×10^9/L	Platelets 1 ATD

↓

Continue cycle of clinical and laboratory monitoring and administration of 'goal-directed' blood component therapy until bleeding stops

Figure 2. Example of a major haemorrhage protocol [20]. *Reproduced with permission from Hunt B, Allard S, Keeling D, et al, of the forthcoming British Committee for Standards in Haematology (BCSH) major haemorrhage guidelines, as published in the Handbook of Transfusion Medicine, 5th ed, 2013 (TSO).*

other support services. Communication with the laboratory should follow a set format that facilitates timely and efficient provision of blood components. Specifically the communication lead should indicate:

- Their name, location and extension number.
- 'This relates to the massive haemorrhage situation'.
- The patient's demographics: surname, forename, unique patient number, date of birth (as tailored to local policies and guidelines).
- Whether group O red cells have been used and the quantity. Whether group-specific or cross-matched red cells will be required.
- Order massive haemorrhage pack(s) as per the MHP and agreed with the team leader — or order specific blood components according to the patient situation.
- Inform the laboratory if blood has been transferred from another hospital or the patient is being transferred.
- Communicate to the laboratory when there is pathway stand down and indicate which components have been used.

The communication lead is responsible for receiving calls from the laboratory indicating the results of urgent investigations and informing when blood components are available for collection. The communication lead is required to communicate with support services, e.g. porters and radiology/endoscopy/theatres, to ensure timely provision of blood products and a coordinated approach to the patient's overall care. They should be a relatively senior member of the team.

The MHP requires a designated 'runner' whose only responsibility is delivering samples to the lab and collecting blood components. This may be a specified porter or a designated member of staff from the clinical area. The runner must have been competency-assessed to collect blood components.

The fourth key member of the team is the 'scribe'. They are responsible for taking blood samples, organising investigations and overall documentation. It is essential that positive patient identification is maintained as a top priority during MHP activation to avoid delays and/or errors in blood provision. The MHP should state which blood tests are required (FBC, cross-match, U&Es, PT/APTT/Clauss fibrinogen, calcium, lactate, ABGs) and specify rules concerning labelling/requesting and minimum patient identification. Documentation in the patient's notes should include clinical events and decisions, vital signs, timings of blood samples taken and blood component administration, in addition to key communications. It is also essential to ensure traceability forms have been completed for all blood components administered. This role should be designated to an appropriate member of staff to ensure compliance with legal requirements (*Blood Safety and Quality Regulations No. 50, 2005*).

Conclusions

Successful recognition and management of massive haemorrhage requires a holistic multidisciplinary approach tailored to the clinical situation. The use of a massive haemorrhage protocol (MHP) or toolkit enables timely provision of blood components, improved communication and global adherence to recommended best practice. Current research into the role of tranexamic acid, fibrinogen concentrate, red cell: plasma ratios and near-point testing in massive haemorrhage ensures evidence-based practice in this field will continue to evolve in the foreseeable future.

Checklist summary

✓ Introduce simulation training for all staff involved in triggering and delivering the massive haemorrhage protocol (MHP).

✓ Ensure an audit system is in place to assess MHP activation, non-activation and blood component wastage to optimise effective use of the toolkit.

✓ Early intervention (endoscopy, surgery, radiology) is essential to stop bleeding so ensure pathways are in place to access these services at all times.

✓ Tailor MHPs to individual clinical departments and laboratories whilst maintaining evidence-based practice.

✓ Allocate four key team roles during each MHP activation (team leader, communication lead, runner and scribe) — to ensure effective communication, action and documentation by the whole team throughout.

References

1. National Patient Safety Agency. The transfusion of blood and blood components in an emergency. Rapid Response Report NPSA/2010/017, 2010.

2. Association of Anaesthetists of Great Britain and Ireland. Blood transfusion and the anaesthetist: management of massive haemorrhage. *Anaesthesia* 2010; 65: 1153-61.

3. CRASH-2 trial collaborators. Effects of tranexamic acid on death, vascular occlusive events, and blood transfusion in trauma patients with significant haemorrhage (CRASH-2): a randomised, placebo-controlled trial. *Lancet* 2010; 376(9734): 23-32.

4. Stansbury LG, Dutton RP, Stein DM, *et al*. Controversy in trauma resuscitation: do rations of plasma to red bleed cells matter? *Transfus Med Rev* 2009; 23(4): 255-65.

5. Spahn DR, Bouillon B, Cerny V, *et al*. Management of bleeding and coagulopathy following major trauma: an updated European guideline. *Crit Care* 2013; 17(2): R76.

6. National Health and Medical Research Council (NHMRC). Patient blood management guideline: module 1 - Critical bleeding/massive transfusion. National Blood Authority, 2011.

7. Villanueva C, Colomo A, Bosch A, *et al*. Transfusion strategies for acute upper gastrointestinal bleeding. *N Engl J Med* 2013; 368(1): 11-21.

8. Carson JL, Carless PA, Hebert PC. Transfusion thresholds and other strategies for guiding allogeneic red blood cell transfusion. *Cochrane Database Syst Rev* 2012; 4: CD002042.

9. Milkins C, Berryman J, Cantwell C, *et al*. British Committee for Standards in Haematology. Guidelines for pre-transfusion compatibility procedures in blood transfusion laboratories. *Transfus Med* 2013; 23(1): 3-35.

10. Brohi K, Singh J, Heron M, *et al*. Acute traumatic coagulopathy. *J Trauma* 2003; 54(6): 1127-30.

11. Mackie IJ, Kitchen S, Machin SJ, *et al*. Haemostasis and Thrombosis Task Force of the British Committee for Standards in Haematology. Guidelines on fibrinogen assays. *Br J Haematol* 2003; 121(3): 396-404.

12. Afshari A, Wikkelsø A, Brok J, *et al*. Thrombelastography (TEG) or thromboelastometry (ROTEM) to monitor haemotherapy versus usual care in patients with massive transfusion. *Cochrane Database Syst Rev* 2011; 3: CD007871.

13. National Institute for Health and Care Excellence (NICE). Detecting, managing and monitoring haemostasis: viscoelastometric point-of-care testing (ROTEM, TEG and Sonoclot systems). London, UK: NICE diagnostics guidance, 2014.

14. Pereira A. Cryoprecipitate versus commercial fibrinogen concentrate in patients who occasionally require a therapeutic supply of fibrinogen: risk comparison in the case of an emerging transfusion-transmitted infection. *Haematologica* 2007; 92(6): 846-9.

15. Hutton B, Joseph L, Fergusson D, *et al.* Risks of harms using antifibrinolytics in cardiac surgery: systematic review and network meta-analysis of randomised and observational studies. *Br Med J* 2012; 345: e5798.

16. Levi M, Levy JH, Andersen HF, *et al.* Safety of recombinant activated factor VII in randomized clincal trials. *N Engl J Med* 2010; 363(19): 1791-800.

17. Collis RE, Collins PW. Haemostatic management of obstetric haemorrhage. *Anaesthesia* 2015; 70 (Suppl.1): 78-86.

18. Ducloy-Bouthors AS, Jude B, Duhamel A, *et al*; EXADELI Study Group. High-dose tranexamic acid reduces blood loss in postpartum haemorrhage. *Crit Care* 2011; 15(2): R117.

19. North West Regional Transfusion Committee. Flow chart outlining management of massive haemorrhage in adults taken, 2013. http://www. transfusionguidelines.org.uk/ uk-transfusion-committees/regional-transfusion-committees/north-west/policies/ massive-haemorrhage-toolkit.

20. Norfolk D, Ed. *Handbook of Transfusion Medicine*, 5th ed. Norwich, UK: TSO, 2013. transfusionguidelines.org.uk.

Chapter 23

Thromboelastography and thromboelastometry

Alastair F. Nimmo MB ChB FRCA
Consultant Anaesthetist, Royal Infirmary of Edinburgh, Edinburgh, UK

- "The delay between taking a blood sample and laboratory haematology test results being available may render the results irrelevant or misleading in patients with severe haemorrhage or shock."

- "Thromboelastography/thromboelastometry analysers enable rapid point-of-care diagnosis of the abnormalities of coagulation that occur as a result of surgery or trauma or in obstetric haemorrhage."

- "When the surgeon complained that 'everything is bleeding' we used to order and give FFP and platelets routinely. Now we can quickly see what the problem is and target the treatment at that."
Anaesthetist after starting to use thromboelastography/thromboelastometry during major surgery.

- "Like night and day."
Operating Department Practitioner in Edinburgh describing the change in management of bleeding patients during thoracoabdominal aortic aneurysm

Background

In bleeding surgical, obstetric and trauma patients, coagulation may be impaired and result in further bleeding. Traditionally, the results of laboratory blood count and coagulation tests have been used to determine whether treatment is required to improve the patient's ability to form blood clot and to decide what treatment should be given. However, if there is heavy bleeding or shock the situation may change rapidly so that by the time laboratory results are available they are no longer relevant. For example, the laboratory results from a sample taken 60 minutes earlier may show an acceptable fibrinogen concentration and platelet count but in the meantime continued heavy bleeding and fluid replacement may have resulted in critically low values. Therefore, refusing to issue blood components for transfusion on the grounds that laboratory results suggest no treatment is required can be inappropriate and dangerous. On the other hand, treatment may have been given in the time between sending a sample to the laboratory and receiving the results, so that the laboratory reports an abnormality that is no longer present and further blood component transfusions are recommended that are not in fact required.

Point-of-care (POC) testing can provide more rapid results and potentially enable more appropriate treatment of impaired haemostasis in bleeding patients. Many clinicians have adopted this technique in recent years and consider that it enables them to diagnose and treat impaired coagulation more rapidly and effectively while avoiding inappropriate over-transfusion of blood components. However, the use of analysers outside the laboratory by clinical staff poses challenges in ensuring that that there is adequate training and quality control so that the results obtained from POC tests are reliable.

Types of POC haemostasis analyser and their main roles (Table 1)

The laboratory tests, prothrombin time (PT) and activated partial thromboplastin time (APTT), measure how long it takes for clot to be detected after the addition of an activator of coagulation to plasma. They are used for the monitoring of anticoagulant therapy and as screening

Table 1. Types of POC haemostasis analyser and their main roles.

Portable whole blood coagulation time analysers:

- PT — monitoring of therapy with coumarin anticoagulants such as warfarin; testing of patients presenting for surgery who have been taking warfarin.
- APTT — measurement of the effect of IV unfractionated heparin.
- ACT — measurement of the effect of larger doses of IV unfractionated heparin, e.g. in cardiac surgery.

Whole blood viscoelastic coagulation analysers:

- Thromboelastography (TEG®); thromboelastometry (ROTEM®); Sonoclot®.
- Rapid diagnosis in bleeding surgical, obstetric and trauma patients.

Platelet function analysers:

- Measurement of the effect on platelets of aspirin and $P2Y_{12}$ inhibitor drugs such as clopidogrel.

tests for coagulation factor deficiencies. Small portable analysers enable these tests and the activated clotting time (ACT) to be rapidly performed on a drop of whole blood beside the patient.

The 'viscoelastic' whole blood coagulation analysers measure the physical properties of a whole blood sample as coagulation occurs and produce a graph of clot 'strength' against time. The abnormalities that commonly occur as the result of haemorrhage and shock can be rapidly detected and quantified.

Standard viscoelastic tests do not detect the effect of antiplatelet drugs such as aspirin and clopidogrel on platelets. However, additional tests of platelet function may be performed for this purpose using either a specific POC platelet function analyser, or the TEG® analyser (PlateletMapping® assay) or an additional module for the ROTEM® analyser (ROTEM® platelet module).

In the remainder of this chapter I will consider the role of the standard viscoelastic thromboelastography/thromboelastometry tests in guiding the management of bleeding patients. Two analysers, TEG® and ROTEM®, are available. The manufacturer of the TEG® analyser (Haemonetics, Braintree, Massachusetts, USA) uses the term thromboelastography and that of the ROTEM® analyser (TEM International, Munich, Germany) uses thromboelastometry, but for convenience I will use the abbreviation "TE" here to refer to both analysers.

Evidence for the use of thromboelastography/thrombo-elastometry

Many users of TE analysers, including the author, believe that they significantly improve the ability to provide effective treatment to bleeding patients with impaired haemostasis while avoiding inappropriate transfusions of blood components. However, there is relatively little evidence from randomised clinical trials on the benefits of either laboratory or POC tests in bleeding patients. In part this is because studies on the management of severe haemorrhage are difficult to undertake. Cases may be infrequent and unpredictable while management is urgent so that there can be difficulties in having a researcher available and in obtaining patient consent. Perhaps the easiest setting in which to study different methods of management of bleeding patients is that of elective complex cardiac surgery and, therefore, it is not surprising that much of the evidence comes from this area.

There are a number of different strategies that can be employed when faced with a bleeding patient who is suspected to have an impaired ability to form blood clot:

- Blood component transfusions may be given in fixed ratios, e.g. one unit of fresh frozen plasma (FFP) to one unit of red cells.
- Transfusions may be given according to the experience and judgement of the clinician.
- Transfusions may be given according to the results of POC tests.
- Transfusions may be given according to the results of laboratory tests.

In clinical practice, a combination of strategies is often used. For example, when faced with a shocked patient with a ruptured abdominal aortic aneurysm, the anaesthetist might request an "aneurysm pack" from the blood bank which contains a fixed ratio of red cells, FFP and platelet concentrate, begin the transfusions on the basis of experience and judgement, and then continue according to the results of POC tests.

It must be remembered that both laboratory and POC tests are diagnostic tests and not treatments. They cannot in themselves make a patient better. Therefore, it is inevitable that a randomised trial of a strategy including POC tests against an alternative strategy is studying not only the tests themselves but also the way in which the results are used to alter patient management. For example, an algorithm for using the results of TE tests may be designed so as to maintain the plasma fibrinogen concentration around the lowest end of the normal reference range or may be designed to achieve a higher fibrinogen concentration.

A randomised trial in coagulopathic cardiac surgery patients[1] compared management using an algorithm based on the results of POC tests with management using an algorithm based on the results of laboratory tests. POC tests were undertaken with a ROTEM® analyser and a Multiplate® platelet function analyser. The POC test group received fewer blood component transfusions, spent less time in ICU and had a lower 6-month mortality rate. A Health Technology Assessment report on the clinical and cost-effectiveness of thromboelastography/thromboelastometry [2] concluded that "The use of TE is recommended in cardiac and liver transplant surgery. There is no published robust, controlled clinical data to support the use of TE in other major surgery associated with a high blood loss. However,... observational evidence supports using TE in such surgical areas." On the other hand, a NICE diagnostics guidance report [3], while stating that "The ROTEM system and the TEG system are recommended to help detect, manage and monitor haemostasis during and after cardiac surgery", considered that further research was needed into the clinical benefits and cost-effectiveness of using viscoelastic point-of-care testing to help in the emergency control of bleeding after trauma or during postpartum haemorrhage. European guidelines on the management of trauma [4] "recommend that viscoelastic methods also be performed to assist in characterising the coagulopathy and in guiding haemostatic therapy", while UK guidelines on Obstetric Anaesthetic Services [5] state that "It is strongly recommended that there should be equipment to enable bedside estimation of coagulation such as thromboelastography (TEG) or thromboelastometry (ROTEM)."

The author's hospital has used ROTEM® analysers for the past 15 years in the management of patients undergoing major vascular surgery, including repair of thoracoabdominal aortic aneurysms (TAAAs). These cases can be associated with very high blood loss and severe disturbance of coagulation. Regular ROTEM® tests are performed during surgery and used to guide treatment of impaired haemostasis while POC testing of haemoglobin using a blood gas analyser is used to guide red cell transfusion. No laboratory tests are performed until admission to the recovery room or critical care unit after surgery. A retrospective case-note, electronic medical record and laboratory result database review of all elective open TAAA repairs between Jan 1st 2013 and Dec 31st 2014 was undertaken to examine whether this intra-operative management resulted in satisfactory postoperative laboratory results. There were 54 cases and the blood loss in theatre is shown in Figure 1. The surgeons' clinical assessment was that coagulation was satisfactory at the end of surgery in all cases. There was one postoperative bleeding complication — a relaparotomy and splenectomy for bleeding from

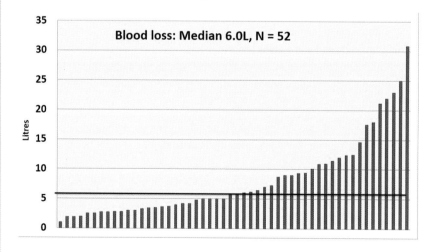

Figure 1. Intra-operative blood loss for each patient who had elective open TAAA repair surgery in 2013 and 2014. (Blood loss data were available for 52 of the 54 cases.) *Figure provided by Dr Euan McGregor.*

a splenic capsular tear. In almost all cases the desired targets for the postoperative laboratory results were achieved (Table 2). It was considered essential to achieve a postoperative fibrinogen concentration over 1g/L and desirable to achieve a postoperative fibrinogen concentration of around 1.5g/L and this was also achieved (Figure 2).

Table 2. Postoperative laboratory results for 54 TAAA operations managed exclusively by POC testing during surgery. The median postoperative haemoglobin was 92g/L (IQR 85-98).

Postoperative lab result target	Achieved in
Hb ≥70g/L	53/54 (98%)
Platelet count ≥50 x 10^9/L	52/54 (96%)
Fibrinogen concentration >1.0g/L	54/54 (100%)
PT ratio to normal of ≤1.5	54/54 (100%)

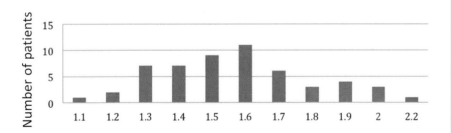

Postoperative fibrinogen concentration g/L

Figure 2. Fibrinogen concentration from the first laboratory result after surgery for the 54 elective open TAAA repair operations performed in 2013 and 2014. *Figure provided by Dr Euan McGregor.*

How do thromboelastometry analysers work?

The original thromboelastograph analyser was described in 1948 by Hartert [6] working in Heidelberg and the principle of operation is shown in Figure 3. Blood is placed in a small cup which is heated to 37°C and slowly rotated backwards and forwards through about 5°. A pin is suspended in the blood sample by a fine wire and is attached to a mirror which deflects a light beam shining onto photographic film moving on a chart recorder. Initially when there is no clot, although the cup rotates, the pin remains stationary and the light produces a straight line on the chart

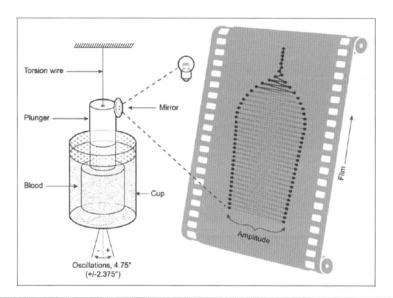

Figure 3. Principle of operation of Hartert's thromboelastograph device — the precursor of the TEG® analyser. The cylindrical container (cup) is rotated through a total angle of 4.75° around the vertical axis. Light from a slit lamp is reflected onto photographic film that moves at a rate of 2mm/min to record rotation of the rod (the film roll is 15m long and 100mm wide). In practice, lines between the dots on the film are not visible because the intensity of the light and photosensitivity of the film are configured so that the film is blackened only when the light is stationary, that is, at the point of maximum rotation of the cup when there is a 1-second pause in the oscillatory movement. *Reproduced from: Hochleitner G, Sutor K, Levett C, et al. Revisiting Hartert's 1962 calculation of the physical constants of thrombelastography. Clin Appl Thromb Hemost 2015; Sep 23 [Epub ahead of print]. © SAGE Publications, Inc., 2015 Reprinted with permission from SAGE Publications, Inc.*

recorder. However, when the blood starts to clot, fibrin strands and platelet aggregates form between the cup and the pin, transmitting some of the cup's movement to the pin which starts to rotate, causing the light beam to move up and down on the paper. Initially, when the clot is weak, the rotation of the pin and deflection of the light beam is slight and the amplitude of the trace on the paper is small. As the clot becomes stronger, the pin rotates more and the amplitude of the trace increases. The trace that is produced has time on the x-axis and clot strength in mm on the y-axis. The modern version of the TEG® analyser uses a mechanical-electrical transducer to detect the movement of the pin rather than a mirror and a computer monitor to display the trace rather than a chart recorder.

The ROTEM® analyser was developed by Calatzis [7] in Munich in the 1990s with the intention of producing an analyser which was less sensitive to movement and vibration. In this analyser it is the pin that rotates while the cup remains stationary (Figure 4). Initially the pin moves freely but as

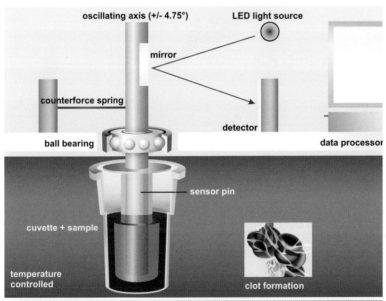

Figure 4. Principle of operation of the ROTEM® analyser. The axis holding the plastic pin is rotated by a spring and as clot forms between the pin and the stationary cup the amount of rotation is reduced. Rotation of the pin is measured by means of light reflected from a mirror on the top of the axis onto a detector. *Reproduced with permission from Tem International GmbH.*

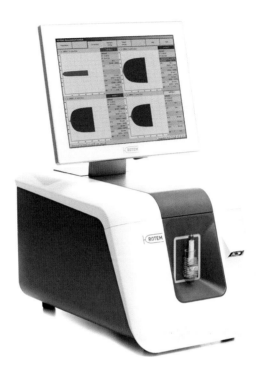

Figure 5. The fully automated ROTEM® *sigma* analyser. Performing the tests simply requires that a standard citrate blood sample tube as used for laboratory coagulation tests is inserted into a disposable cartridge on the front of the analyser. *Reproduced with permission from Tem International GmbH.*

clot forms, the movement of the pin is reduced and, the stronger the clot becomes, the less the pin rotates. A computer converts the rotation of the pin into a curve of clot strength against time similar to that produced by the TEG® analyser.

Until recently, undertaking a TE test has required that plastic pins and cups are carefully positioned in the analyser and a pipette is used to add blood plus or minus reagents to the cups. However, the latest version of the ROTEM® analyser, the ROTEM® *sigma* (Figure 5), is a fully automated thromboelastometry analyser. The cups, pins and reagents are all contained in a disposable cartridge and it is only necessary to insert a blood sample tube into the cartridge to perform the test.

Haemonetics has also developed an automated analyser, the TEG® 6s (Figure 6), in which blood is added to a disposable cartridge. The TEG® 6s does not use the traditional thromboelastography/thromboelastometry method of measuring clot strength and does not have rotating cups or pins. The measurement technique is described by the manufacturer as "the measurement of clot viscoelasticity using the resonance method. To measure the clot strength with the resonance method, the sample is exposed to a fixed vibration frequency. With LED illumination, a detector

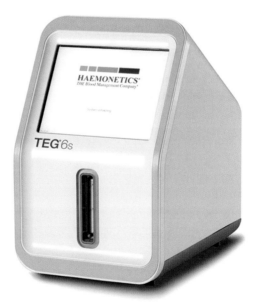

Figure 6. The automated TEG®6s haemostasis analyser. A disposable cartridge is inserted into the analyser and then blood is transferred from a sample tube to the analyser using a syringe or pipette. The analyser uses a "resonance method" rather than a rotating cup or pin. *Reproduced with permission from Haemonetics Corporation.*

measures up/down motion of the blood meniscus. Frequency leading to resonance is identified and then converted to a TEG readout. Stronger clots have higher resonant frequencies and higher TEG readouts." The signal is processed to derive the same type of curve as produced by previous TEG® analysers.

TE analysers may be used with samples of venous or arterial blood. Different tests, involving the addition of different reagents, may be performed simultaneously on a blood sample in order to give additional information.

How to interpret the results

There are three important pieces of information to derive from the thromboelastography/thromboelastometry trace:

- Clot strength — shown by the width or amplitude of the trace.
- Time until clot is first detected — shown by the length of the straight line at the start of the trace.
- Clot stability — whether clot strength is maintained after it reaches a maximum.

The strength of the clot

This is indicated by the maximum width of the trace in mm (known as the maximum clot firmness or MCF in ROTEM® and maximum amplitude or MA in TEG®). A measure of clot strength can be obtained more rapidly by measuring the width of the trace 10 minutes after clot is first detected and in the ROTEM® this is known as the amplitude at 10 minutes or A10 (Figure 7). An even more rapid assessment of clot strength is provided by the width of the trace 5 minutes after clot is first detected (A5).

Clot is composed primarily of platelets and fibrin, and clot strength is reduced by thrombocytopenia or a low fibrinogen concentration or a combination of the two. These abnormalities occur commonly in bleeding surgical, obstetric and trauma patients. However, the effect of drugs such

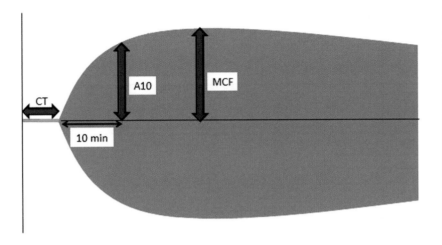

Figure 7. Measurements of clot strength and of the time until clot is first detected on the ROTEM® analyser (see text).

as aspirin or clopidogrel is not seen on standard thromboelastometry tests because the thrombin that forms when blood clots is a very powerful stimulus to platelet aggregation. Tests for the effect of these drugs on platelet function have to be performed on anticoagulated samples in which the production of thrombin is prevented.

In order to distinguish between a reduction in clot strength resulting from thrombocytopenia and that resulting from a low fibrinogen concentration (or impaired fibrin polymerisation), an additional test is performed in which a reagent is added to prevent platelet aggregation (ROTEM® FIBTEM test; TEG® functional fibrinogen test). The resulting clot consists predominantly of fibrin with relatively few platelets and has a reduced amplitude compared to a test in which the clot consists of both fibrin and platelets such as the EXTEM test (Figure 8).

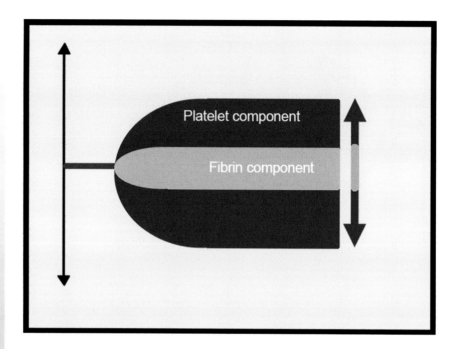

Figure 8. The amplitude of a TE trace may be regarded as having a platelet component and a fibrin component. When a test is performed that includes a reagent to prevent platelet aggregation, the resulting clot is composed primarily of fibrin and has a reduced amplitude (ROTEM® FIBTEM test/TEG® functional fibrinogen test).

Comparison of the fibrin clot strength with that of the platelet plus fibrin clot enables a diagnosis of the cause of reduced clot strength to be made. For example, Figure 9 shows the diagnostic algorithm used by the author for surgical, obstetric and trauma patients. This is designed to be used to diagnose and treat a plasma fibrinogen concentration that is below the normal range, i.e. below approximately 1.5g/L. Some authors believe that it is desirable in some groups of bleeding patients not only to maintain a plasma fibrinogen concentration around the lowest end of the normal range but to increase the concentration further and in that case the threshold values for the FIBTEM A10 result in Figure 9 would be higher.

An alternative approach to distinguishing between an abnormal trace caused by thrombocytopenia and one caused by a low fibrinogen concentration does not use the additional test in which platelet aggregation is inhibited. Instead it attempts to use additional measurements of the speed of development of clot strength from the early

CLOT FIRMNESS		A10 in EXTEM		
		< 22 mm	22-38 mm	≥ 39 mm
A10 in FIBTEM	< 5 mm	Low fibrinogen Low platelets	Low fibrinogen (*platelets - see below)	Low fibrinogen
	5-7 mm	Low platelets Low fibrinogen	Low platelets Low fibrinogen	Clot firmness appears satisfactory
	≥ 8 mm	Low platelets	Low platelets	

* Typically, fibrinogen <1.5g/L and platelets 50-100 x 10^9/L.
Also consider giving platelets if ongoing bleeding.

Figure 9. Diagnostic algorithm used by the author to determine the cause of a reduced clot strength in ROTEM®. The appropriate row is selected according to the A10 result from the FIBTEM test (in which the clot contains fibrin but few platelets) and the column is selected according to the result from a test containing both fibrin and platelets such as the EXTEM test. The cell that lies at the intersection of the selected row and column contains a description of the abnormality present. Red indicates a severe abnormality of haemostasis that would normally require treatment in the context of surgery, trauma or obstetric haemorrhage. Yellow indicates a less severe impairment of haemostasis that might not require treatment if there are no clinical signs of bleeding. The result from another test in which the clot contains both fibrin and platelets (INTEM, HEPEM, APTEM) may be used instead of the result from the EXTEM test.

part of a single TE trace for this purpose. When clot strength is reduced, the time between clot first being detected and the amplitude of the trace reaching 20mm (ROTEM® clot formation time, CFT; TEG® Koagulationszeit, K-time) is increased and the angle made by a line drawn at a tangent to the first part of the thromboelastometry curve (alpha angle, α angle) is decreased. It has been suggested that these abnormalities are produced predominantly by a reduced fibrinogen concentration whereas reductions in the amplitude of the trace are caused by thrombocytopenia and therefore that the CFT/K-time or α angle can be used to distinguish between a low fibrinogen concentration and thrombocytopenia. However, thrombocytopenia and low fibrinogen can give similar values for these variables and treatment algorithms based on this approach may result in the transfusion of platelets when the main problem is a reduced fibrinogen concentration [8, 9].

In addition to their use in guiding treatment for impaired haemostasis, measures of clot strength may be used to provide early diagnosis of acute traumatic coagulopathy (ATC) in patients who have suffered major trauma [10].

The time it takes for detectable clot to form

This is indicated by the length of the straight line at the start of the TE trace (Figure 7) and is analogous to laboratory coagulation tests such as the APTT and PT (though with different normal values). This time is known as the clotting time (CT) in the ROTEM® analyser and the Reaktionszeit (R-time) in the TEG®. The time taken for clot to be detected depends on the reagents used to activate coagulation and their concentration.

Tissue factor (as in a PT test) is used in the ROTEM® EXTEM test and the CT is relatively short, enabling information on clot strength to be obtained more quickly. The CT is prolonged by deficiencies of coagulation factors of the classical extrinsic pathway of coagulation.

A contact activator of coagulation (as in an APTT test) is used in the ROTEM® INTEM test and in the TEG kaolin and Celite® tests. The normal value of the CT or R-time is longer than in the EXTEM test and it is prolonged by deficiencies of coagulation factors of the classical intrinsic pathway of coagulation and by heparin.

In the TEG® RapidTEG test, a combination of tissue factor and kaolin is used.

It is important to remember that fibrinogen is a coagulation factor (factor 1) and fibrinogen deficiency also prolongs the CT/R-times. Also, because much of the activity of coagulation factors occurs on the surface of platelets, marked thrombocytopenia can produce some prolongation of these times. Therefore, the significance of a prolonged CT/R-time result should be interpreted in the light of the estimate of fibrinogen concentration and platelet count obtained from assessing clot amplitude as described above.

The ROTEM® INTEM test and TEG® kaolin or Celite® tests may be used to detect and quantify the effect of standard (unfractionated) heparin. These tests are often performed along with a simultaneous test in which the enzyme heparinase is added to break down any heparin in the blood sample (ROTEM® HEPTEM test and TEG® heparinase test).

Whilst other anticoagulants may sometimes prolong the CT/R-time in ROTEM® or TEG® tests, the standard tests which are commercially available at present are not designed for their monitoring and should not be used to quantify the effect of anticoagulation with low-molecular-weight heparin, coumarin anticoagulants such as warfarin, or the newer oral anticoagulants. Indeed, the standard ROTEM® and TEG® tests may show normal results in patients therapeutically anticoagulated with warfarin.

Whether the clot remains strong or breaks down.

A small decrease in the width of the trace after it reaches its maximum occurs as a result of clot retraction. However, a marked reduction in clot strength indicates that excessive breakdown of the clot by fibrinolysis is occurring (Figure 10). This can be confirmed using a test in which an antifibrinolytic drug is added to the blood sample in the analyser (ROTEM® APTEM test). Hyperfibrinolysis may be treated by giving the patient intravenous tranexamic acid or epsilon-aminocaproic acid.

Post-partum haemorrhage

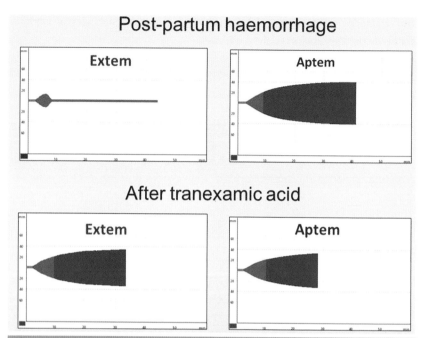

After tranexamic acid

Figure 10. ROTEM® traces during a postpartum haemorrhage. The upper EXTEM trace shows severe hyperfibrinolysis. This is not present in the APTEM test in which aprotinin is added to the blood sample to prevent fibrinolysis. The patient was given intravenous tranexamic acid and repeat ROTEM® tests no longer showed fibrinolysis (lower traces). *Figure provided by Dr Sarah Thompson.*

How to set up a successful thromboelastometry service

Many hospitals have successfully set up a point-of-care thromboelastometry service and report that the information from the analysers is extremely useful in guiding the management of bleeding patients. However, in other hospitals, analysers have been purchased but are rarely used because of lack of interest from the staff managing bleeding patients, lack of availability of a trained staff member to perform the tests or concerns about quality control and compliance with point-of-care testing policies. Point-of-care testing policies should ensure that testing of haemostasis is carried out to a high standard but not make unrealistic demands that render point-of-care testing impractical. It should be remembered that while the alternative standard laboratory tests of coagulation may be performed very reliably, the time to obtain the results may render them irrelevant or misleading in patients with severe haemorrhage or shock.

The greatest benefits from thromboelastometry are likely to be obtained when the tests are available 24 hours a day and can be rapidly performed close to the patient. However, in some hospitals, staff who have been trained to perform the tests are only available during week-day daytimes and/or the analyser is situated remotely in the hospital laboratory (sometimes with a link to a screen in the clinical area displaying the results).

Rapid diagnosis of the cause and severity of impaired haemostasis is only of value if it leads to rapid and appropriate therapy. Therefore, arrangements should be in place for the rapid supply of blood components to clinical areas managing a bleeding patient with thromboelastometry monitoring, without the need for confirmatory laboratory tests or the routine need for discussion with a haematologist. In hospitals where fibrinogen concentrate is used to treat hypofibrinogenaemia, that should be immediately available.

The National Institute for Health and Care Excellence has produced a resource [11] with practical information and advice for staff planning to start using thromboelastometry.

Conclusions

Thromboelastography/thromboelastometry analysers enable rapid point-of-care diagnosis of the abnormalities of coagulation that occur as a result of surgery or trauma or in obstetric haemorrhage — a low plasma fibrinogen concentration, thrombocytopenia, a deficiency of coagulation factors and excessive fibrinolysis. They may also be used to assess the effect of standard (unfractionated) heparin on coagulation and to determine whether the effect of heparin has been reversed. However, the standard TE tests do not detect the effect on platelets of aspirin or $P2Y_{12}$ inhibitor drugs such as clopidogrel and are not appropriate for the assessment of the effect of low-molecular-weight heparin or oral anticoagulants. The latest analysers are automated so that the tests are easier to perform than was previously the case. A good understanding of the principles behind TE and of how to interpret the results is required if the use of TE analysers is to lead on to appropriate patient management.

Checklist summary

Desirable characteristics of a point-of-care thromboelastometry service:

✓ Led by a 'clinical champion' — typically, a doctor treating bleeding surgical, trauma or obstetric patients.

✓ Supported by a 'co-ordinator' who ensures that the analyser(s) are maintained and repaired, that consumables are ordered, that formal documented training of staff on performing the tests and their interpretation is undertaken and that regular quality control is undertaken.

✓ Staff trained in performing the tests are available 24 hours a day — depending on local circumstances, tests may be performed by nurses, operating department practitioners, perfusionists or doctors. (Comparatively little training is required for the new generation of automated analysers.)

✓ Doctors interpreting the results have undergone training in interpretation and guidelines on interpretation are readily available.

✓ Regular quality control tests are performed as recommended by the device's manufacturer.

✓ Participation in an external quality assurance scheme.

✓ Rapid availability of blood components/fibrinogen concentrate if the thromboelastometry results indicate these are required.

References

1.   Weber CF1, Görlinger K, Meininger D, *et al*. Point-of-care testing: a prospective, randomized clinical trial of efficacy in coagulopathic cardiac surgery patients. *Anesthesiology* 2012; 117(3): 531-47.

2.   Craig J, Aguiar-Ibanez R, Bhattacharya S, *et al*. The clinical and cost effectiveness of thromboelastography/thromboelastometry. Health Technology Assessment Report 11. NHS Quality Improvement Scotland, 2008.

3.   National Institute for Health and Care Excellence. Detecting, managing and monitoring haemostasis: viscoelastometric point-of-care testing (ROTEM, TEG and Sonoclot systems). NICE diagnostics guidance, DG13. London, UK: NICE, 2014. https://www.nice.org.uk/Guidance/DG13.

4.   Spahn DR, Bouillon B, Cerny V, *et al*. Management of bleeding and coagulopathy following major trauma: an updated European guideline. *Crit Care* 2013; 17(2): R76.

5.   OAA/AAGBI guidelines for obstetric anaesthetic services, 2013. https://www.aagbi.org/sites/default/files/obstetric_anaesthetic_services_2013.pdf.

6.   Hartert H. Blutgerinnungsstudien mit der Thrombelastographie, einem neuen Untersuchungsverfahren [Blood coagulation studies with thrombelsatography: a new evaluation technique]. *Klin Wochenschr* 1948; 26: 577-83.

7.   Calatzis An, Calatzis Al, Fritzsche P. Weiterentwicklungen der thrombelastographie: automatische computerauswertung und neuentwicklung eines thrombelastographen. [Further development of thromboelastography: automatic computer analysis and development of a new thrombelastograph.] *Biomedizinische Technik/Biomedical Engineering* 1995; 40(s1): 393-94.

8.   Larsen OH, Fenger-Eriksen C, Christiansen K, *et al*. Diagnostic performance and therapeutic consequence of thromboelastometry activated by kaolin versus a panel of specific reagents. *Anesthesiology* 2011; 115(2): 294-302.

9.   Solomon C1, Schöchl H, Ranucci M, *et al*. Can the viscoelastic parameter α-angle distinguish fibrinogen from platelet deficiency and guide fibrinogen supplementation? *Anesth Analg* 2015; 121(2): 289-301.

10.   Davenport R, Khan S. Management of major trauma haemorrhage: treatment priorities and controversies. *Br J Haematol* 2011; 155(5): 537-48.

11.   National Institute for Health and Care Excellence. NICE diagnostic support for viscoelastometric point-of-care testing (ROTEM, TEG and Sonoclot systems). London, UK: NICE, 2014. https://www.nice.org.uk/guidance/dg13/resources/nice-diagnostic-support-for-viscoelastometric-pointofcare-testing-rotem-teg-and-sonoclot-systems-99757.

Chapter 24

Military management of massive haemorrhage

Heidi Doughty MBA FRCP FRCPath
Consultant Adviser in Transfusion Medicine, Centre of Defence Pathology, Royal Centre of Defence Medicine, Queen Elizabeth Hospital Birmingham, UK and NHS Blood and Transplant, Birmingham, UK

- "The priority in massive haemorrhage is to stop the bleeding."

- "Damage control resuscitation encompasses haemostatic techniques right from the point of wounding."

- "Transfusion support should consider the continuity of transfusion care."

- "In mass casualty events, all blood counts."

Background

Massive haemorrhage is the most immediate threat to the injured service-person. The mortality rate after massive haemorrhage in trauma is high unless actively managed from the point of wounding. Trauma also results in a complex disturbance of coagulation which is a marker of poor survival and must be addressed [1]. The pathophysiology of these mechanisms continues to be explored. Hypoperfusion, hyperfibrinolysis, activation of protein C and upregulation of the thrombomodulin pathways are thought to contribute significantly [2]. In addition, the integrity of the vascular endothelium may be lost in hypoxia [3]. Treatment requires haemorrhage control and prevention of shock.

The conflicts in Iraq and Afghanistan have been a stimulus to develop new paradigms of treatment. These have been supported by structured practice guidelines and a total quality system approach to the care of combat casualties. The initial management of the casualty with massive haemorrhage became <C>ABC, where C stands for catastrophic haemorrhage. This includes rapid control of bleeding using tourniquets and haemostatic dressings, judicious use of fluids during resuscitation, and mitigation of hypothermia. The approach is similar to that of patient blood management in that the priority in massive haemorrhage is to stop the bleeding.

In 2007, the range of advances in pre-hospital and hospital care were drawn together into a coherent doctrine — damage control resuscitation (DCR) [4]. DCR encompasses haemostatic techniques from the point of wounding through to damage control surgery (DCS). Techniques include in-flight intervention and resuscitation by a medical retrieval team, consultant-led trauma teams and an aggressive approach to coagulopathy — referred to as haemostatic resuscitation (HR). HR introduced the pre-emptive use of plasma to be given before evidence of a coagulopathy. Haemostatic resuscitation now precedes surgery and may reduce overall blood use.

Evidence

The evidence for the change in transfusion practice was initially based on retrospective analysis of military and civilian trauma databases [5]. Despite the limitations, the clinical outcomes of the whole combat care system were impressive. The rationale for plasma-based therapy remains uncertain. However, randomised controlled trials, such as PROMMTT published in 2013 and PROPPR published in 2015 [6, 7], has led to national transfusion guidelines supporting the early use of plasma in ratios of 3:2 to 1:1 [8]. The UK trauma community have recently proposed the routine use of 1:1 red cell concentrate (RCC) and plasma for traumatic haemorrhage. However, uncertainty demonstrates the need for research to be embedded into routine practice. In addition, the impact of changes must be analysed through the systematic use of trauma registries.

Massive transfusion initially developed within the context of deployed, centralised hospital care. However, transfusion support is now delivered throughout most of the patient care pathway. The expeditionary nature of military operations requires a more flexible mobile medical response. This implies a reduction in the logistic burden and confidence in the evidence for practice. Recent experience has led to a partial implementation of the massive transfusion protocol (MTP) in a pragmatic approach that seeks to combine clinical best practice with real-world operational constraint [9].

How to do it

Management of massive haemorrhage

Haemorrhage control starts in the pre-hospital environment as part of DCR and the <C>ABC approach to first aid. The haemostatic elements of DCR are shown in a haemostasis ladder overleaf (Figure 1).

Haemorrhage control and haemostatic support continues during hospital-based resuscitation and damage control surgery. The physiological management of bleeding is managed through optimal resuscitation and may be supported by transfusion therapy.

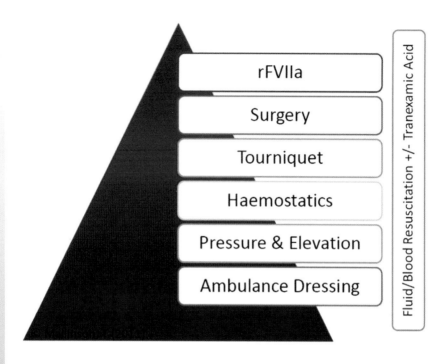

Figure 1. Ladder of haemostasis. *Reproduced from: Mallison T, 2011. This file is licensed under the Creative Commons Attribution — Share Alike 3.0 Unported license. https://creativecommons.org/licenses/by-sa/3.0/deed.en.*

Massive transfusion policy

The massive transfusion protocol (MTP) provides a joint clinical and laboratory framework for the delivery of multi-component "massive transfusion" support (Table 1). The definition of massive transfusion has evolved over time. Whereas it once referred to the replacement of a blood volume during a 24-hour period, the concept now is more about early and timely transfusion; modern rapid infusers can transfuse normothermic blood as fast as a unit per minute. The speed challenges laboratory support but saves lives.

Table 1. General clinical and transfusion goals in massive transfusion.

- Clinical evaluation and treatment strategy.
- Resuscitate and stop bleeding (<C>ABC).
- Tranexamic acid within 3 hours of injury (loading dose of 1g over 10 minutes followed by 1g infusion).
- Normal temperature.
- Systolic pressure 80-90mmHg in the initial phase without brain injury with a mean arterial pressure >80mmHg in patients with combined haemorrhage and brain injury.
- Urine output >40ml/h.
- Central venous pressure (CVP) 0-5mmHg.
- ABO and RhD blood groups.
- Haemoglobin (Hb) >90g/L until stable. Suggest 90-100g/L for air evacuation or patients with cardiorespiratory disease.
- Platelets >50 x 10^9/L. Give one pool of platelets when the platelet count is falling below 75 x 10^9/L. A target of 100 may be considered in patients with ongoing bleeding and/or traumatic brain injury.
- Prothrombin time (PT) ratio <1.5. Give fresh frozen plasma (FFP) at a standard dose, e.g. 12-15ml/kg when prothrombin time is greater than 1.5.
- Fibrinogen 1.5g-2g/L. Give fibrinogen supplementation (50mg/kg) if fibrinogen level falls below 1.5g/L or as guided by TEG®/ROTEM®. Use a starting dose of cryoprecipitate at a dose of two 5-pools or fibrinogen concentrate of 4g.
- Normalise serum base excess (BE) and lactate.
- Monitor and manage serum calcium and potassium.
- Start thromboprophylaxis with low-molecular-weight heparin (LMWH) once haemorrhage is controlled.

The current MTP aims to use near physiological blood replacement therapy based on a fixed formula protocol which is then tailored to individual patient requirements guided by clinical and laboratory results [10]. The UK protocol uses fresh frozen plasma (FFP) and red cell concentrate (RCC) in a 1:1 ratio as soon as practicable, together with the early use of cryoprecipitate as a source of fibrinogen and platelet support. The delivery is in the form of a 'shock pack' based on RCC and pre-thawed plasma. The use of pre-thawed plasma with a shelf life of 5 days was introduced in 2008 to support rapid delivery and pre-hospital emergency care (PHEC). FFP may be substituted with other plasmas.

Tranexamic acid (TXA) is given during PHEC within 3 hours of blood loss, followed by a second dose as an infusion. The CRASH protocol for TXA was a loading dose of 1g over 10 minutes followed by 1g in 500ml in normal saline over 8 hours [11]. In military practice this may be modified to use smaller volumes of fluid and syringe drivers. The transfusion policy includes the use of fresh whole blood and recombinant activated factor seven (rFVIIa). Recombinant FVIIa use is in line with European guidelines [12]. The fibrinogen level, calcium, temperature and pH should be normalised before use of rFVIIa. Viscoelastometry (ROTEM®) is used alongside conventional coagulation and haematology studies to support goal-directed therapy [10].

Taking transfusion forward

Continuity of care

Military transfusion support assumes the continuity of transfusion care. Transfusion may be needed throughout the patient journey from the pre-hospital arena to ongoing care in the home base. The immediate success of DCR is determined by the pre-hospital physiological optimisation of the critically injured, whereas the definitive control of bleeding is delivered through DCS. The requirement for ongoing care continues during medical evacuation. Careful preparation and 'packaging' of the patient is required during each transfer to minimise further bleeding or physiological deterioration.

Most of the interventions used are those of patient blood management and do not specifically require blood transfusion. Air evacuation, however, requires a higher haemoglobin reserve and haemostatic competence. The choice and timing of haematological support is dependent on the scenario and access to blood components. The immediate risk of ABO incompatibility may be managed by the use of universal components. However, the reliance on using 'universal' blood components may compromise not only sufficiency of supply but also blood grouping. In addition, the repeated use of red cells may occasionally lead to the development of atypical red cell antibodies which must be taken into consideration when selecting blood to cover revision surgery.

Blood on board

Civilian air ambulances are currently considering the pros and cons of carrying blood on board. In military practice and in the context of catastrophic haemorrhage or critical injury, blood has been life-saving in the pre-hospital arena. During operations in Iraq and Afghanistan, transfusion support in the form of RCC and pre-thawed FFP together with TXA was used successfully. The use of blood in pre-hospital care was used to support severely injured patients recovered by helicopter-borne medevac teams with short transfer times of 1-2 hours (Figure 2). The introduction of phase-change materials (substances with a high heat of fusion) revolutionised air-borne transfusion logistics for both PHEC and medical evacuation. Retrospective studies of blood transfusion en route

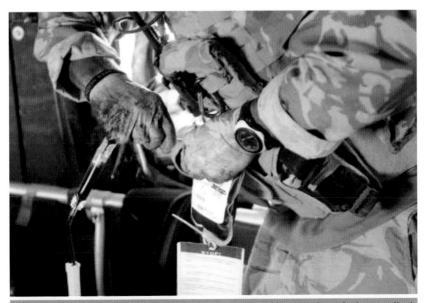

Figure 2. Blood on board. Transfusion preparation on board the medical emergency response team (MERT).

suggest a survival advantage from this advanced care in transit [13]. Civilian practitioners have recently extended these systems to offer not just blood, but a wide range of haemostasis products.

Blood far forward

Transfusion in the field has traditionally not been considered as part of routine ground-based pre-hospital care. However, this may require review in the context of prolonged evacuation times or where there is entrapment. Component-based transfusion has been successfully used by military GP-led teams with a high level of clinical governance. Cold chain management systems support the storage of pre-hospital blood by both vehicles and foot patrols. Blood can be kept at 2-8°C within phase-change containers, but many containers are still relatively heavy and bulky and require regular reconditioning of the thermal insulation elements by freezing. These logistic constraints have driven the search towards alternative blood components and haemostatic solutions.

Alternative components

The supply and storage of standard blood components places considerable logistic demands particularly if large amounts of frozen material are required. Dried and liquid blood products offer 'freedom from frozen' when delivering haemostatic support.

Lyophilised plasma

Lyophilised plasma products are useful alternatives to frozen plasma due to their ability to be stored at ambient temperature. There has been a recent upsurge of interest in the use of whole dried plasma, with a number of products in development. Products vary in their clotting factor content, solubility, donor exposures, and licensing maturity. The German Red Cross has introduced a single donor whole plasma product, LyoPlas N-w, in both civilian and military units (Figure 3). The French military have described their clinical experience with a pathogen-inactivated, lyophilised product based on a mini-pool of plasma to provide a universal plasma [14]. Currently, however, lyophilised plasma is only presented in medicinal glass which is less attractive for forward resuscitation.

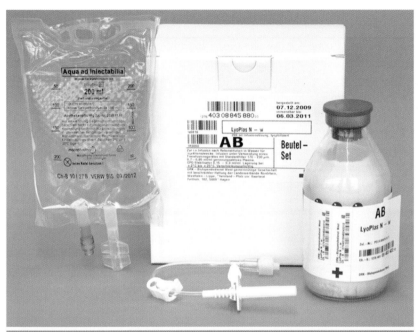

Figure 3. LyoPlas N-w set showing water for injection, lyophilised plasma and transfer set for reconstitution. *Reproduced with permission from DRK Blutspendedienst West.*

Fibrinogen concentrate

Fibrinogen levels fall following traumatic haemorrhage and these are an independent predictor of mortality. Fibrinogen is now considered central to clot strength and stability so there is a good rationale for fibrinogen replacement [15]. Fibrinogen concentrate is an alternative source of fibrinogen but it is not currently licensed for use in acquired coagulopathies in all countries. The current evidence does not support the superiority of one source of fibrinogen over another. Further trials are required to demonstrate the optimal timing and source of fibrinogen. However, it is increasingly used off-licence especially where cryoprecipitate is not available.

Cold storage for platelets

Storing platelets for transfusion at room temperature increases the risk of microbial infection and decreases platelet functionality. Cold storage may be a better alternative, but it leads to rapid platelet clearance after transfusion, initiated by changes in glycoprotein Ibα, the receptor for von Willebrand factor. This pre-activation of platelets during cold storage which reduces post-transfusion circulation may offer an advantage for immediate haemorrhage control. If this is the case then whole blood could be stored at 4°C, maintaining some platelet function for up to 10 days permitting 1:1:1 transfusion straight out of the box [16].

Whole blood

Few mature civilian blood services provide fresh whole blood (FWB) but it is used in many countries and may be applied in the military context. FWB not only addresses concern about the 'storage lesion', but also provides a supply of fresh plasma and a small dose of platelets. Whereas the use of multiple components results in higher volumes of infused anticoagulant during resuscitation, fresh whole blood provides a physiological replacement therapy with less anticoagulant. Military experience has shown that the widespread collection of FWB can be done safely, ironically returning to the days before modern blood banks existed.

There is increasing interest in the use of whole blood in trauma, both as fresh and stored whole blood. Whole blood may be the best transfusion support in massive haemorrhage. There is some evidence that the complementary use of FWB alongside components may be associated with a survival advantage. There are, however, a number of perceived obstacles to the reintroduction of whole blood. These include cold storage, platelet-sparing leucodepletion and haemolysins [17].

The major concern with the use of FWB is the risk of infectious disease, especially when using an emergency donor panel (EDP) who are volunteers pre-screened in accordance with national guidelines to donate whole blood or platelets by apheresis in emergency situations. Any of the risks can be mitigated by avoiding unnecessary blood use through optimal PHEC and transfusion triage. However, full donor testing should be available in civilian practice. Civilian practice has already made use of an EDP for support during a mass casualty event [18].

Mass casualty events

Transfusion demand and capability planning should be an integrated part of medical planning for both deployments and overseas training exercises. Blood supply should be part of civilian emergency planning [18]. Military and civilian hospitals have both benefited from investment in the transfusion infrastructure. However, training in transfusion safety and patient blood management remains essential. Elements should include the introduction of haemorrhage control, transfusion triage, haemostatic adjuncts and the greater use of point-of-collection testing (POCT).

Mass casualty events (MCE) may result in a demand for blood that cannot be immediately met. Whereas sporting events and other mass gatherings can be planned for, MCEs such as bombings require resilience within the health service system. The planning for the London Olympics 2012 [19] included a 100-year worldwide literature review of blood use following mass casualty events. The 2013 review provided RCC use for 51 events all occurring within the last 30 years and involving over 11,000 casualties. A significant relationship ($r2 = 0.75$, $p = 0.01$) was observed between number of casualties with injury severity scores greater than 15 (ISS >15) and RCC use in terrorist MCEs. The number of units of RCC in the severely injured varied from 2-8. The numbers varied due to the use of different denominators and blood components.

Most developed transfusion systems can meet the initial surge in demand through redeployment of stored components. A collaborative approach with good communication between transfusion providers, treatment units and the community is essential. Higher readiness donors may be used; however, most donors will be encouraged to keep their future appointments to ensure continuity of supply; whereas, the application of DCR, transfusion triage and patient blood management should reduce unnecessary demand. In mass casualty events, all blood counts.

Conclusions

Transfusion has emerged as an essential element of combat care. The success must be placed in the context of injury severity and the whole healthcare system, especially pre-hospital care. Combat has always stimulated innovation; military developments are based on both emerging evidence and pragmatism. The ongoing challenge is delivery of transfusion support forward without the logistic tail. Many of the lessons identified from military medical and transfusion care have already been adopted into civilian practice and planning. Military practice has informed both pre-hospital emergency care and medical support to mass casualty events. Combat care has in turn benefited from civilian transfusion expertise including all elements of patient blood management. The continued military-civilian collaboration and innovation in transfusion practice has the potential to benefit not only the military, but also the wider healthcare community.

Checklist summary

✓ Stop the bleeding with pre-hospital haemorrhage control and early surgery (<C>ABC).

✓ Start haemostatic resuscitation (1:1:1) early in the critically injured.

✓ Actively manage transfusion and blood safety.

✓ Be prepared to conduct transfusion triage especially if there are multiple patients.

✓ Include transfusion support and logistics as part of medical planning.

References

1.   Brohi K, Singh J, Heron M, Coats T. Acute traumatic coagulopathy. *J Trauma* 2003; 54(6): 1127-30.

2.   Brohi K, Cohen MJ, Ganter MT, *et al.* Acute traumatic coagulopathy: initiated by hypoperfusion: modulated through the protein C pathway? *Ann Surg* 2007; 245(5): 812-8.

3.   Ganter MT, Cohen MJ, Brohi K, *et al.* Angiopoietin-2, marker and mediator of endothelial activation with prognostic significance early after trauma? *Ann Surg* 2008; 247(2): 320-6.

4.   Hodgetts TJ, Mahoney PF, Kirkman E. Damage control resuscitation. *J R Army Med Corps* 2007; 153(4): 299-300.

5.   Borgman MA, Spinella PC, Perkins JG, *et al.* The ratio of blood products transfused affects mortality in patients receiving massive transfusions at a combat support hospital. *J Trauma* 2007; 63(4): 805-13.

6.   Holcomb JB, del Junco DJ, Fox EE, *et al.* The Prospective, Observational, Multicenter, Major Trauma Transfusion (PROMMTT) Study. Comparative effectiveness of a time-varying treatment with competing risks. *JAMA* 2013; 148(2): 127-36.

7.   Holcomb JB, Tilley BC, Baraniuk S, *et al.* Transfusion of plasma, platelets, and red blood cells in a 1:1:1 vs a 1:1:2 ratio and mortality in patients with severe trauma: the PROPPR randomized clinical trial. *JAMA* 2015; 313(5): 471-82.

8.   Hunt BJ, Allard S, Keeling D, *et al*, on behalf of the British Committee for Standards in Haematology. A practical guideline for the haematological management of major haemorrhage. *Br J Haematol* 2015; 170(6): 788-803.

9.   Jenkins D, Stubbs J, Williams S, *et al.* Implementation and execution of civilian remote damage control resuscitation programs. *Shock* 2014; 41(Suppl 1): 84-9.

10. Doughty HA, Woolley T, Thomas GOR. Massive transfusion. *J R Army Med Corps* 2011; 157(Suppl 3): S277-83.

11. CRASH-2 trial collaborators. Effects of tranexamic acid on death, vascular occlusive events, and blood transfusion in trauma patients with significant haemorrhage (CRASH-2): a randomised, placebo-controlled trial. *Lancet* 2010; 376(9734): 23-32.

12. Spahn DR, Bouillon B, Cerny V, *et al.* Management of bleeding and coagulopathy following major trauma: an updated European guideline. *Crit Care* 2013; 17(2): R76.

13. O'Reilly DJ, Morrison JJ, Jansen JO, *et al.* Special report: initial UK experience of prehospital blood transfusion in combat casualties. *J Trauma Acute Care Surg* 2014; 77(3)Suppl 2: S66-S70.

14. Martinaud C, Ausset S, Deshayes AV, *et al.* Use of freeze-dried plasma in French intensive care unit in Afghanistan. *J Trauma* 2011; 71(6): 1761-5.

15. Rourke C, Curry N, Khan S, *et al.* Fibrinogen levels during trauma hemorrhage, response to replacement therapy, and association with patient outcomes. *J Thromb Haemost* 2012; 10(7): 1342-51.

16. Pidcoke HF, Spinella PC, Ramasubramanian AK, *et al.* Refrigerated platelets for the treatment of acute bleeding: a review of the literature and reexamination of current standards. *Shock* 2014; 41(Suppl 1): 51-3.

17. Spinella P, Strandenes G, Hervig T, *et al.* Whole blood for hemostatic resuscitation of major bleeding. *Transfusion* 2016; in press.

18. Doughty H, Glasgow S, Kristoffersen E. Mass casualty events: pre-hospital care and emergency system transfusion preparedness across the continuum of care. *Transfusion* 2016; in press.

19. Glasgow SM, Allard S, Rackham R, Doughty H. Going for gold: blood planning for the London 2012 Olympic Games. *Transfus Med* 2014; 24(3): 145-53.

Chapter 25

Obstetric haemorrhage

Barbara Macafee BSc MBChB FRCA
Consultant Anaesthetist, Belfast Health and Social Care Trust, Belfast, UK
Bernard Norman MB BS FRCA
Consultant Anaesthetist, Chelsea and Westminster NHS Foundation Trust, London, UK

- "Obstetric haemorrhage remains the leading cause of maternal mortality and severe morbidity in resource-poor and resource-rich countries, respectively." [1]

- "The first essential factor in predicting haemorrhage is knowledge of the pathology. This is best remembered under the headings of the 4 'Ts'." [2]

- "Saving Lives, Improving Mothers' Care." [3]

- "The good physician treats the disease; the great physician treats the patient who has the disease." [4]

Background

Obstetric haemorrhage remains a leading cause of morbidity and mortality around the world, despite significant advances in monitoring haemostasis, early targeted treatment of massive haemorrhage and team organisation and training, with the introduction of massive haemorrhage protocols (MHP), team simulation training and drills. In successive Confidential Enquiries into Maternal Deaths and Morbidity (CEMD), substandard care in the recognition and treatment of haemorrhage has been identified. The most recent enquiry by MBRRACE-UK [3] identified adequate fluid replacement in haemorrhage as one of the key anaesthetic lessons. Meanwhile, there has been a shift in attitude towards greater blood conservation, protection of limited blood resources, employment of restrictive transfusion policies and greater patient protection from inappropriate transfusions.

A large number of definitions of obstetric haemorrhage exist [1]. A commonly used definition of moderate postpartum haemorrhage (PPH) is between 1000 and 2000ml blood loss and severe PPH greater than 2000ml. On average major haemorrhage constitutes blood loss after delivery of the placenta of greater than 500ml for vaginal delivery and 1000ml for Caesarean section. Other parameters used to define haemorrhage include a fall in haemoglobin concentration (Hb) of $\geq$40g/L, transfusion of one blood volume (70ml/kg) over 24 hours, packed red blood cell transfusion of greater than 4 units or transfusion of 10 units over 24 hours, or the need for an invasive surgical procedure [1]. The lack of a standard definition makes direct comparison of the effectiveness of treatment difficult, as the literature lacks a standardisation of definitions.

In order to improve the care we give to mothers, we need to focus our attention on decreasing the morbidity from postpartum haemorrhage. We can achieve this by focusing on three areas — prevention, treatment and rescue from haemorrhage [5]. Typically, obstetricians play a major role in prevention with antenatal strategies and active management of the third stage of labour with uterotonic drugs and controlled cord traction. Involvement of anaesthetists in the treatment and rescue stages influences fluid resuscitation and treatment of coagulation problems, as well as ongoing critical care [5].

The initial estimate of blood loss can have major implications on the direction of treatment and management of the patient and thus outcome. Clinicians are known to be poor at this estimation, typically underestimating blood loss by up to 30% [5]. Any unexplained tachycardia and hypotension postpartum should be assumed to be blood loss until this is excluded.

The first essential factor in predicting haemorrhage is knowledge of the pathology, which is best remembered under the headings of the four 'Ts' [2]:

- Tone (uterine atony or inflammation).
- Tissue (placental complications).
- Trauma (physical injury or previous trauma).
- Thrombin (congenital, or more commonly, acquired coagulation abnormalities).

An early predictor clinical tool for PPH that is entering the obstetric literature is the shock index (SI) — heart rate/systolic blood pressure (HR/SBP) [6]. It is an early assessment of hypovolaemic or non-hypovolaemic shock. It may help to predict ICU admission, blood transfusion >4 units, Hb <70g/L and the need for invasive surgical procedures. Normal values in non-pregnant females range between 0.5-0.7 and in pregnant females between 0.7-0.9. Nathan *et al* (2015) [6] found that an SI >1.7 was a good predictor of ICU admission and need for blood transfusion >4 units in women who had a PPH >1500ml. However, this did not take into account ongoing resuscitative measures which could have changed the parameters at any time.

Current research interest is aimed at prediction of likely bleeding in PPH and severity of haemorrhage, with a key focus on relative hypofibrinoginaemia and its implications as a valid biomarker in PPH. Recurring topics of discussion include rapid point-of-care testing and targeted blood component correction of coagulopathies. Evidence is emerging of the heterogeneous nature of obstetric haemorrhage, ranging from uterine atony, genital tract trauma and placental adhesion to various different coagulopathies. Current thinking is that the cause of obstetric bleeding influences the type and time of onset of coagulopathies (Table 1).

Table 1. Mechanisms of coagulopathy dependent on the aetiology of obstetric bleed. Late onset is abnormal coagulation usually only after 2000ml blood loss [1]. *Reproduced with permission from John Wiley & Sons Ltd.*

| | | | | Mechanism of coagulopathy | |
| | | | | | Consumptive |
Aetiology of bleed	Likelihood of coagulopathy (% transfused FFP)	Time of onset of coagulopathy	Dilution	Local to uterus and placenta	Disseminated intravascular
Uterine atony	14	Late	Severe cases	Severe cases	Very rare
Genital tract or surgical trauma	4	Late	Severe cases	Severe cases	Very rare
Placental abruption	42	Early (often before blood loss observed)	Severe cases	Main cause in mild and moderate cases	Severe cases
Retained and adherent placenta	8	Early or late	Most cases	Some cases	Rare unless associated with infection
Uterine rupture	66	Early	Main cause because large bleeds are common	Some cases	-
AFE	100	Early	Large bleeds	-	Main cause
Pre-eclampsia/ HELLP	ND	Early (often before labour)	Large bleeds	Some cases	Some cases

AFE = amniotic fluid embolism; FFP = fresh frozen plasma; ND = not determined

Placental abruption, uterine rupture and amniotic fluid embolism (AFE) can be seen to cause early onset of coagulopathy, with a dilution coagulopathy seen mainly in uterine rupture and AFE. Volume replacement leads to dilution of all coagulation factors, which leads to a fall in fibrinogen levels and platelet counts and affects thrombin generation [1]. Colloids, especially hydroxyethyl starches, may interfere with fibrin clot strength [7]. Consumptive coagulopathy is seen with placental abruption. Normal coagulation tends to exist with uterine atony and genital tract trauma, unless the blood loss is uncontrolled, which can result in a late-onset dilution and consumptive coagulopathy. Disseminated intravascular coagulopathy is an uncommon event. It is mainly observed in amniotic fluid embolus, severe pre-eclampsia or HELLP syndrome and more severe cases of abruption [8].

Knowledge of the changes in maternal physiology during pregnancy is vital in order to interpret results appropriately and act effectively. Early in the pregnant state, mothers tend towards hypercoagulability. Coagulation factors are all increased in pregnancy, except for factor XI [9]. Antithrombin III levels are depressed. The increased levels of procoagulant factors in pregnancy are particularly marked in factor VIII, fibrinogen and von Willebrand factor. The interpretation of hypofibrinogenaemia, as a marker of severity of PPH, is currently a hot topic of discussion [10]. Fibrinogen is a plasma glycoprotein, and its conversion to fibrin, catalysed by thrombin, plays a key role in clot formation and stabilisation. Fibrinogen also induces platelet activation and aggregation. Fibrinogen levels in pregnancy tend to be double the levels seen in non-pregnant females [11], ranging from 4-6g/L at term, compared to 2-4g/L in the non-pregnant state [12]. Studies have shown that in PPH, many women display normal coagulation studies despite massive haemorrhage. In contrast, fibrinogen levels were seen to drop progressively with increasing blood loss [13], subsequently reaching significant low levels well before changes were visible in other coagulation factors [14]. A number of studies have concluded that a fibrinogen level <3g/L and especially <2g/L, in the early phase of PPH, is associated with progression, whilst a fibrinogen >4g/L is not [1]. It is important to note that the Clauss assay for fibrinogen level testing should be used as it is the most sensitive and accurate of all the fibrinogen tests. Other assays are PT-derived and are not as accurate.

Evidence

Many clinical guidelines and current management of obstetric haemorrhage are derived from research into blood loss in major trauma, extrapolation from secondary outcomes and clinical audit, and much of this work is carried out in the non-pregnant population [9, 11]. Continuous review of emerging evidence requires an adaptive approach to these protocols in order to get the best outcome for our obstetric patients.

Monitoring haemostasis

Three main strategies are currently employed in obstetric units to assess haemostasis:

- Laboratory-based coagulation studies — prothrombin time (PT), activated partial thromboplastin time (APTT), and fibrinogen levels.
- Point-of-care (POC) or 'near-patient' testing.
- Clinical observation with blood product replacement.

The main limitation of traditional laboratory-based assessment of coagulation is speed of testing, and the relative slow production of results (45-minute turnaround time in the average lab) in a rapidly evolving clinical situation. There is limited sensitivity to developing coagulopathy resulting in often normal laboratory results despite massive haemorrhage [1].

POC testing, in the form of thromboelastography (TEG®; Haemonetics, Braintree, MA, USA) or thromboelastometry (ROTEM®; TEM International, Munich, Germany), is a relatively new form of monitoring in the obstetric environment, and with the additional expense of equipment and consumables, many units do not have this facility available to them. Increasingly, it is being used to supplement laboratory testing, giving more rapid assessment of an emerging haemorrhage situation, but may in the future replace traditional laboratory testing. When available, the main advantage is rapid identification of abnormal coagulation (average turnaround time 10-15 minutes), thus allowing early institution of targeted treatment with component blood products. ROTEM® FIBTEM A5 assay is a potential early tool in diagnosing coagulation abnormalities and evidence has suggested it can be used instead of Clauss fibrinogen [1].

Management strategies

A number of learned bodies have released guidelines for the management of postpartum haemorrhage. The Royal College of Obstetricians and Gynaecologists (RCOG) Green-top guideline No 529 and the Association of Anaesthetists of Great Britain and Ireland (AAGBI) [11] are the main sources of guidance for clinicians in the UK, and both these support primary monitoring with a coagulation screen, supported by POC monitoring when available. There are also European guidelines that exist along with guidelines issued by the World Health Organisation (WHO) [15, 16]. Six other management strategies form the mainstay of treatment – empirical fresh frozen plasma (FFP), goal-directed FFP, fibrinogen, platelets, tranexamic acid and recombinant factor VIIa. These strategies are generic in nature, and do not distinguish between the different causes of PPH, which require slightly different management plans in order to optimise outcome.

Uterotonics

Oxytocic drugs, usually in the form of an oxytocin analogue, such as syntocinon and ergometrine, aim to encourage uterine contractions and aid placental separation in the third stage of labour. These are usually administered as first-line treatment on delivery of the anterior shoulder during vaginal delivery or following delivery of baby during Caesarean section. Manual 'rubbing up' of the uterus works alongside these drugs to encourage uterine contraction. Retained products of conception may hinder uterine contraction and further examination of the uterus is required if it remains relaxed. If PPH continues, administration of an oxytocin infusion may be indicated. Prolonged use of an infusion is associated with an antidiuretic effect, which can result in water retention, leading to hyponatraemia and seizures. Prostaglandins such as misoprostol are used to induce labour but can also be used in the management of PPH. They can be administered orally, vaginally, rectally, sublingually and by the intrauterine route. Carboprost, another prostaglandin, is used as a second-line treatment in PPH, associated with uterine atony. Given intramuscularly, it is indicated if there is a poor response to more traditional oxytocics.

Red cell transfusion

Transfusion of red cells should always involve a blood warming system to prevent the triad of hypothermia, acquired coagulopathy and acidosis, which can worsen ongoing haemorrhage. Ideally, cross-matched blood is the blood of choice, but if time is of the essence, group-specific blood or Group O Rh negative Kell negative blood should be given. Major haemorrhage is deemed >4 unit blood transfusion.

Cell salvage

Intra-operative cell salvage (ICS) has been recommended as a method of blood replacement, in which red blood cells lost during surgery are recovered, washed and reinfused into the patient. It is now a recognised technique in massive obstetric haemorrhage management protocols. ICS avoids the risk of conventional allogeneic blood transfusion such as infection, allergic reactions, development of antibodies, cost and scarcity of supply. Potential risks of ICS are amniotic fluid embolism (AFE) and sensitisation to foetal red cells but the evidence appears to suggest these risks are mostly theoretical. A trained operator is required to operate the equipment — this may be a limiting factor in the out-of-hours situation. This should not delay the start of a procedure unless ICS is crucial to the care of the patient.

Fresh frozen plasma

Much of the work related to fresh frozen plasma has been extrapolated from trauma care and there is no evidence to support its use in postpartum haemorrhage. The more traditional empirical approach, whereby 1 unit of FFP is given for every 6 units of red cells, or in the event of >4500ml PPH, or if massive transfusion is anticipated, has been followed for many years. The limitations of FFP are that it needs cross-matching and takes 20-30 minutes to thaw prior to administration. A more recent approach taken from the work in military medicine, encompasses the idea of 'shock packs', transfusing FFP:red blood cells in a ratio of 1:1 [17]. Some advocate the additional use of platelets in a 1:1:1 ratio [18]. The aim of these packs is to pre-empt the ensuing coagulopathy and thrombin degradation by replacing coagulation factors early. However, the obstetric population are different to the trauma population, in that in most PPHs, the women maintain normal coagulation until later on in the haemorrhage process. This results in them receiving blood products with fewer coagulation factors or fibrinogen than they are circulating at that current time, thus leading to potential dilution of their own circulating factors and potential over-transfusion. Donated fresh frozen plasma contains a fibrinogen level of around 2g/L, as it is taken from the non-pregnant population [1]. In contrast to this approach, the guidelines also advocate 'goal-directed' FFP administration based on a formula, whereby 15ml/kg is given if the PT/APTT ratio >1.5 x normal [9]. The AAGBI guidelines [11] take a more aggressive approach by aiming to treat early to prevent the coagulation ratio reaching >1.5 x normal or advise giving more FFP if the coagulation ratio is above this. Coagulation values of this level represent severe derangement, resulting in a more reactive management strategy being adopted. Most units would advocate a more proactive plan whereby coagulation values do not reach this level of haemostatic impairment.

Prothrombin complex concentrates (PCCs)

Prothrombin complex concentrates are intermediate-purity pooled plasma products containing a mixture of vitamin K-dependent proteins and may contain the natural coagulation inhibitors, protein C and protein S. After removal of antithrombin and factor XI, PCCs are produced by ion-exchange chromatography from the cryoprecipitate supernatant of large plasma pools [19]. Most PCCs contain heparin, to prevent other factors in the concentrates, either three- or four-factor complexes (II, IX, X + VII), from being activated. PCCs were primarily produced to treat patients with haemophilia B, but are increasingly being seen as a replacement for fresh frozen plasma. Their role has now diversified into replacement therapy of congenital and acquired deficiency of vitamin K-dependent clotting factors, but they are occasionally used off-licence to treat postpartum haemorrhage. Overall clotting factor concentration can reach levels approximately 25 times higher than normal plasma and PCCs have been associated with thrombotic events in the non-obstetric population [1]. Studies are ongoing looking at its use in severe PPH but caution is advised in the obstetric population in view of this thrombotic association [1].

Cryoprecipitate

The use of cryoprecipitate is recommended to keep fibrinogen levels >1-1.5g/L [9, 11]. This is advised only if FFP has not been successful in raising the fibrinogen levels. On average, one pool of cryoprecipitate raises the fibrinogen level by 0.5g/L [1]. Cryoprecipitate will also help to restore some coagulation factors, chiefly factor VIII, von Willebrand factor and factor XIII.

Fibrinogen concentrate

Fibrinogen replacement therapy is indicated as prophylaxis and therapy of haemorrhage in congenital and acquired fibrinogen deficiency [20]. It has been used in the management of PPH, as a replacement for cryoprecipitate, but this indication is unlicensed in many countries [1]. Most of the evidence in obstetrics is based on case reports. Fibrinogen supplementation can be provided by FFP transfusion, cryoprecipitate or by fibrinogen concentrate. Fibrinogen concentrate (RiaSTAP™; CSL Behring, King of Prussia, PA, USA)[1] is produced from pooled human plasma. The concentration of fibrinogen is standardised. It can be reconstituted quickly with sterile water and infusion volumes are low, allowing rapid administration as a stat dose without delays for thawing or cross-matching [21]. Multiple studies state that a fibrinogen of at least 2g/L is required for adequate haemostasis in ongoing obstetric bleeding [1]. Anecdotal reports state that improved clinical haemostasis is achieved due to the higher fibrinogen levels. In order to raise the fibrinogen level by 1g/L, 70mg/kg fibrinogen is required [22]. Four prospective trials are currently ongoing looking at the role of fibrinogen in the management of PPH [1]. Of those, the FIB-PPH trial, a double-blind, placebo controlled study of women with a clinical diagnosis of PPH, has just published [23]. They were randomised to receive either fibrinogen concentrate or placebo and the primary outcome was the need to receive a blood transfusion. No difference in transfusion rates was seen between the two groups.

Platelets

Platelets provide a vital role in haemostasis, therefore in ongoing haemorrhage, adequate levels of platelets must be maintained in order to form platelet plugs (primary haemostasis), which in turn activate the coagulation cascade with resultant fibrin deposition and linking (secondary haemostasis). It has been suggested that the platelet count should be kept >50 x 10^9/L during progressive PPH, and that a platelet transfusion should be given when the count drops to below 75 x 10^9/L [9, 11]. Platelet transfusions are more likely in conditions such as severe pre-eclampsia, placental abruption and amniotic fluid embolism, which present with early-onset coagulopathy.

Tranexamic acid

Tranexamic acid is an antifibrinolytic agent. Studies in the non-obstetric population have shown strong evidence of reduced bleeding and transfusion requirement when tranexamic acid has been used in massive haemorrhage. The majority of studies have been carried out in trauma patients. It is known to show a modest decrease in estimated blood loss (EBL) in both the peri-operative setting and in prophylactic administration in elective Caesarean and routine vaginal deliveries. Caution is recommended in obstetrics due to the already procoagulant state of the parturient. In fact, the RCOG states that the consensus view regarding this agent is that it seldom has a place in the management of obstetric haemorrhage [9]. Further research is required, and the World Maternal Antifibrinolytic Trial (WOMAN) trial (www.thewomantrial.lshtm.ac.uk) aims to answer some questions regarding the role of tranexamic acid in early PPH [1].

Recombinant factor VIIa

The RCOG advises that recombinant factor VIIa (NovoSeven®; Novo Nordisk, Bagsvaerd, Denmark) may be used in life-threatening bleeding [9]. Alongside its unlicensed use in PPH, fibrinogen levels should be kept >1g/L and platelet count >20 x 10^9/L [9]. Standardised protocols for the use of recombinant factor VII in the obstetric setting are recommended by the

AAGBI [11] and in agreement with NICE guidelines [24], fibrinogen and other coagulation factors should be normal before its use.

How to do it

Identification of massive obstetric haemorrhage

Pay close attention to early warning scoring systems. Recognise the likelihood of concealed haemorrhage and a tendency to underestimate the amount of blood loss. Look for early signs of shock — tachycardia, tachypnoea, anxiety — and remember that a young pregnant woman can conceal almost 30% blood loss before she displays hypotension. Other clinical signs to recognise are poor capillary return, sweating, pallor and poor urinary output. Start primary resuscitation of the patient — airway, breathing, circulation (ABC), high-flow oxygen, large-bore IV access, fluid resuscitation, warm blood transfusion, blood products as soon as possible and keep the patient warm. Resuscitation should be ongoing as monitoring is applied, bloods and further investigations carried out and medical treatment, in the form of manual compression and uterotonics, administered. Activate the Massive Obstetric Haemorrhage (MOH) protocol when blood loss is 1500ml or there are clinical signs of shock. An example of a MOH protocol is provided in Figure 1.

Multidisciplinary team

Senior staff should be present early on from the three main specialties — obstetrics, anaesthesia and midwifery. Early communication with a senior haematologist can help to set the scene from the outset, allowing clear lines of communication between theatre and laboratories and efficient sanctioning of specialist haematology products when required. Trained anaesthetic assistance rostered solely for the obstetric suite is vital to keep abreast of the ongoing resuscitation. A dedicated porter for taking samples to the laboratories and bringing blood products to theatre is essential, with instructions to only step down once senior clinicians are satisfied that the situation in theatre has stabilised. Consider the need for a trained operator for cell salvage at this point, as time may be needed to locate appropriate staff. Allocate a scribe who firstly notes the time of

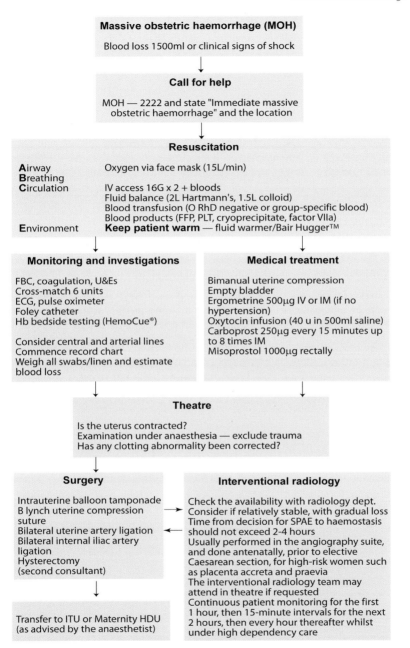

Massive obstetric haemorrhage (MOH)

Blood loss 1500ml or clinical signs of shock

↓

Call for help

MOH — 2222 and state "Immediate massive
obstetric haemorrhage" and the location

↓

Resuscitation

Airway   Oxygen via face mask (15L/min)
Breathing
Circulation   IV access 16G x 2 + bloods
      Fluid balance (2L Hartmann's, 1.5L colloid)
      Blood transfusion (O RhD negative or group-specific blood)
      Blood products (FFP, PLT, cryoprecipitate, factor VIIa)
Environment   **Keep patient warm** — fluid warmer/Bair Hugger™

Monitoring and investigations

FBC, coagulation, U&Es
Cross-match 6 units
ECG, pulse oximeter
Foley catheter
Hb bedside testing (HemoCue®)

Consider central and arterial lines
Commence record chart
Weigh all swabs/linen and estimate
blood loss

Medical treatment

Bimanual uterine compression
Empty bladder
Ergometrine 500µg IV or IM (if no
hypertension)
Oxytocin infusion (40 u in 500ml saline)
Carboprost 250µg every 15 minutes up
to 8 times IM
Misoprostol 1000µg rectally

Theatre

Is the uterus contracted?
Examination under anaesthesia — exclude trauma
Has any clotting abnormality been corrected?

Surgery

Intrauterine balloon tamponade
B lynch uterine compression
suture
Bilateral uterine artery ligation
Bilateral internal iliac artery
ligation
Hysterectomy
(second consultant)

↓

Transfer to ITU or Maternity HDU
(as advised by the anaesthetist)

Interventional radiology

Check the availability with radiology dept.
Consider if relatively stable, with gradual loss
Time from decision for SPAE to haemostasis
should not exceed 2-4 hours
Usually performed in the angiography suite,
and done antenatally, prior to elective
Caesarean section, for high-risk women such
as placenta accreta and praevia
The interventional radiology team may
attend in theatre if requested
Continuous patient monitoring for the first
1 hour, then 15-minute intervals for the next
2 hours, then every hour thereafter whilst
under high dependency care

NB: Resuscitation, monitoring, investigation and treatment should occur simultaneously.

Figure 1. Flow chart outlining the management of massive obstetric haemorrhage
taken from Chelsea and Westminster Hospital NHS Foundation Trust. *Reproduced with
kind permission from Womens Services, Chelsea and Westminster Hospital NHS Foundation Trust.*

activation of the MOH protocol, and then is responsible for all documentation and timings during the resuscitation.

Early identification of the cause of haemorrhage

Identification of the likely cause of haemorrhage can allow some pre-emptive decision-making regarding the need for specific blood products. This can result in earlier action and more successful resuscitation.

Surgical intervention

A number of interventions can be proposed — packing the uterus, intrauterine balloon insertion (balloon tamponade), e.g. Bakri™ balloon, BT-Cath® balloon, Belfort-Dildy balloon, compression (B-Lynch) sutures or ligation or embolisation of the uterine or internal iliac arteries. Emerging evidence is that balloon tamponade is a very effective temporising measure which is effective in itself. Early recourse to hysterectomy is recommended, especially where bleeding is associated with placenta accreta or uterine rupture [9]. Hysterectomy should not be delayed until the woman is in extremis [9].

Interventional radiology

Depending on availability in your hospital, this tends to be organised antenatally for planned Caesarean sections in high-risk women such as placenta accreta and praevia. Factors to keep in mind are delivery of anaesthesia and surgical intervention in a less familiar environment, usually the angiography suite, and staffing issues. Requests can be made for the radiology team to attend theatre instead.

Maternal critical care

The postoperative management of these high-risk women needs to be considered early on in massive obstetric haemorrhage, as the appropriate teams, either maternity high dependency unit (HDU) or intensive therapy unit (ITU) teams, need to be notified and can provide valuable input into the ongoing resuscitation.

Audit and simulation training

Regular review and audit of local MOH protocols is vital if we are going to improve morbidity and mortality figures from postpartum haemorrhage. Representatives from all the multidisciplinary team should be involved in the drafting of guidelines, to ensure all feedback is listened to and acted upon.

Conclusions

Prevention, treatment and rescue from haemorrhage remain the key focus areas in the management of obstetric haemorrhage. By determining the pathology behind the haemorrhage, predictions can be made regarding the type and time of onset of coagulopathies. In clinical practice, traditional management strategies of blood products, tranexamic acid and recombinant factor VIIa are being complemented by the emerging concentrate products. Current research is aimed at the prediction of PPH, focusing on hypofibrinogenaemia as a possible biomarker in PPH, and targeted blood component correction of coagulopthies.

Checklist summary

✓ Determine the cause of haemorrhage early — PPH is heterogeneous.

✓ Note fibrinogen levels as a marker of severity of bleeding.

✓ Employ point-of-care testing as a useful supplementation to laboratory testing.

✓ Use goal-directed FFP and targeted correction of coagulopathies.

✓ Adopt regular real-time on-site simulation training for members of staff involved in activating and implementing MOH protocols with debrief sessions.

References

1. Collis RE, Collins PW. Haemostatic management of obstetric haemorrhage. *Anaesthesia* 2015; 70 (Suppl. 1): 78-86.

2. Dyer RA, Vorster AD, Arcache MJ. New trends in the management of postpartum haemorrhage. *South Afr J Anaesth Analg* 2014; 20(1): 44-7.

3. MBRRACE-UK. Saving Lives, Improving Mothers' Care - Lessons learned to inform future maternity care from the UK and Ireland Confidential Enquiries into Maternal Deaths and Morbidity 2009-12. Oxford, UK: National Perinatal Epidemiology Unit, University of Oxford, 2014: 45-55. https://www.npeu.ox.ac.uk/mbrrace-uk.

4. Osler W. Aequanimitas London. P. Blakiston's Sons & Co., 1904.

5. Weeks A. The prevention and treatment of postpartum haemorrhage: what do we know, and where do we go to next? *Br J Obstet Gynecol* 2015; 122: 202-12.

6. Nathan HL, El Ayadi A, Hezelgrave NL. Shock index: an effective predictor of outcome in postpartum haemorrhage? *Br J Obstet Gynecol* 2015; 122: 268-75.

7. Fenger-Eriksen C, Moore GW, Rangarajan S, *et al.* Fibrinogen estimates are influenced by methods of measurement and hemodilution with colloid plasma expanders. *Transfusion* 2010; 50: 2571-6.

8. Levi M. Pathogenesis and management of peripartum coagulopathic calamities (disseminated intravascular coagulation and amniotic fluid embolism). *Thromb Res* 2013; 131: S32-4.

9. Royal College of Obstetricians and Gynaecologists. Prevention and management of postpartum haemorrhage. Green-top guideline No. 52, 2009. http://www.rcog.org.uk/files/rcog-corp/GT52PostpartumHaemorrhage0411.pdf.

10. Butwick AJ. Postpartum haemorrhage and low fibrinogen levels: the past, present and future. *Int J Obstet Anesth* 2013; 22: 87-91.

11. Thomas D, Wee M, Clyburn, *et al.* Blood transfusion and the anaesthetist: management of massive haemorrhage. *Anaesthesia* 2010; 65: 1153-61.

12. Szecsi PB, Jorgensen M, Klajnbard A, *et al.* Haemostatic reference intervals in pregnancy. *Thromb Haemost* 2010; 103: 718-27.

13. De Lloyd L, Bovington R, Kaye A, *et al.* Standard haemostatic tests following major obstetric haemorrhage. *Int J Obstet Anesth* 2011; 20: 135-41.

14. Allard S, Green L, Hunt BJ. How we manage the haematological aspects of major obstetric haemorrhage. *Br J Haematol* 2014; 164: 177-88.

15. Winter C, Macfarlane A, Deneux-Tharaux C, *et al.* Variations in policies for management of the third stage of labour and the immediate management of postpartum haemorrhage in Europe. *Br J Obstet Gynecol* 2007; 114(7): 845-54.

16. World Health Organisation. WHO guidelines for the management of postpartum haemorrhage and retained placenta. Geneva, World Health Organisation, 2012. http://apps.who.int/iris/bitstream/10665/75411/1/9789241548502_eng.pdf.

17. Pasquier P, Gayat E, Rackelboom T, *et al.* An observational study of the fresh frozen plasma:red blood cell ratio in post-partum hemorrhage. *Anesth Analg* 2013; 116: 155-61.

18. Saule I, Hawkins N. Transfusion practice in major obstetric haemorrhage: lessons from trauma. *Int J Obstet Anesth* 2012; 21: 79-83.

19. Franchini M, Lippi G. Prothrombin complex concentrates: an update. *Blood Transfus* 2010; 8(3): 149-54.

20. Franchini M, Lippi G. Fibrinogen replacement therapy: a critical review of the literature. *Blood Transfus* 2012; 10(1): 23-7.

21. Fenger-Erikson C, Ingerslev J, Sorenson B. Fibrinogen concentrate - a potential universal haemostatic agent. *Expert Opin Biol Ther* 2009; 9: 1325-33.

22. Glover NJ, Collis RE, Collins P. Fibrinogen concentrate use during major obstetric haemorrhage. *Anaesthesia* 2010; 65: 1229-30.

23. Wikkelsoe AJ, Afshari A, Stensballe J, *et al.* The FIB-PPH trial: fibrinogen concentrate as initial treatment for postpartum haemorrhage: study protocol for a randomised controlled trial. *Trials* 2012; 13: 110.

24. National Institute for Health and Care Excellence. Kenyon S. Intrapartum care: care of healthy women and their babies during childbirth, CG55. London, UK: NICE, 2007. http://www.nice.org.uk/ guidance/cg55/chapter/guidance.

Chapter 26

Cancer patients — blood health and surgery

M. Ann Benton MA FRCP FRCPath
Consultant Haematologist ABMU Health Board, Wales and National Clinical Lead for Transfusion, Welsh Blood Service, UK

- "It is expected that annual cancer cases will rise from 14 million in 2012 to 22 million within the next two decades."

- "Worldwide, almost 32.5 million people diagnosed with cancer from 2007 were alive at the end of 2012."

- "Fatigue affects between 7 and 9 out of 10 people with cancer."

- "Between 30% and 90% of patients with cancer have anaemia."

- "When used correctly, blood saves lives and improves health."

- "In patients with colorectal cancer undergoing surgery, allogeneic blood transfusions are associated with adverse clinical outcomes, including increased

Background

For many of us, cancer will be an inevitable part of our lives, either for ourselves, our family members or our friends. An estimated 14 million people across the world were diagnosed with cancer in 2012, and it is predicted that there will be a 70% increase in new cases over the next 20 years [1]. Ageing is well recognised as a risk factor for the development of cancer, a consequence of failing cellular repair mechanisms and aberrant regulation of the immune system. Ageing is also a major risk factor for receiving a blood transfusion, with up to 76% of blood transfusions being given to those over 65 years of age in high-income countries, usually as supportive care in surgery, trauma, or therapy for solid organ and haematological cancers [2] (Figure 1) [3].

Unfortunately, ageing is one risk factor none of us can avoid, and surgery is often the key to cure for many solid organ cancers. Anaemia at

Blood use by age and specialty

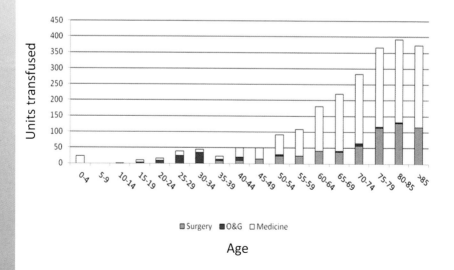

Figure 1. Red cell units transfused by age and specialty during a 2-week audit of blood use in Wales, 2014 [3].

presentation may be due to iron deficiency as a consequence of tumour-related bleeding (gastrointestinal, gynaecological and renal tumours) and/or chronic disease due to systemic cytokine effects from the tumour. Surgery may be complex and extensive, increasing the risk of bleeding and hence the need for red blood cell transfusion support. Careful assessment, including thrombotic risk and the benefit of anticoagulation, with collaboration between anaesthetist and surgeon, is essential to avoid adding risks from bleeding and transfusion to those from the cancer itself.

In addition, fatigue is a major symptom of both cancer and its treatment, even in the absence of what would usually be considered clinically significant anaemia, and some solid organ cancer therapies require near normal haemoglobin concentrations to ensure efficacy and best outcomes. Bone marrow suppression is an inevitable consequence of many combination chemotherapy regimes, and in the blood cancers may be a consequence of both the disease and its treatment (Figure 2) [3].

Units transfused as a percentage of overall use

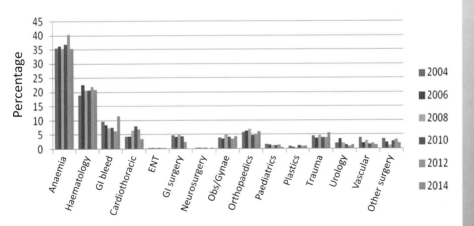

Figure 2. Anaemia and haematological disorders account for 55% of blood transfused [3].

Episodic neutropenia and thrombocytopenia may add complications of infection, sepsis and bleeding on top of symptoms from anaemia, necessitating platelet and, rarely, granulocyte transfusion in addition to red cells.

Luckily, increasing numbers of patients are now cured or living with their cancer. An estimated 32.5 million people diagnosed with cancer since 2007 were still alive in 2012 [1]. Early detection, correct diagnosis, new chemotherapeutic agents, immune modulation, and an increasing understanding of molecular signalling pathways leading to specific targeted therapy have a significant part to play in this success. However, good supportive care with safe blood component therapy is also a key factor as it facilitates complex surgery and intensive chemotherapy/radiotherapy regimes even in those with significant comorbidities. As our understanding of the mechanisms of cancer and the availability of targeted therapy expands, the emphasis for high-income countries is moving towards individualised care, maximising benefit and minimising risk, which must include any potential risks from blood component transfusion. Alongside the recognised risks of acute immune-related reactions and adverse events, process errors and physiological implications, longer-term immune-modulator factors gain greater significance in relation to tumour recurrence. There is increasing evidence that this tumour-related immune-modulator effect (TRIM) has a significant impact on outcome in relation to cancer therapy [4]. The identified benefit from the immediate use of blood component support must therefore outweigh the impact of a potential reduction in the effectiveness of the anti-tumour intervention, and an increased risk of cancer recurrence (Figure 3).

Although an eye to the future may initially seem less relevant in the context of cancer, the evidence suggests that long-term survival will increasingly be the expectation following treatment. This means the possibility of immune-related late effects of blood component use increasing the risk of tumour recurrence must be carefully considered in the risk/benefit assessment of all therapeutic interventions, even prior to confirmation of a diagnosis of cancer.

Potential adverse impact of red cell transfusion on the risk of cancer recurrence

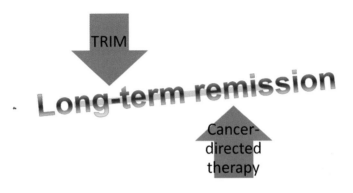

Figure 3. Transfusion-related immune modulation reducing the effectiveness of chemotherapy.

The evidence

The incidence of cancer and the incidence of red cell transfusion both increase with ageing [1, 3]; ageing is inevitable, and hence the longer we live, the more likely it is that both will occur. Up to 60% of red cell transfusion in developed countries is given to people over 70 years of age [3]. Only about 25% of all red cells used support surgical interventions, but 30% of red cell transfusions are given to support patients with haematological disorders, and a further 10% for those with non-haematological cancers [3]. Many patients with solid organ cancers may well require complex surgery as the primary intervention to achieve cure, and are likely to be older, have additional comorbidities, and reduced tolerance of anaemia, making the risk of transfusion support for surgery greater [5]. Overall, up to 40% of patients with cancer will be anaemic at presentation, as a consequence of iron deficiency due to tumour-associated bleeding (gastrointestinal, urological and gynaecological malignancy), or the anaemia of chronic disease due to tumour-associated cytokines [6]. This burden of anaemia increases significantly with treatment, rising to 90% in those treated with chemotherapy [7], and has been shown to be an independent prognostic factor for survival [8], as well as having major implications for quality of life [9].

In addition, curative radiotherapy for solid organ cancers relies on adequate haemoglobin concentration for a successful outcome [7] and so managing anaemia is crucial to maximise treatment benefit, quality of life, outcome and overall survival.

Appropriate and effective management of anaemia requires correct diagnosis of the cause followed by implementation of therapy. As with all clinical scenarios, if there is a requirement for an immediate increase in haemoglobin level, then transfusion of red cells will be the only option available. Acute life-threatening gastrointestinal bleeding as a presentation of stomach or colon cancer may rarely occur. Blood loss during complex surgery may be anticipated from the staging investigation scans, and sophisticated imaging techniques are now able to provide much more detailed information on the nature, extent and invasiveness of tumour masses. Excellent surgical technique to address large- and small-vessel bleeding, along with the back-up of interventional radiology support if needed, the use of intra-operative cell salvage, and greater tolerance of low haemoglobin concentrations can all limit, or negate the need for allogeneic red cell use [10].

However, unexpected complications may still arise leading to life-threatening blood loss and the need for essential emergency blood transfusion support. In such a scenario, the impact of any potential adverse longer-term effect from transfusion may be justified, but adopting a restrictive transfusion strategy (Hb trigger of <70g/L) appears not to be associated with adverse outcomes [11-13]. This is important, as a significant body of evidence is accumulating which indicates that both disease-free survival and long-term outcome in some cancers may be worse in patients receiving blood transfusion as part of their cancer therapy [14-16].

A relatively recent large meta-analysis looking at blood transfusion in colorectal surgery (n = 20,795) confirmed the earlier findings reported by Amato and Pescatori showing that transfused patients had a higher risk for all-cause mortality (odds ratio [OR]: 1.72), cancer-related mortality (OR:

1.71) and recurrence/metastasis/death (OR: 1.66) compared to non-transfused controls [17, 18].

Allogeneic blood transfusion may be avoidable in cases of either anticipated or unscheduled surgical bleeding if cell salvage is available to allow autologous red cell collection and return[19]. Concerns over the theoretical possibility of adverse consequences from tumour cell or bacterial contamination related to cancer and/or 'dirty' surgery remain, although evidence to date suggests that the risk of either is minimal if recommended wash protocols and appropriate cell filters are employed.

In haematological malignancy, bone marrow function may be suboptimal as a consequence of both infiltration by disease and the impact of marrow-directed chemotherapy. The tolerance for lower haemoglobin thresholds rather than reflex blood transfusion in response to numbers in the absence of clinical symptoms will limit donor exposure and harmful immune modulator effects. In addition to anaemia, often bleeding and neutropenic infection cause significant morbidity. The use of prophylactic platelets in haematological malignancy and stem cell transplants has become standard practice but there is no evidence that platelet dose affects the number of patients with significant bleeding, or that it affects the incidence of WHO grade 4 bleeding [20]. Increasing evidence that even intensive marrow-directed regimes can be safely implemented without blood component support is accruing from centres willing to manage blood cancers with intensive therapy of curative intent for those patients who decline blood and component therapy [21].

How to do it

Consider the patient, not just the cancer

The diagnosis, staging and management of any form of cancer is a complex and intense process for both clinician and patient (Figure 4). Time appears to pass incredibly slowly during the initial stages, making this a hugely stressful and psychologically challenging time. Ensuring adequate information is given, and patient choice is allowed to contribute to decision-making about the cancer and the treatment options may not be

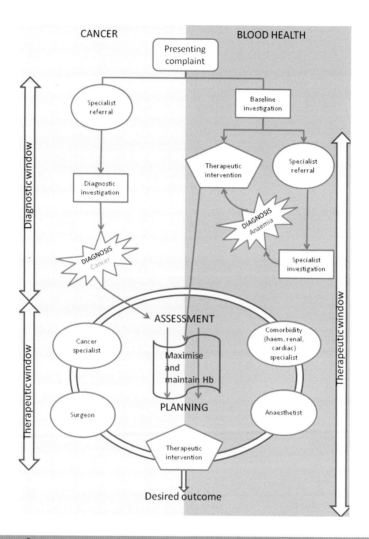

Figure 4. A management pathway, including blood health, for patients presenting with cancer-related symptoms.

as easy to achieve as perceived. It is understandable that making time for proper consideration of support-related issues may not be high on the priority list, and a 'blood health' assessment may seem trivial to the patient desperate to start cancer treatment at the earliest opportunity. However, minimising risks from treatment, including those associated with blood component therapy, will provide optimum care both acutely and in the long term. Introducing such an approach into management can be achieved by applying the following steps outlined below.

Think blood health and cancer — careful clinical assessment and appropriate investigation

This is a key aspect during the identification, diagnosis and staging of malignancy, and offers an ideal opportunity to explore the current blood health status of the patient and maximise their own bone marrow potential. Patients presenting to primary care with anaemia and low mean cell volume (MCV) should have baseline ferritin, C-reactive protein and iron studies, and be started on oral iron therapy whilst awaiting appropriate investigation for the cause of blood loss (Figure 5).

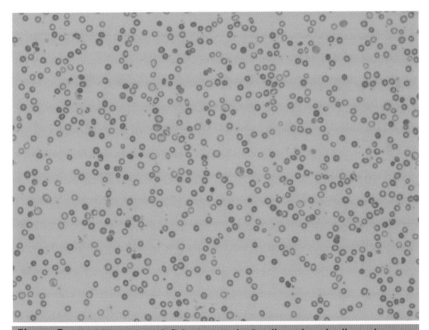

Figure 5. Blood film — iron-deficient anaemia. Smaller pale red cells can be seen, indicating a lack of enough iron to form sufficient haemoglobin to fill the cell cytoplasm during the development of the red cells.

If the patient has ongoing bleeding and therefore a degree of reticulocytosis (young red cells in the blood), the MCV may be in the normal range despite the presence of iron deficiency due to a mixed population of cells of variable size. In this case a blood film will be informative and indicate an iron-deficient population (small pale red cells)(Figure 6). Ask your haematologist to check the film.

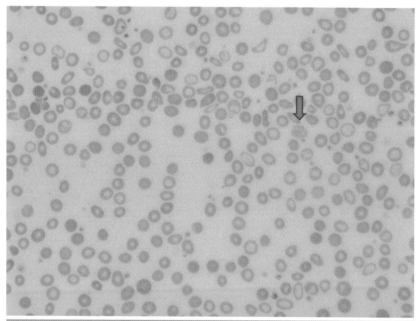

Figure 6. Blood film. Background of small pale cells (iron deficient) with polychromasia indicating an increase in young red cells released from the bone marrow earlier than usual and which contain more RNA. These cells pick up the blue dye during the film-staining process, creating a mix of pink mature red cells and slightly larger, bluish immature red cells. These reticulocytes increase the mean cell volume and can 'hide' the presence of iron deficiency through a normal MCV.

In the presence of a normally functioning bone marrow, compliance with iron replacement therapy and no ongoing bleeding, haemoglobin concentration should improve at the rate of 10g/L per week. Intravenous total iron therapy offers the benefit of confirmed compliance, immediate correction of iron deficit, and minimal side effects, balanced against the need for in-hospital intervention, an invasive procedure and a small risk of acute allergic reaction. In addition, the IV route may be able to overcome the functional iron deficiency caused by the cytokine effects of the cancer [22].

If there is evidence of chronic kidney disease, consider a renal dose of erythropoietin (EPO) in addition to iron therapy to maximise marrow erythroid function.

Poor nutritional status, cachexia and tumour burden can all cause folate deficiency. Oral supplementation is straightforward, but vitamin B12 status should be assessed to avoid precipitating neurological complications (sub-acute combined degeneration of the cord). If in doubt, give one dose of 1000mg hydroxycobalamin IM to ensure adequate B12 levels before initiating oral folate therapy.

A full clinical assessment with due consideration of comorbidity, particularly cardiac reserve, will allow a relative cardiac risk to be determined. From this, a haemoglobin tolerability trigger can be defined and applied to the management plan supporting either surgery or chemotherapy/radiotherapy. This should be discussed with the clinical team and shared with the patient along with the rationale for red cell transfusion avoidance if clinically safe to do so.

Adequate preparation and planning — pre-surgery or pre-chemotherapy/radiotherapy

Working through the following key areas will ensure consideration of all relevant issues, engagement of all necessary personnel, and delivery of optimum patient care:

- Optimise the available time for improving individual blood health, complete investigations and liaise with other specialists as appropriate, i.e. haematologists, renal physicians, surgeons, anaesthetists and radiologists.
- Initiate appropriate therapy (iron, folate, B12, EPO).
- Utilise technology and imaging to inform regarding the risks of bleeding. Consider interventional radiology input pre- or peri-operatively.

- Assess thrombotic risk and the use of prophylactic anticoagulants. Seek advice regarding bridging therapy if necessary.
- Investigate the cause of low platelets or an abnormal coagulation screen and agree an intra-operative management plan with a haematologist, or appropriate thresholds for prophylactic support post-chemotherapy. Treat on a clinical basis rather than purely on numbers.
- Plan complex surgery with experienced surgeons and anaesthetists, and ensure that adequate time is available for full pre-op assessment with the operating anaesthetist to plan anaesthetic technique, patient positioning and cell salvage if required. Apply a 'bloodless' surgery approach [21].
- Consider the use of antifibrinolytics for both prophylaxis and in the event of excessive bleeding. Use topical sealants and other appropriate haemostatic technology such as diathermy, lasers, and arterial embolisation.
- Consider cell salvage, discuss the potential risks and benefits with the patient, book the equipment and operator, and confirm that the appropriate white cell filters are available.
- Agree a haemoglobin tolerability trigger with the team and patient, and document the assessment outcome and rationale as part of the case notes [22].

Establish multidisciplinary review for high-risk cases

The concept of a multidisciplinary team approach is fundamental to best practice and good patient care in cancer. It brings together the key healthcare professionals involved in the care of the individual allowing for a wide range of specialist expertise and knowledge to contribute to the decision-making process. Current focus is usually restricted to confirming the tumour type, and debating the most effective therapy for that tumour, either for curative intent or palliation. This is also an excellent opportunity to address aspects of blood health, identify opportunities to maximise bone marrow function, establish an individualised management plan and implement therapy to minimise requirement for blood product use. Such a multidisciplinary-type approach has been adopted for 'bloodless' surgery programs, and for managing blood cancers in those declining blood and component therapy, without adverse impact on outcome [21]. The allocation of a key worker with specialist knowledge of blood health issues and management provides additional opportunities to ensure personalised care and informed patient choice.

The key principles above are outlined in Figure 7.

How to do it

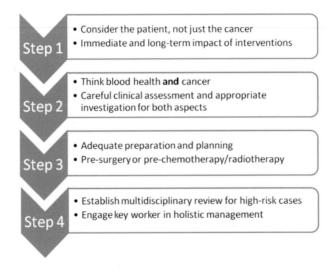

Step 1
- Consider the patient, not just the cancer
- Immediate and long-term impact of interventions

Step 2
- Think blood health **and** cancer
- Careful clinical assessment and appropriate investigation for both aspects

Step 3
- Adequate preparation and planning
- Pre-surgery or pre-chemotherapy/radiotherapy

Step 4
- Establish multidisciplinary review for high-risk cases
- Engage key worker in holistic management

Figure 7. Key principles for optimum patient management, addressing both blood health and cancer.

Conclusions

As we grow older, the population as a whole ages, and as our ability to manage cancer continues to advance, increasing numbers of us will have our own personal experience of cancer. For some of us, blood transfusion support may be essential and life-saving, making any potential increased

411

risk of cancer recurrence acceptable. However, those of us able to optimize our own blood health and maintain adequate levels of haemoglobin rather than rely on an acute injection of haemoglobin by a tissue transplant of donated red cells stand to gain maximum benefit from our cancer therapy. There is much that can be done to reduce unnecessary blood component transfusion and it is the responsibility of all healthcare professionals to support patients in achieving care that is optimal for them both immediately and for their future.

Acknowledgement

My thanks go to Karen Shreeve for the data and diagrams.

Checklist summary

✓ Evaluate and maximise blood health at the earliest opportunity.

✓ Seek expert advice from multidisciplinary sources.

✓ Consider the implications of all therapeutic interventions, immediate and longer term.

✓ Define individualised trigger thresholds in collaboration with the patient (Hb and platelets).

✓ Think future, plan, phone a friend.

References

1. Stewart B, Wild CP. World cancer report (epub). The International Agency for Research on Cancer (IARC), 2014. ISBN-13 9789283204329.

2. WHO top ten facts on blood transfusion. http://www.who.int/features/factfiles/blood_transfusion/blood_transfusion/en/index1.html.

3. Shreeve K, Benton MA, El-Hack W. Where does blood go? A review of 5 data collection cycles. BBT WBS, 2014: personal communication.

4.   Cata JP, Wang H, Gottumukkala V, *et al.* Inflammatory response, immunosuppression, and cancer recurrence after perioperative blood transfusions. *Br J Anaesth* 2013; 110(5): 690-701.

5.   Shander A, Knight K, Thurer R, *et al.* Prevalence and outcomes of anemia in surgery: a systematic review of the literature. *Am J Med* 2004; 116 Suppl 7A: 58S-69S.

6.   Knight K, Wade S, Balducci L. Prevalence and outcomes of anaemia in cancer: a systematic review of the literature. *Am J Med* 2004; 116 Suppl 7A: 11S-26S.

7.   Tas F, Eralp Y, Basaran M, *et al.* Anaemia in oncology practice: relation to diseases and their therapies. *Am J Clin Oncol* 2004; 2 Suppl 1: 11-26.

8.   Caro JJ, Salas M, Ward A, *et al.* Anaemia as an independent prognostic factor for survival in patients with cancer: a systematic, quantitative review. *Cancer* 2001; 91: 2214-21.

9.   Stasi R, Abriani L, Beccaglia P, *et al.* Cancer-related fatigue: evolving concepts in evaluation and treatment. *Cancer* 2003; 98: 1786-801.

10. Cata JP, Gottumukkala V. Blood transfusion practices in cancer surgery. *Indian J Anaesth* 2014; 58(5): 637-42.

11. Salpeter SR, Buckley JS, Chatterjee S. The impact of more restrictive blood transfusion strategies on clinical outcomes: a meter analysis and systematic review. *Am J Med* 2014; 127(2): 124-31.e3.

12. Kim Y, Spolverato G, Lucas DJ, *et al.* Red cell transfusion triggers and postoperative outcomes after major surgery. *J Gastrointest Surg* 2015; 19(11): 2062-73.

13. Padhi S, Kemmis-Betty S, Rajesh S. Blood transfusion: summary of NICE guidance. *Br Med J* 2015; 351: 30-2.

14. Liu L, Wang Z, Jiang S, *et al.* Perioperative allogenenic blood transfusion is associated with worse clinical outcomes for hepatocellular carcinoma: a meta-analysis. *PLoS One* 2013; 8(5): e64261.

15. De Oliveira GS Jr, Schink JC, Buoy C, *et al.* The association between allogeneic perioperative blood transfusion on tumour recurrence and survival in patients with advanced ovarian cancer. *Transfus Med* 2012; 22(2): 97-103.

16. Boehm K, Beyer B, Tennstedt P, *et al.* No impact of blood transfusion on oncological outcome after radical prostatectomy in patients with prostate cancer. *World J Urol* 2015; 33(6): 801-6.

17. Amato A, Pescatori M. Perioperative blood transfusions for the recurrence of colorectal cancer. *Cochrane Database Syst Rev* 2006; 1: CD005033.

18. Acheson AG, Brookes MJ, Spahn DR. Effects of allogeneic red blood cell transfusions on clinical outcomes in patients undergoing colorectal cancer surgery: a systematic review and meta-analysis. *Ann Surg* 2012; 256: 235-44.

19.   Waters JH, Yazer M, Chen YF, Kloke J. Blood salvage and cancer surgery: a meta-analysis of available studies. *Transfusion* 2012; 52: 2167-73.

20.   Estcourt L, Stanworth S, Doree C, *et al.* Prophylactic platelet transfusion for prevention of bleeding in patients with haematological disorders after chemotherapy and stem cell transplantation. *Cochrane Database Syst Rev* 2012; 5: CD004269.

21.   Frank SM, Wick EC, Dezern AE, *et al.* Risk adjusted clinical outcomes in patients enrolled in a bloodless program. *Transfusion* 2014; 54 (10 0 2): 2668-77.

22.   Gilreath JA, Stenehjem DD, Rodgers GM. Diagnosis and treatment of cancer-related anemia. *Am J Hematol* 2014; 89(2): 203-12.

Chapter 27

Acute upper gastrointestinal bleeding

Abhishek Chauhan MRCP
Specialty Trainee Gastroenterology, Queen Elizabeth Hospital, Birmingham, UK
Tariq Iqbal MD FRCP
Consultant Gastroenterologist, Queen Elizabeth Hospital, Birmingham, UK

- "Upper gastrointestinal bleeding accounts for 14% of red blood cell tranfusions in England."

- "Arguably the most significant change in the management of gastrointestinal bleeding revolves around newly favoured restrictive transfusion targets."

- "Mortality from acute upper gastrointestinal bleeding increases with age. Independent of age the presence of significant comorbidity also increases mortality rates from upper GI haemorrhage."

- "Scoring systems allow one to triage patients based on clinical parameters at presentation."

Background

Acute upper gastrointestinal bleeding (AUGIB) remains a common medical emergency with a sizeable mortality. An audit conducted in the United Kingdom in 2007 found the overall mortality from GI bleeding to be 7% in hospital inpatients [1].

Although the incidence of AUGIB generally seems to be declining in the West, owing arguably to improved treatment (and detection) of *Helicobactor pylori* as well as better prevention strategies during non-steroidal anti-inflammatory drug use, recent studies still suggest an annual incidence of 90-100 per 100,000 of the population [2]. Pertinently, upper GI bleeding is a frequent indication for transfusion of blood components and it has been estimated that this indication alone accounts for 14% of red blood cell (RBC) transfusions in England [3].

The last 10 years have seen a shift in the landscape regarding the aetiology and management of acute upper GI haemorrhage. Whilst better patient outcomes due to advances in both radiological and endoscopic intervention coupled with wider use of powerful ulcer healing drugs and less invasive surgical intervention have developed [4], newer 'irreversible' anticoagulants such as dabigatran and rivaroxaban pose novel treatment dilemmas [5]. Although the FDA has now given idarucizumab (Praxbind®), a humanized monoclonal antibody fragment that binds to dabigatran (Pradaxa®; both Boehringer Ingelheim), accelerated approval on October 16, 2015, for use in patients who require emergency surgery or other urgent procedures or who have life-threatening or uncontrolled bleeding.

Perhaps the most significant change in the management of GI bleeding revolves around newly favoured restrictive transfusion haemoglobin targets.

Studies as far back as 1999 revealed the non-inferiority of a conservative versus liberal transfusion strategy in terms of patient outcome [6], albeit in a cohort of critically ill patients not specifically bleeding from the GI tract. A similar study in critically ill children a few years later yielded a haemoglobin target of 70g/L for red cell transfusion as adequate to reduce transfusion requirements whilst not adversely affecting patient outcome [6]. Although these studies in themselves did not influence gastrointestinal bleeding transfusion practice, they helped lay the foundations for the paradigm shift we have recently seen. Villanueva *et al* demonstrated improved patient outcomes with a restrictive transfusion regimen (aiming to transfuse when the haemoglobin level fell to 70g/L haemoglobin) versus liberal transfusion thresholds (90g/L) [7] in patients with AUGIB. It should be noted that in this seminal study, patients with significant ischaemic heart disease, vascular disease and stroke were excluded. Nevertheless, we are in the midst of observing a potentially major shift in transfusion practice for the management of gastrointestinal haemorrhage.

Evidence

There is a distinct lack of adequately powered studies assessing initial assessment in AUGIB. Data from the British GI bleed steering consortium in 1995 revealed a very high fatality rate (42.5%) from upper GI haemorrhage amongst inpatients [8]. The more recent follow-up audit by the British Society of Gastroenterologists and National Blood Transfusion Service reported an improved but still sizeable mortality in this cohort of 26% [1]. This is probably because of improved management of the associated comorbidities and improvements in therapeutic endoscopy in the decade between the two studies.

Risk factors associated with poor outcome

Taking account of relevant risk factors in patients with suspected upper GI haemorrhage allows clinical triage regarding not only urgency of endoscopic evaluation/treatment but also in deciding patient suitability for discharge and potential outpatient management.

Age and premorbid status

The mortality associated with GI bleeding increases with age [9]. Importantly, there are some crucial differences to take into account when assessing or treating an acute upper gastrointestinal bleed in a patient over the age of 60. Notably, the odds ratio (OR) for mortality goes from 1.8 to 3 for over 60-year-olds (compared to patients aged 45-59 years), and from 3 to 4.5 to 12 for patients over the age of 75 years (compared to younger cohorts) [4]. Additionally, there are differences in presentation, with elderly people describing fewer antecedent symptoms such as abdominal pain or dyspepsia, being more likely to be on aspirin or NSAIDs and more likely to have significant comorbidity. These factors contribute to higher rates of rebleeding, hospitalization and ultimately death in this cohort [10].

Independent of age, the presence of significant comorbidity such as heart failure or disseminated malignancy also increases mortality rates from upper GI haemorrhage [8].

Volume of the bleed

In keeping with other forms of haemorrhagic shock, larger volumes of blood loss are associated with poorer outcomes. Melaena associated with a bleeding source proximal to the ligament of Treitz (a band of smooth muscle extending from the junction of the duodenum and jejunum to the left crus of the diaphagm and functioning as a suspensory ligament) may signify brisk upper GI bleeding and almost doubles mortality [11]. It is therefore unsurprising that the presence of shock or hypotension at presentation increases the risk of death by 20% compared to haemodynamically insignificant GI bleeding [4].

Liver disease

Patients with bleeding varices and underlying chronic liver disease have appreciably different outcomes compared to patients with non-variceal haemorrhage. Although the overall mortality with variceal haemorrhage is 14% [12], considerable variation mirroring the severity of the underlying liver disease is seen. A patient with Child's grade A cirrhosis for instance has a 1 in 10 chance of dying at index presentation with a variceal bleed compared to an almost 1 in 2 risk of mortality in an individual with Child's grade C cirrhosis [13].

Scoring systems

Scoring systems (with varying levels of validation) that stratify patients at risk of death due to rebleeding after an upper GI bleed are widely in use. Such scores effectively allow one to triage patients based on clinical parameters at presentation and make decisions regarding the urgency of endoscopic intervention. It must, however, be stressed that no scoring system is totally predictive and care must be taken to interpret these scores in the context of the individual patient.

Arguably the most commonly used scoring systems are the Rockall and Glasgow-Blatchford scores. The Rockall score is often divided into a pre-endoscopic or initial score and then a composite final score (Table 1), which takes into account endoscopic findings [4, 14]. Although the Rockall score has been externally validated and at conception was intended as a tool for predicting both mortality and rebleeding risk, subsequent studies have demonstrated that it is better at predicting mortality rather than rebleeding risk [15]. Although the Glasgow-Blatchford score (Table 2) has

Table 1. Rockall table [16].

Variable	Score 0	Score 1	Score 2	Score 3
Age	<60	60-79	>80	
Shock	No shock	Pulse >100 SBP >100mmHg	SBP <100mm Hg	
Comorbidity	Nil major		CHF, IHD, major morbidity	
Diagnosis	Mallory-Weiss	All other diagnoses	GI malignancy	Renal failure, liver failure, metastatic cancer
Stigmata of recent haemorrhage	None		Blood, adherent clot, spurting vessel	

SBP = systolic blood pressure; CHF = congestive heart failure; IHD = ischaemic heart disease; GI = gastrointestinal.

Table 2. Glasgow-Blatchford score [16].

Admission risk marker	Score component value
Blood urea (mmol/L)	
6.5-8.0	2
8.0-10.0	3
10.0-25	4
>25	6
Haemoglobin (g/L) for men	
12.0-12.9	1
10.0-11.9	3
<10.0	6
Haemoglobin (g/L) for women	
10.0-11.9	1
<10.0	6
Systolic blood pressure (mm Hg)	
100-109	1
90-99	2
<90	3
Other markers	
Pulse ≥100 (per min)	1
Presentation with melaena	1
Presentation with syncope	2
Hepatic disease	2
Cardiac failure	2

been shown to be superior to the initial Rockall score in predicting the need for treatment and rebleeding risk in upper GI bleeds [16-18], external validation assessing the performance of the Glasgow-Blatchford score in predicting mortality and applicability as a tool to triage patients to outpatient endoscopy [19] is still required.

A patient with a Rockall score of 0 identifies 15% of patients with AUGIB at presentation who have an extremely low risk of death (0.2%)

and rebleeding (0.2%), and therefore may be suitable for early discharge or non-admission [4].

The colloid versus crystalloid debate

The management of hypovolaemic or indeed any type of shock has, in recent years, been dominated by the issue of whether crystalloids are superior to colloids for volume replacement.

Since colloids theoretically stay in the intravascular space longer than crystalloids, these fluids were traditionally thought of as superior than their crystalloid counterparts for the purposes of intravascular fluid replacement.

The SAFE study in 2004 was perhaps the first study to directly compare the two fluid types and demonstrated non-inferiority of a crystalloid solution (normal saline) when compared to a colloid (4% albumin) in the treatment of shocked patients on intensive care [20]. A 2007 Cochrane review again suggested no statistical difference in the two groups [21].

More recently, however, the CRISTAL trial showed colloids to improve 90-day mortality compared to crystalloids [22] in critically unwell patients. For the purposes of resuscitation in the shocked GI bleed patient, no data are available comparing the two fluids and as such no specific recommendations favouring one over the other can currently be made.

Coagulopathy

Historically, chronic liver disease has been thought of as the epitome of acquired bleeding disorders; recent evidence, however, highlights this as a rather monochromatic perspective. Complex haemostatic abnormalities encompassing prolonged prothrombin time, consumptive thrombocytopaenia, secondary hyperfibrinolysis and chronic coagulation activation characterize the 'coagulopathy' of chronic liver disease [23] and as such traditional notions of merely an increased bleeding diathesis is an oversimplification [24]. Nevertheless, the presence of coagulopathy on admission in patients with variceal haemorrhage significantly increases the risk of rebleeding and mortality [25]. The situation in non-variceal upper GI bleeds is more complicated with a prolonged International Normalised Ratio (INR) not influencing the rates of rebleeding but increasing mortality [25].

Tranexamic acid (TXA) is a drug that reduces clot breakdown by inhibiting the action of plasmin, which is involved in fibrinolysis. There has been recent interest in the potential of this drug to help achieve haemostasis during AUGIB. A 2014 systematic review suggested a mortality benefit in patients with AUGIB treated with TXA [26]; the general consensus is that discrepancies in current data make it hard to recommend TXA as routine in the management of acute upper GI bleeding just yet [26, 27]. A large, multi-national, randomised controlled trial (RCT) to address this question is, however, currently in progress [28].

Novel anticoagulants (NOAC)

Direct thrombin inhibitors (dabigatran) and factor Xa blocking agents (apixaban and rivaroxaban) comprise a new generation of oral anticoagulation agents (NOAC). Whilst being at least as efficacious as warfarin in reducing the risk of thromboembolic stroke in patients with atrial fibrillation [29-31], these drugs have been shown to almost halve the incidence of intracranial bleeding [32]. Owing to far more predictable pharmacodynamics and pharmacokinetic profiles and hence a reduced need for monitoring, these drugs are rapidly replacing warfarin as the anticoagulant of choice to reduce the risk of thromboembolic stroke.

A recent retrospective, propensity matched cohort study showed there to be no difference in the risk of GI bleeding (in patients under 75) when comparing dabigatran or rivaroxaban to warfarin [5]. A heavily criticized (due to selection bias) systematic review analysing 43 RCTs, however, suggested an increased risk of GI bleeding in patients on NOACs compared to conventional care [33, 34].

Although no specific reversal agents are widely in use to counteract the action of NOACs in the context of GI bleeding, new reversal agents are under development and currently in trials to manage bleeding in this cohort. A recombinant factor Xa competitive decoy is currently under investigation [35], and the most promising data comes from the RE-VERSE AD trial where idarucizumab, an antibody fragment, has been shown to completely reverse the anticoagulant effects of dabigatran [36].

Given the short half-lives of these drugs, supportive care including optimum resuscitation coupled with endoscopic (or surgical) haemostasis and close observation for rebleeding is probably the most pragmatic method of managing gastrointestinal bleeding in patients on NOACs. Due to the novel pharmacology of the NOACs, hospital-specific management plans to deal with major GI bleeding in such patients should be developed through joint collaborations between gastroenterologists, emergency department physicians, cardiologists, haematologists, and nephrologists [32]. Given the paucity of data on reversal agents, it is hard to currently recommend any agents to reverse NOAC-related GI bleeding, apart from idarucizumab, although clinical data are awaited.

How to do it

Resuscitation and initial management

Airway, Breathing, Circulation (ABC)

Staff competent in airway assessment and basic airway manoeuvres should assess patients presenting with acute upper gastrointestinal bleeding in a timely manner. These patients are at particular risk of airway compromise so regular airway reassessment is critical [4]. The next steps in management involve establishing intravenous access ideally using wide-bore cannulae and fluid resuscitation.

Volume resuscitation

The presence of haemodynamic shock negatively influences patient outcome after a GI bleed. The key to effective management in a shocked patient is early assessment, prompt recognition of shock, fluid resuscitation and regular reassessment. The degree of shock and response to therapy will guide the amount and rate of fluid administration. The choice of non-red blood cell-containing fluid used for resuscitation should be governed by local availability; in massive haemorrhage, rapid volume expansion to maintain critical end-organ perfusion is paramount. Early goal-directed therapy in shock effectively minimizes the duration of organ hypoperfusion and robust evidence highlights significant benefit to patient outcomes [37]. A point to note is the need to tailor fluid regimens in patients with comorbidities such as cardiac or renal failure, in order to avoid the risk of fluid overload.

The Scottish Intercollegiate Guidelines Network (SIGN) guidelines recommend red cell transfusion after 30-40% of circulating volume is lost [4]. However, determining the degree of shock on the basis of clinical parameters alone can be subjective at the best of times and therefore we do not recommend this as a means for determining whether an individual patient requires a red cell transfusion. Checking the haemoglobin level provides a more objective method of determining the need for a red cell transfusion, although in a patient with very acute haemorrhage the haemoglobin level may be erroneously reassuring (due to lack of adequate haemodilution in the time period immediately following blood loss).

Villanueva *et al* reported improved patient outcomes in gastroenterological haemorrhage where conservative targets for haemoglobin (transfuse at 7g/dL) are followed [7]. It is important to note that this study involved 8-hourly haemoglobin testing and endoscopy within 6 hours of presentation, which may not be practical. This study also excluded patients with exsanguinating haemorrhage and comorbidities such as significant vascular disease; in other words conditions where significant blood transfusion may have actually improved outcome. A pragmatic management strategy would be to transfuse at a threshold of 7g/dL in suitable patients (no cardiac or vascular disease) in suitable facilities (where 8-hourly haemoglobin measurement is feasible — in high dependency or intensive care facilities for instance). Until further studies are conducted, local protocol should dictate transfusion practice in gastrointestinal haemorrhage. The TRIGGER trial in fact revealed that favouring a restrictive strategy in AUGIB results in a non-significant reduction in RBC transfusion with no significant difference in clinical outcomes [38].

Coagulopathy management

Blood samples should be sent to the laboratory at the earliest opportunity. In the presence of active bleeding, the British Committee for Standards in Haematology (BCSH) recommend a platelet transfusion threshold of 75×10^9/L, but also suggest that in conditions of abnormal platelet function (in patients on antiplatelet drugs for instance), platelets should be transfused empirically [39].

Volume replacement therapy with crystalloids or colloids and red cell transfusion will dilute coagulation factor levels. Therefore, regular reassessment of coagulation indices, particularly in massive haemorrhage requiring large amounts of volume replacement, is essential.

Fibrinogen level, prothrombin time (PT) and activated partial thromboplastin time should be monitored at regular intervals and specialist haematology input may be required to help guide coagulopathy treatment. Most hospitals will have protocols in place for dealing with massive haemorrhage and local guidance should be followed. It is important to note that although fresh frozen plasma (FFP) is recommended and routinely used during bleeding, the evidence for it being clinically efficacious is relatively weak [40]. FFP in large enough quantities will correct fibrinogen levels and most clotting factor levels; however, failure to correct fibrinogen levels using solely FFP should prompt consideration of cryoprecipitate [39]. When bleeding is due to oral anticoagulation overdose, prothrombin complex concentrate (Octaplex® or Beriplex®) should be considered, as this has been shown to be superior to FFP alone [41].

Pre-endoscopic management

Proton pump inhibitors (PPIs)
The pre-endoscopic use of proton pump inhibitors is not routinely recommended as there is no discernable benefit to clinical outcomes

including mortality, rebleeding or the need for surgery [42]. The exception to this is situations where endoscopic haemostatic treatment is not available, as PPI therapy in such situations has been shown to reduce the risk of rebleeding and the need for surgery [43]. The use of PPIs is not recommended when the cause of an AUGIB is due to gastro-oesophageal varices, except in situations where post-variceal ligation ulcer healing is a concern or simultaneous peptic ulcer disease is present [44].

Variceal bleeds

In cases of suspected or confirmed variceal bleeding, broad-spectrum antibiotics should be administered. Antibiotics lower the rebleed risk and rate of bacterial infections, thus decreasing mortality [45]. Although local policy and patterns of resistance will dictate the choice of antibiotic, oral quinolones or a third-generation cephalosporin are recommended [46].

Lowering portal pressures pharmacologically improves outcomes in acute variceal bleeding. Medical options for this include vasoconstrictors such as vasopressin (or one of its analogues such as terlipressin) or somatostatin (or one of its analogues) [47]. These medications should be started as soon as a variceal bleed is suspected [47], and continued until cessation of bleeding or up to 5 days [47].

Timing of endoscopy

Patients presenting with likely AUGIB should generally undergo upper GI endoscopy within 24 hours of presentation, provided they are adequately resuscitated [48]. It should be noted that a cut-off time point for endoscopy of 12 hours is reasonable in high-risk patients (significant shock or bloody emesis at presentation) [49]. Continuing haemodynamic instability despite adequate resuscitation should prompt hyper-urgent endoscopic examination, especially when bleeding varices are thought culpable [47]. The modes and methods of achieving haemostasis endoscopically are beyond the scope of this chapter, but suffice it to say variceal band ligation with the use of intravenous terlipressin to reduce portal pressure is the treatment of choice in variceal bleeding. In ulcer-related AUGIB, the use of two modes of endoscopic therapy are recommended in each case to improve outcome [47, 48]. In variceal bleeds where haemostasis is not achieved through variceal band ligation, continued resuscitation with variceal balloon tamponade is the next step. In situations of uncontrolled variceal bleeding and rebleeding, a covered transjugular intrahepatic portosystemic shunt (TIPSS) insertion is recommended (provided the portal vein is patent) [47]. Transarterial embolisation (TAE) should be available for non-resolving ulcer bleeding [48].

Post-endoscopic management

Intravenous PPI therapy in the form of an 80mg bolus followed by 8mg/hour for 72 hours should be given to all patients with high-risk ulcers after endoscopic haemostasis (adherent clot, non-bleeding visible vessel or actively bleeding ulcer). Oral therapy is adequate for ulcers with clean bases [48]. After satisfactory haemostasis in the case of variceal bleeds and depending on local resources, early covered TIPSS (<72 hours after index variceal bleed) can be considered in selected patients with Child's B cirrhosis and active bleeding or Child's C cirrhosis with a Child's score of <14 [47].

Conclusions

Acute upper gastrointestinal haemorrhage is a common medical emergency, with an appreciable morbidity and mortality. The key to effective management is early and regular assessment with aggressive fluid resuscitation. Coagulopathy in upper GI bleeding is common and should always be investigated. Although restrictive targets for blood transfusion have been shown to improve patient outcomes, caution must be exercised when using these targets in clinical practice especially where access to intensive monitoring and emergent endoscopy is not available.

A management algorithm for AUGIB is shown overleaf (Figure 1).

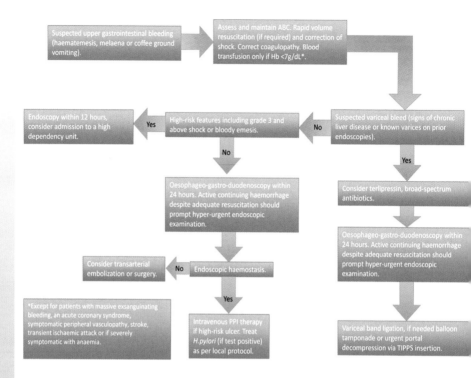

Figure 1. Management algorithm for AUGIB.

Checklist summary

✓ AUGIB is common and is associated with a high mortality rate.

✓ The high mortality is dependent upon the cause of the bleeding and the patient's comorbidities.

✓ Careful assessment of the patient at presentation is critical.

✓ Many patients with AUGIB have coagulopathy.

✓ Initial volume replacement should not be with blood.

✓ Recent RCT data suggest that restrictive blood transfusion is associated with a better outcome in AUGIB.

References

1. St. Elsewhere's NHS Foundation Trust. UK Comparative Audit of Upper Gastrointestinal Bleeding and the Use of Blood, 2007. http://www.bsg.org.uk/clinical/general/uk-upper-gi-bleeding-audit.html.

2. Hreinsson JP, Kalaitzakis E, Gudmundsson S, Björnsson ES. Upper gastrointestinal bleeding: incidence, etiology and outcomes in a population-based setting. *Scand J Gastroenterol* 2015; 48(4): 439-47.

3. Jairath V, Kahan BC, Stanworth SJ, *et al.* Prevalence, management, and outcomes of patients with coagulopathy after acute nonvariceal upper gastrointestinal bleeding in the United Kingdom. *Transfusion* 2012; 53(5): 1069-76.

4. Scottish Intercollegiate Guidelines Network (SIGN). Management of acute upper and lower gastrointestinal bleeding. SIGN Guideline No. 105, 2008; Sep 15: 1-64.

5. Abraham NS, Singh S, Alexander GC, *et al.* Comparative risk of gastrointestinal bleeding with dabigatran, rivaroxaban, and warfarin: population-based cohort study. *Br Med J* 2015; 350: h1857-7.

6. Lacroix J, Hébert PC, Hutchison JS, *et al.* Transfusion strategies for patients in pediatric intensive care units. *N Engl J Med* 2007; 356(16): 1609-19.

7. Villanueva C, Colomo A, Bosch A, *et al.* Transfusion strategies for acute upper gastrointestinal bleeding. *N Engl J Med* 2013; 368(1): 11-21.

8. Rockall TA, Logan R, Devlin HB, Northfield TC. Incidence of and mortality from acute upper gastrointestinal haemorrhage in the United Kingdom. *Br Med J* 1995; 311(6999): 222-6.

9. Zimmerman J, Siguencia J, Tsvang E, *et al.* Predictors of mortality in patients admitted to hospital for acute upper gastrointestinal hemorrhage. *Scand J Gastroenterol* 1995; 30(4): 327-31.

10. Yachimski PS, Friedman LS. Gastrointestinal bleeding in the elderly. *Nat Clin Pract Gastroenterol Hepatol* 2008; 5(2): 80-93.

11. Wilcox CM, Alexander LN, Cotsonis G. A prospective characterization of upper gastrointestinal hemorrhage presenting with hematochezia. *Am J Gastroenterol* 1997; 92(2): 231-5.

12. Blatchford O, Davidson LA, Murray WR, *et al.* Acute upper gastrointestinal haemorrhage in west of Scotland: case ascertainment study. *Br Med J* 1997; 315(7107): 510-4.

13. Palmer K. Acute upper gastrointestinal haemorrhage. *Br Med Bull* 2007; 83(1): 307-24.

14. Rockall TA, Logan RF, Devlin HB, Northfield TC. Risk assessment after acute upper gastrointestinal haemorrhage. *Gut* 1996; 38(3): 316-21.

15. Vreeburg EM, Terwee CB, Snel P, *et al.* Validation of the Rockall risk scoring system in upper gastrointestinal bleeding. *Gut* 1999; 44(3): 331-5.

16. National Clinical Guideline Centre (NCGC). Clinical guideline: Methods, evidence and recommendations. Acute upper gastrointestinal bleeding - management. London, UK: National Institute for Health and Clinical Excellence, 2012: 1-285.

17. Pang SH, Ching JYL, Lau JYW, *et al.* Comparing the Blatchford and pre-endoscopic Rockall score in predicting the need for endoscopic therapy in patients with upper GI hemorrhage. *Gastrointest Endosc* 2010; 71(7): 1134-40.

18. Stanley AJ, Dalton HR, Blatchford O, *et al.* Multicentre comparison of the Glasgow Blatchford and Rockall scores in the prediction of clinical end-points after upper gastrointestinal haemorrhage. *Aliment Pharmacol Ther* 2011; 34(4): 470-5.

19. Subramanian V, Hawkey CJ. Assessing bleeds clinically: what's the score? *Lancet* 2009; 373(9657): 5-7.

20. Finfer S, Bellomo R, Boyce N, *et al.* A comparison of albumin and saline for fluid resuscitation in the intensive care unit. *N Engl J Med* 2004; 350(22): 2247-56.

21. Perel P, Roberts I, Ker K. Colloids versus crystalloids for fluid resuscitation in critically ill patients. *Cochrane Database Syst Rev* 2013; 2: CD000567.

22. Annane D. Effects of fluid resuscitation with colloids vs. crystalloids on mortality in critically ill patients presenting with hypovolemic shock. *JAMA* 2013; 310(17): 1809-9.

23. Basili S, Raparelli V, Violi F. The coagulopathy of chronic liver disease: is there a causal relationship with bleeding? Yes. *Eur J Intern Med* 2010; 21(2): 62-4.

24. Tripodi A, Mannucci PM. The coagulopathy of chronic liver disease. *N Engl J Med* 2011; 365(2): 147-56.

25. Jairath V, Rehal S, Logan R, *et al.* Acute variceal haemorrhage in the United Kingdom: patient characteristics, management and outcomes in a nationwide audit. *Dig Liver Dis* 2014; 46(5): 419-26.

26. Bennett C, Klingenberg SL, Langholz E, Gluud LL. Tranexamic acid for upper gastrointestinal bleeding. *Cochrane Database Syst Rev* 2014; 11: CD006640.

27. Manno D, Ker K, Roberts I. How effective is tranexamic acid for acute gastrointestinal bleeding? *Br Med J* 2014; 348: g1421-1.

28. Roberts I, Coats T, Edwards P, *et al.* HALT-IT - tranexamic acid for the treatment of gastrointestinal bleeding: study protocol for a randomised controlled trial. *Trials* 2014; 15(1): 450.

29. Connolly SJ, Ezekowitz MD, Yusuf S, *et al.* Dabigatran versus warfarin in patients with atrial fibrillation. *N Engl J Med* 2009; 361(12): 1139-51.

30. Patel MR, Mahaffey KW, Garg J, *et al.* Rivaroxaban versus warfarin in nonvalvular atrial fibrillation. *N Engl J Med* 2011; 365(10): 883-91.

31. Granger CB, Alexander JH, McMurray JJV, *et al*. Apixaban versus warfarin in patients with atrial fibrillation. *N Engl J Med* 2011; 365(11): 981-92.

32. Desai J, Granger CB, Weitz JI, Aisenberg J. Novel oral anticoagulants in gastroenterology practice. *Gastrointest Endosc* 2013; 78(2): 227-39.

33. Holster IL, Valkhoff VE, Kuipers EJ, Tjwa ETTL. New oral anticoagulants increase risk for gastrointestinal bleeding: a systematic review and meta-analysis. *Gastroenterology* 2013; 145(1): 105-15.

34. Westendorf JB, Pannach S. Increase of gastrointestinal bleeding with new oral anticoagulants: problems of a meta-analysis. *Gastroenterology* 2013; 145(5): 1162-3.

35. Lu G, DeGuzman FR, Hollenbach SJ, *et al*. A specific antidote for reversal of anticoagulation by direct and indirect inhibitors of coagulation factor Xa. *Nat Med* 2013; 19(4): 446-51.

36. Pollack CV, Reilly PA, Eikelboom J, *et al*. Idarucizumab for dabigatran reversal. *N Engl J Med* 2015; 373(6): 511-20.

37. Rivers E, Nguyen B, Havstad S, *et al*. Early goal-directed therapy in the treatment of severe sepsis and septic shock. *N Engl J Med* 2001; 345(19): 1368-77.

38. Jairath V, Kahan BC, Gray A, *et al*. Restrictive versus liberal blood transfusion for acute upper gastrointestinal bleeding (TRIGGER): a pragmatic, open-label, cluster randomised feasibility trial. *Lancet* 2015; 386(9989): 137-44.

39. Stainsby D, MacLennan S, Thomas D, *et al*; British Committee for Standards in Haematology. Guidelines on the management of massive blood loss. *Br J Haematol* 2006; 135(5): 634-41.

40. Stanworth SJ, Brunskill SJ, Hyde CJ, *et al*. Is fresh frozen plasma clinically effective? A systematic review of randomized controlled trials. *Br J Haematol* 2004; 126(1): 139-52.

41. Hickey M, Gatien M, Taljaard M, *et al*. Outcomes of urgent warfarin reversal with frozen plasma versus prothrombin complex concentrate in the emergency department. *Circulation* 2013; 128(4): 360-4.

42. Sreedharan A, Martin J, Leontiadis GI, *et al*. Proton pump inhibitor treatment initiated prior to endoscopic diagnosis in upper gastrointestinal bleeding. *Cochrane Database Syst Rev* 2010; 7: CD005415.

43. Leontiadis GI, Sharma VK, Howden CW. Proton pump inhibitor therapy for peptic ulcer bleeding: Cochrane collaboration meta-analysis of randomized controlled trials. *Mayo Clin Proc* 2007; 82(3): 286-96.

44. Lo EAG, Wilby KJ, Ensom MHH. Use of proton pump inhibitors in the management of gastroesophageal varices: a systematic review. *Ann Pharmacother* 2015; 49(2): 207-19.

45.   Hou M-C, Lin H-C, Liu T-T, *et al.* Antibiotic prophylaxis after endoscopic therapy prevents rebleeding in acute variceal hemorrhage: a randomized trial. *Hepatology* 2004; 39(3): 746-53.

46.   Rajoriya N. Historical overview and review of current day treatment in the management of acute variceal haemorrhage. *World J Gastroenterol* 2014; 20(21): 6481-15.

47.   Tripathi D, Stanley AJ, Hayes PC, *et al.* UK guidelines on the management of variceal haemorrhage in cirrhotic patients. *Gut* 2015; 64(11): 1680-704.

48.   Laine L, Jensen DM. Management of patients with ulcer bleeding. *Am J Gastroenterol* 2012; 107(3): 345-60.

49.   Lim LG, Ho KY, Chan YH, *et al.* Urgent endoscopy is associated with lower mortality in high-risk but not low-risk nonvariceal upper gastrointestinal bleeding. *Endoscopy* 2011; 43(4): 300-6.

Chapter 28

Accommodating patients who are Jehovah's Witnesses and their choice of treatment without blood transfusion

Paul M. Stevenson
Hospital Liaison Committee, Exeter, UK

- "There are some patients who will die without transfusions and there are some that will die because of transfusion." [1]

- "Each patient who is one of Jehovah's Witnesses will make a personal and individual choice."

- "There are no stereotypical Witness patients."

- "Central to avoiding transfusion is a well-planned and multidisciplinary team approach."

- "It is important, where possible, to discuss ahead of time a patient's preferences and decisions."

Background

The term "bloodless medicine and surgery" refers to medical and surgical care performed in such a way that allogeneic blood transfusion is avoided. However, we do understand that the practice of bloodless surgery is not limited to withholding blood transfusion: rather, it involves a comprehensive approach to avoiding allogeneic blood transfusion by optimizing a patient's haemoglobin levels, minimizing blood loss, and tolerating and managing anaemia [2]. This is accomplished in surgical patients by using pharmacological agents, blood conservation devices, and blood management techniques during the pre-operative, intra-operative, and postoperative periods of the care of patients [3] and it also requires a well-planned multidisciplinary approach. Some of the methods in bloodless surgery date back to the 1950s and earlier [4-6]. These approaches are now embraced worldwide by an increasing number of clinicians.

One of the pioneers of bloodless cardiovascular surgery was Dr. Denton Cooley of the Texas Heart Institute in the United States. In 1977, he published a report on his surgical team's 20 years' experience in which bloodless open-heart surgery was safely performed in 542 patients, ranging in age from 1 day to 89 years. Noting the positive outcome and the avoidance of transfusion complications, Cooley's team recommended a broader application of the bloodless techniques [7]. The work of Dr. Cooley and his team provided the impetus for others to develop and refine bloodless surgery techniques. Surgeons in several countries became skilled in providing bloodless open-heart surgery. In Britain we noted the pioneering work of the editors of this book. In the late 1970s and early 1980s, a hospital in California established a program with a dedicated medical and surgical team providing bloodless care to thousands of Jehovah's Witnesses [8].

During the last half century, clinicians have acquired considerably more experience in bloodless medicine, and have produced an abundance of scientific, ethical, and legal documentation in this field. At leading medical centres throughout Europe, including the UK, all manner of medical treatment is being provided to Jehovah's Witnesses without the use of allogeneic blood transfusions with good clinical and economic outcomes [9, 10]. The benefits and cost savings of bloodless medicine — and the avoidance of the hazards, complications, and societal costs of blood transfusions — are being recognised by a growing number of medical professionals [11, 12]. Care without transfusion is also offered to patients who have non-religiously-based objections to blood transfusion and who are not Witnesses. Medical and surgical care is now possible for major surgical and medical procedures including cardiac, orthopaedic, and transplant surgery. In Europe, approximately 50 hospitals have established programmes to provide non-blood medical and surgical care. A surgical team in Ireland with experience using patient blood management strategies stated that "bloodless surgery has come to represent good practice, and in the future, it may well be the accepted standard of care" [13].

In order for the medical community and patients to benefit from the accumulated experience in managing patients without blood transfusion, some centres of excellence have developed blood conservation guidelines and patient blood management protocols[14-17]. It has also been suggested that the subject be included in the curriculum at medical schools and postgraduate centres [18].

The position of Jehovah's Witnesses

Blood transfusion

"Jehovah's Witnesses love and cherish life. They consider it holy, a gift from their God, which needs to be handled with care. . . They consider blood to be as holy as life itself. Jehovah's Witnesses consider friendship with God a precious good and a violation of this relationship by disobedience to Biblical laws a great loss" [19].

The Royal College of Surgeons of England correctly noted that our religious position to abstain from blood is "a deeply-held core value" [20]. As Jehovah's Witnesses, we believe that allogeneic blood transfusion is prohibited by Biblical passages such as the one found in the Acts of the Apostles where first-century Christians were exhorted to "keep abstaining . . . from blood" (Acts 15:29; 21:25). We view this scriptural injunction as ruling out transfusion of whole blood and component transfusion (packed red cells, white blood cells, platelets, and plasma). We also refuse stored autologous blood. These are not transient emotional concerns: our insistence on treatment using transfusion-alternative strategies is our informed choice.

Plasma derivatives

Each patient who is one of Jehovah's Witnesses will, as a matter of personal, individual choice, decide whether he/she wishes to accept plasma derivatives (such as albumin, immunoglobulins, clotting factors, prothrombin complex concentrates and fibrinogen concentrate) as shown in Figure 1. It is therefore important to discuss ahead of time a patient's preferences and decisions. There are no stereotypical Witness patients.

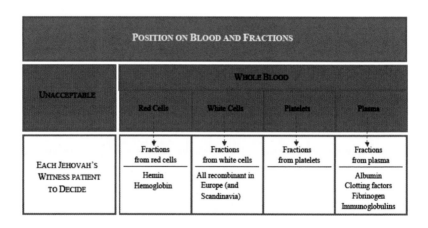

POSITION ON BLOOD AND FRACTIONS				
	WHOLE BLOOD			
UNACCEPTABLE	Red Cells	White Cells	Platelets	Plasma
	↓	↓	↓	↓
EACH JEHOVAH'S WITNESS PATIENT TO DECIDE	Fractions from red cells	Fractions from white cells	Fractions from platelets	Fractions from plasma
	Hemin Hemoglobin	All recombinant in Europe (and Scandinavia)		Albumin Clotting factors Fibrinogen Immunoglobulins

Figure 1. Jehovah's Witnesses and their position on blood and fractions.

Autologous techniques

Jehovah's Witnesses do not accept pre-operative autologous blood donation. Regarding intra-operative and postoperative blood management, each patient makes an informed decision about autologous (autotransfusion) techniques such as haemodilution, blood salvage, heart-lung machine, and haemodialysis (pumps primed with non-blood fluids). The same is true regarding epidural blood patches, plasmapheresis, and autologous platelet gel. (See Figure 2.) The treating team should determine pre-operatively what products or procedures are acceptable to each patient [21].

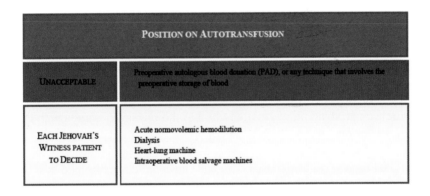

POSITION ON AUTOTRANSFUSION	
UNACCEPTABLE	Preoperative autologous blood donation (PAD), or any technique that involves the preoperative storage of blood
EACH JEHOVAH'S WITNESS PATIENT TO DECIDE	Acute normovolemic hemodilution Dialysis Heart-lung machine Intraoperative blood salvage machines

Figure 2. Jehovah's Witnesses and their position on autotransfusion.

Advance decision documents

As Jehovah's Witnesses, we carry on our person a document complying with the Mental Capacity Act 2005 and directing that no blood transfusions be administered to us under any circumstances. In Britain, a copy of this document is generally lodged with the patient's GP (as recommended by the British Medical Association, BMA) [22]. It is normal practice for doctors to discuss the implications of this directive with each patient prior to elective surgery. In the event of our being rendered unconscious, or in any other circumstances losing competence, it is designed to convey our healthcare choices.

In a recent paper, Wheeler stated: "Adult patients anticipating such a time when they may lack capacity can make arrangements to avoid being given a specified treatment that they choose not to have. This can be done by making an 'advance decision', which is a statutory construct that has evolved from the 'living wills' and 'advance directives' that were created by the common law. The statute that created advance decisions is the Mental Capacity Act 2005" [23].

Seeber and Shander in *Basics of Blood Management* stated: "Healthcare professionals often do not consult with the advance directive or tend to engage in 'soft' paternalism by making decisions that they think are in the best interests of the patient. Nevertheless, advance directives are binding, no matter whether the physician agrees with their content or not" [24].

Clinicians in the United Kingdom (UK) have already respected this legal right for decades, and as Witnesses we have been intensely grateful for their honouring of our fundamental right of bodily self-determination in medical decisions and respecting the principles of patient autonomy and informed choice.

Blood-saving surgical equipment, techniques and strategies

Providing a complete list of transfusion-alternative strategies is beyond the scope of this chapter and are discussed elsewhere in this book. Bloodless surgery is a global concept that includes all available techniques and strategies to avoid exposing a patient to risks of allogeneic blood transfusion. Clinical strategies to avoid blood transfusion have been summarized elsewhere [25-28]. Central to avoiding transfusion is a well-planned and multidisciplinary team approach employing the three key principles mentioned earlier. This can be accomplished by careful planning, judicious use of blood-saving surgical techniques, equipment and devices, pharmaceuticals, haemostatic agents (topical and systemic), arterial embolisation, staging complex surgical procedures, maintaining normovolaemia and normothermia (in most cases), blood micro-sampling for laboratory analysis, and blood salvage, combined and tailored individually to each patient.

Hospital Liaison Committee network: a free resource for healthcare practitioners

In the previous edition of this publication, Virge James and Dorothy Stainsby made the kind (and flattering) observation: "The empowerment of patients has led to many patient organisations and the production of information . . . The most co-ordinated and successful international effort has been that of Jehovah's Witnesses. They produce educational literature and videos of high quality. All are available from their Hospital Liaison Committee network" [29].

We understand that at times our choices can pose a challenge for clinicians who are treating us. In an effort to alleviate this we have established an international network of Hospital Liaison Committees *. Members of these groups are trained to facilitate communication between medical staff and patients who are Jehovah's Witnesses.

The *Handbook of Transfusion Medicine* (2013) stated: "Where appropriate, the patient and clinical team may find it helpful to contact the local Hospital Liaison Committee" [30]. The BMA add: "Lists of centres of excellence in bloodless surgery and of doctors experienced in

---

* To access this arrangement in the United Kingdom, please contact Hospital Information Services, London (Tel: 020 8906 2211; Email: his.gb@jw.org).

working constructively with Jehovah's Witnesses are held by the UK-wide network of Jehovah's Witnesses Hospital Liaison Committees" [31].

My colleagues are available to make presentations, facilitate workshops, and answer questions regarding the treatment of patients who are Jehovah's Witnesses to consultants, doctors, nurses, midwives, and groups studying medicine at all levels. There is no charge for any of these services.

We can share information pertaining to blood conservation techniques and transfusion alternative strategies. We endeavour to maintain a specialised database of relevant medical articles, papers, and abstracts dealing with non-blood management strategies, researched from the world's medical literature. We can put clinicians in touch with specialists (nationally or internationally), many with extensive experience in treating patients who seek alternatives to blood transfusion.

Conclusions

The Bible commands Christians to "abstain. . . from blood", so we do not accept transfusions of whole blood or its primary components. We also do not donate or store our own blood. The Bible obviously does not give specific direction on the subject of derivatives extracted through fractionation, so each of us makes a personal choice whether to accept this. Similarly, each of us makes an informed decision as to whether to accept such autologous procedures as cell salvage, haemodilution, dialysis or plasmapheresis. Most Witnesses carry with them their own Advance Decision to Refuse Specific Medical Treatment document as a record of their personal decisions. The fact that individual patient choices may differ from one Witness to another does not mean that the issue is inconsequential. We appreciate efforts to provide quality medical care, and we weigh carefully the risk/benefit ratio of any treatment. The simple fact is that we "abstain from blood".

Checklist summary

✓ Jehovah's Witnesses absolutely refuse transfusion of both whole blood and such major blood components as red and white blood cells, platelets, and plasma. They also refuse stored autologous blood.

✓ They carry an Advance Decision to Refuse Specified Medical Treatment document with them. This directive is in proper form and is binding.

✓ Judicious use of blood-saving surgical techniques, equipment and devices, pharmaceuticals, haemostatic agents (topical and systemic), arterial embolisation, staging complex surgical procedures, maintaining normovolaemia and normothermia (in most cases), blood micro-sampling for laboratory analysis, and cell salvage, can be combined and tailored individually to each patient.

✓ A network of Hospital Liaison Committees for Jehovah's Witnesses offers a service that is a free resource for the patient and the hospital and is available 24 hours a day.

✓ A protocol for treating Jehovah's Witnesses might include discussion with the patient, treating without allogeneic blood, consulting with other surgeons or transferring the patient to a cooperative hospital before the patient's condition deteriorates.

References

1. Anthes E. Save Blood, Save Lives. *Nature* 2015; 520: 25-6. [Professor Ian Roberts, quoted in].

2. Martyn V, Farmer SL, Wren MN, *et al.* The theory and practice of bloodless surgery. *Transfus Apheresis Sci* 2002; 27: 29-43.

3. Goodnough LT, Shander A, Spence R. Bloodless medicine: clinical care without allogeneic blood transfusion. *Transfusion* 2003; 43: 668-76.

4. Stovner J, Lindell S. Controlled hypotension in prevention of surgical hemorrhage. *Nord Med* 1952; 47: 206-9.

5. Voorhoeve HC, Okker JJ. Bloodless surgery by hypotension. *Ned Tijdschr Geneeskd* 1953; 97: 1348-54.

6.   Burket WC, Ed. *Surgical Papers by William Stewart Halsted*. Baltimore, MD: Johns Hopkins Press, 1924.

7.   Ott DA, Cooley DA. Cardiovascular surgery in Jehovah's Witnesses. Report of 542 operations without blood transfusion. *JAMA* 1977; 238: 1256-8.

8.   Spence RK. Brief history of bloodless medicine and surgery. In: *Transfusion Medicine and Alternatives to Blood Transfusion*. Paris, France: R & J Éditions Médicales, 2000: 23-8.

9.   Gombotz H, Hofmann A. Patient blood management: three pillar strategy to improve outcome through avoidance of allogeneic blood products. *Anaesthesist* 2013; 62: 519-27.

10.   Spahn DR, Theusinger OM, Hofmann A. Patient blood management is a win-win: a wake-up call. *Br J Anaesth* 2012; 108: 889-92.

11.   Isbister JP, Shander A, Spahn DR, *et al*. Adverse blood transfusion outcomes: establishing causation. *Transfus Med Rev* 2011; 25: 89-101.

12.   Shander A, Fink A, Javidroozi M, *et al*; for the International Consensus Conference on Transfusion Outcomes Group. Appropriateness of allogeneic red blood cell transfusion: The International Consensus Conference on Transfusion Outcomes. *Transfus Med Rev* 2011; 25: 232-46.

13.   Adelola OA, Ahmed I, Fenton JE. Management of Jehovah's Witnesses in otolaryngology, head and neck surgery. *Am J Otolaryngol* 2008; 29: 270-8.

14.   Ferraris VA, Brown JR, Despotis GJ, *et al*. 2011 update to the Society of Thoracic Surgeons and the Society of Cardiovascular Anesthesiologists blood conservation clinical practice guidelines. *Ann Thorac Surg* 2011; 91: 944-82.

15.   Leal-Noval SR, Muñoz M, Asuero M, *et al*. Spanish Consensus Statement on alternatives to allogeneic blood transfusion: the 2013 update of the "Seville Document". *Blood Transfus* 2013; 11: 585-610.

16.   Goodnough LT, Maniatis A, Earnshaw P, *et al*. Detection, evaluation, and management of preoperative anaemia in the elective orthopaedic surgical patient: NATA guidelines. *Br J Anaesth* 2011; 106: 13-22.

17.   Muñoz M, García-Erce JA, Villar I, Thomas D. Blood conservation strategies in major orthopaedic surgery: efficacy, safety and European regulations. *Vox Sang* 2009; 96: 1-13.

18.   Thomas JM. The worldwide need for education in nonblood management in obstetrics and gynaecology. *J Soc Obstet Gynaecol Can* 1994; 16: 1483-7.

19.   Seeber P, Shander A. Law, ethics, religion, and blood management. In: *Basics of Blood Management*. UK: John Wiley & Sons Ltd., 2013: 291.

20.   The Royal College of Surgeons of England. Code of Practice for the Surgical Management of Jehovah's Witnesses. London, UK: Council of The Royal College of

Surgeons of England; 2002: §2. Available at: http://www.rcseng.ac.uk/publications/docs/jehovahs_witness.html.

21.   Norfolk D. Management of patients who do not accept transfusion (Appendix 12). In: *Handbook of Transfusion Medicine*, 5th ed. UK: TSO, 2014.

22.   British Medical Association. Advance Statements About Medical Treatment. London, UK: BMJ Publishing Group, 1995; Pt 9.1: 27.

23.   Wheeler R. Adults who refuse blood transfusion in emergency, urgent and elective circumstances. *Ann R Coll Surg Engl* 2014; 96: 568-70.

24.   Seeber P, Shander A. Law, ethics, religion, and blood management. In: *Basics of Blood Management*. UK: John Wiley & Sons Ltd., 2013: 289.

25.   Shander A. Surgery without blood. *Crit Care Med* 2003; 31(12 Suppl): S708-14.

26.   Shander A, Van Aken H, Colomina MJ, *et al*. Patient blood management in Europe. *Br J Anaesth* 2012; 109: 55-68.

27.   Shander A, Moskowitz DM, Javidroozi M. Blood conservation in practice: an overview *Br J Hosp Med* 2009; 70: 16-21.

28.   Gohel MS, Bulbulia RA, Poskitt KR, *et al*. Avoiding blood transfusion in surgical patients (including Jehovah's Witnesses). *Ann R Coll Surg Engl* 2011; 93: 429-31.

29.   James V, Stainsby D. "Regulatory Framework". *A Manual for Blood Conservation*. Shrewsbury, UK: tfm publishing Ltd., 2005: 284.

30.   Norfolk D. Management of patients who do not accept transfusion (Appendix 12). In: *Handbook of Transfusion Medicine*, 5th ed. UK: TSO, 2014.

31.   Medical Ethics Department, BMA. *Medical Ethics Today*, 3rd ed. Chichester, UK: Wiley-Blackwell, 2012: 79.

Chapter 29

Planning and running a study day

Karen Shreeve RN RM MA
Manager, Better Blood Transfusion, Welsh Blood Service, Cardiff, UK
Andrea Harris RGN BSc MSc
Regional Lead, Patient Blood Management, NHS Blood and Transplant, Birmingham, UK

- "If you fail to plan, you plan to fail."
  Benjamin Franklin

- "Individual commitment to a group effort — that is what makes a team work."
  Vince Lombardi

- "Education is the most powerful weapon you can use to change the world."
  Nelson Mandela

- "Organize, don't agonize."
  Nancy Pelosi

- "Feedback is a dish best served hot."
  Mark Engelbos, Checkmarket.com
  Event Marketing: 7 tips to evaluate your event

Background

A well planned, focused study day offers enormous benefit to the attendees, whatever their background or discipline. It will address continuing professional development (CPD), offer new knowledge, reinforce best practice, promote wider thinking and creativity, and facilitate networking. Conversely, a badly planned day will leave the attendees feeling that their precious time has been wasted with no benefit to themselves or their organisation. Additionally, it may bring loss of reputation and standing to the organisers. Therefore, there is every incentive to get it right.

This chapter offers some simple ideas for planning, delivering and evaluating your study day. We begin with planning, which will include assembling your planning team, selecting the venue, identifying the subject matter and content, approaching and briefing your speakers, agreeing the timing and format for the day, and importantly, coordinating your trusted colleagues as the day draws near. These helpers will also be essential on the day itself to ensure its smooth running. This will include organisation of people, resources, equipment, space, and, of course, refreshments. Finally, when the day is over you will need to evaluate and reflect in preparation for the next event. The chapter concludes with a summary for success in the checklist.

Planning the study day

Benjamin Franklin is quoted as saying, "If you fail to plan, you are planning to fail". You may have been tasked by your manager with planning a study day or you may have come up with the idea yourself. Whichever it is, success is reliant upon your actions at the very start in relation to the key elements shown in Figure 1 and expanded in the text that follows.

These steps should serve as a basic guide and may occur in an order other than they appear. Additionally, the list is not exhaustive and there may be other elements that you will include in your planning. Ultimately, the essential element is to have a plan that matches your timescale!

Planning team	•Multidisciplinary •Thinkers and doers
Selecting a venue	•Size and cost •Location and access
Funding the event	•Cost to delegates •Internal and external funding sources
Target audience	•Multidisciplinary or specific •Qualified, non-qualified or mixed
Subject matter	•Aims and objectives •Link to national theme /event /current issues
Format for the day	•'Talk and chalk', interactive or combined •Full day or half a day
Choose speakers	•Experts in field •Inspiring, enthusiastic and willing
Resources needed	•Presentation equipment •Facilitation resources
Refreshments	•Tea, coffee and snacks •Lunchtime buffet
Volunteers	•Immediate colleagues •Wider networks
Publicity	•Posters and flyers, inter/intranet •Booking requests

Figure 1. Key elements in planning a study day.

Assemble the planning team

There are recognisable benefits in working as a team. Belbin's theory identifies the different roles of team members and the benefits to be gained (Table 1) [1].

Table 1. Characteristics of team roles. *Adapted from Belbin.* *(http://www.belbin.com/rte.asp?id=8).*

Role	Benefit
Co-ordinator	• focus on the team's objectives. • draw out team members. • delegate work appropriately.
Shaper	• challenging individuals. • provide drive to keep things moving. • helps retain focus and momentum.
Plant	• highly creative. • good at solving problems in unconventional ways.
Monitor-evaluator	• provides a logical eye. • makes impartial judgements where required. • weighs up options in a dispassionate way.
Implementer	• good for planning a practical, workable strategy. • carries it out as efficiently as possible.
Resource investigator	• avoids isolation and inward-focus. • ensures that the idea will carry to the world outside.
Team worker	• helps the team to gel. • versatile. • able to identify the work required and complete it on behalf of the team.
Finisher	• most effective at the end of a task. • skills to 'polish' and scrutinise the work for errors. • subjects work to the highest standards of quality control.

It may not be possible to include all roles in the planning team but aim for a mix of people in terms of background and skills that will include both 'thinkers' and 'doers'. The benefits of working with others in planning the day will be realised through:

- Enhanced creativity.
- Satisfaction associated with working towards a common aim.
- Mutual support.
- A broader skills set.
- Better productivity than lone working/planning.

(Adapted from Live Recruitment [2].)

Select the venue

You may be lucky enough to work in an organisation that has a suitable educational facility. If not, then there are a number of factors to take into account depending on the format of the day (Table 2).

Make arrangements to visit the venue and the rooms that you will be using. Think about the shape and size of the room(s) and whether they are fit for purpose. For example, will delegates who sit at the back be able to see the screen? Consider what type of audio equipment is available. Microphones are often mounted on a lectern, but this is not always the case; some venues offer lapel microphones while others may only supply handheld microphones. Depending on the size of the room and the number of delegates you may decide that an additional roving microphone (or more than one) is needed for delegate questions or debate.

Check whether the room has temperature control, as there is nothing worse than a room that is too hot or too cold. A cloakroom may be useful, especially if the event is being held in the winter so that delegates don't have to carry round heavy coats.

Table 2. Venue requirements.

Item	Factors to consider
Venue layout	Will you need: • Dedicated area for registration? • Refreshment area? • Single lecture room? • Multiple breakout rooms? • Theatre style or 'round table'? • Area for trade and sponsors? • Any areas that can be combined (or dual purpose)?
Capacity	Will it accommodate: • Number of delegates overall? • Number and size of any simultaneous sessions?
Catering	• Does the venue have a catering facility or will you need to source externally?
Cost	• Is the cost of the venue within budget? • If they offer catering is it included in overall price? • Are there any hidden costs for 'extras', e.g. flip charts and pens, audio and visual equipment? • Is VAT included in the quote?
Access and location	Check as required: • Disability access. • Links to public transport. • Parking facilities. • Proximity to overnight accommodation.
Facilities	Does the venue offer (if required): • Projectors and screens? • Designated IT support? • Flipcharts and pens? • Interactive voting handsets? • Access to internet (in presentations)? • Video conferencing? • Simulation suite? • Delegate Wi-Fi?

Funding the event

With purse strings pulled tighter in both public and privately funded organisations there may be limited resources to finance your study day. Even if you have access to a dedicated education budget you may need to supplement it to provide an attractive event. One way of achieving this is to charge the delegates, another is to look for sponsorship from relevant companies who in return might wish to take the opportunity to showcase their products and engage with the delegates.

Plan in advance what will happen if you fall short of budget — will you cancel the event (in which case how will you inform the delegates) or is there another budget you can fall back on in reserve? Also consider what you will do if you make a profit.

Delegate fees

There is a fine balance in setting the fee for delegate attendance. Set the price too high and you might not fill all places, set it too low and you may be oversubscribed but still not cover your costs. Remember that employers will also have limited study budgets so realistic pricing based on content and the benefits of attending is essential. Take a look on-line at other similar study events to get a feel for pricing structures.

Sponsorship

Be sure to include relevant trade companies and agree a fee for the stand that reflects the benefits to the trade. In return make sure that the trade stands are located close to the delegates at break times and encourage them to visit the trade. A practical way of achieving this is to place trade and refreshments in the same room; this will of course depend on your venue facilities.

Factors to consider include:

- Agree in advance the size of the stand, and how many company personnel will be attending (remember, you will need to include them in catering numbers).

- Do the sponsors need access to Wi-Fi?
- Will they need an electrical point — check your venue can provide sufficient electrical points without the danger of trailing leads.

Find out if you will need to disclose any sponsorship to your employing organisation.

Target audience

It is essential to consider your target audience. In many transfusion study days the attendees will be multidisciplinary as shown in Figure 2.

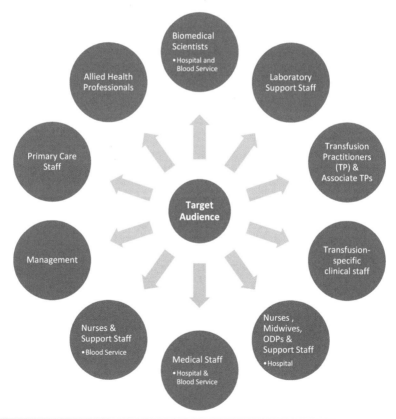

Figure 2. Example of a multidisciplinary audience.

The diversity of the audience will therefore dictate the content and style of the day, so keep this in mind as you plan the programme.

Subject matter: avoid information overload

You and your planning team may have decided upon the target audience before setting the overall theme for the day, or vice versa. There may be a particular initiative, campaign or recently published work that you would like to use as a central theme; new clinical or laboratory guidelines for example. Alternatively, you might wish to address a broader subject area such as blood conservation or a national blood management programme. Whether you plan to focus in detail on a specific topic or wish to look more broadly at a range of issues, do avoid the trap of trying to fit too much into the day.

Consider the key elements and headline messages of your chosen subject. Herein lie your aims and objectives, and therefore your focus for planning. What message do you really want to get across and why? It is impossible to cover everything in one study day so be selective and eliminate random, unrelated pieces of information that someone thinks might be interesting or 'nice to include'. By maintaining focus you will facilitate flow and maintain delegate engagement.

Format for the day

Based on a 1976 publication, the attention span of an adult learner is often quoted as 15-20 minutes [3] with recall being best from the first 10 minutes of any lecture, and reaching its lowest level during the last 10 minutes of the lecture. However, if you watch an audience in front of an exciting film, theatre production or comedian, for example, the attention span is much longer, suggesting that if the topic is of sufficient interest, attention will be held for longer. How then can you be certain that your audience will remain attentive and gain the most from the day?

A review of some of the literature around attention span in lectures suggests that it is important to 'break-up' lectures with periods of active learning [4]. Bearing this in mind, it is advisable that you break the day into manageable segments and using a range of different styles that will include some of the following or other novel methods not listed here:

- Structured lectures.
- Interactive lectures with audience participation.
- Use of video clips.
- Interactive workshops.
- Practical simulation sessions.
- Role play.
- Debate.
- Questions to an expert panel.
- Simultaneous sessions.

Timing	Session	Organiser notes
09:00 – 09:50	Registration and trade stands	
09:50 – 10:00	Welcome and housekeeping	Fire alarms, exits, toilets
10:00 – 10:50	Opening plenary	Two speakers, 20 minutes each with 10 minutes questions at end
10:50 – 11:10	Comfort break and refreshments	
11:10 – 12:00	Simultaneous sessions	A number of simultaneous sessions focusing on different themes
12:00 – 12:45	Debate and discussion	Two debaters
12:45 – 13:45	Lunch break and trade stands	
13:45 – 14:30	Interactive workshops	Solution finding, creative thinking (flip charts, pens, post-it notes)
14:30 – 15:00	Feedback session	Each sub-group presents back to full group
15:00 – 15:30	Final plenary	One speaker with Q&A/discussion time
15:30 – 15:45	Closing remarks	Round-up of day Evaluation forms, certificate of attendance

Figure 3. Example of a multi-method study day.

The day will usually begin with all delegates together following registration but they may be divided into smaller groups for simultaneous sessions as the day progresses, particularly useful for a multidisciplinary audience. Depending on the topic, these sessions may be single lectures, groups of short lectures, interactive discussion groups or practical workshops. Maintain interest by varying the style of sessions but retain a central theme that all can return to later in plenary sessions marking the end of the period or end of the day. Make sure the programme includes sufficient time for audience discussion or 'Questions and Answers', and interspace the sessions with comfort/refreshment breaks as required. An outline example for a multi-method study day is shown in Figure 3.

Speakers, chairpersons and facilitators

Getting the right people to speak increases your chance of running a successful study day. Being an expert in the field does not necessarily equate with being a good speaker so you may wish to approach people on reputation. Your planning team and other colleagues may suggest someone who can not only speak with authority but is also engaging, interesting and entertaining. You will also need capable people to chair each session and facilitate the practical or interactive sessions.

If you personally know your intended speakers, chairpersons and facilitators, you may make an informal approach but there are some key steps in engaging the right people.

Approach the speakers

Follow-up on any verbal approach with an email and/or a letter to confirm dates, times and availability, even if you know the person well. This serves as a prompt to add to their diary and avoid double booking.

Brief the speakers

Provide the speakers with a brief of what you would like them to cover. Supply an explanation of the overall theme and plan for the day that includes topics covered by other speakers or in workshops, and list the key points that you expect each person to cover. This will help avoid duplication and enable your speakers to balance and complement each other's contribution. Inform the speakers when questions and answers are planned, so they accommodate time for this if needed in their presentation. Provide the study day chairperson or facilitators with similar instructions.

Fees and expenses

Ascertain if your speakers require a fee, and calculate any anticipated expenses including travel and the possibility of an overnight stay. This will need to be factored into your overall expenditure.

Speaker biography

Request a short biography from each speaker; a paragraph of 50-100 words is usually sufficient. This can be included in a delegate pack to provide some background on the specialist area of the speaker, and can be used by the chairperson to introduce them.

Resources

You will need to confirm the resources required by the speaker and check on those available at your chosen venue. Be prepared to bring along additional flip charts, pens, post-it notes, etc., according to the type of sessions you have planned. If the venue does not have facilities to display the presentations you will also need to consider if you have access to a laptop and projector. Check if speakers will need access to the internet, if their presentations include any animation or video footage, and aim to have all presentations sent to you at least 1 week before the day so that you can check compatibility with the IT equipment. Inevitably there will be a few late submissions that will need to be loaded and checked on the day!

Prepare the delegate list and delegate pack beforehand to streamline the registration process on the day. The delegate pack will generally contain as a minimum:

- Name badge.
- Programme.
- List of sponsors.
- Certificate of attendance.
- Evaluation form.
- Feedback form.

You may consider retaining the certificate of attendance for delegates to collect as they leave as this deters premature departures!

It is debatable whether or not you should include copies of the presentation slides. This could incur a lot of printing and administration time when compiling the delegate packs, and some speakers would prefer their slides not to be made available in advance. You could instead provide the key learning outcomes, or ask the speakers to summarise the key points or any technical information. Alternatively, just provide some plain paper for delegates to take their own notes.

Refreshments

A full day will usually require up to two refreshment periods and a lunch break, whereas a half day may only require a mid-morning or mid-afternoon refreshment break. Do bear in mind the time allotted for breaks in conjunction with the number of delegates and the number of stations to access refreshments. It is incredibly frustrating to be standing in a long queue to collect your food as the clock moves around towards the start of the next session.

Depending on your start time it is perfectly acceptable to offer refreshments on arrival during registration, then continue through to an earlier lunch followed by an afternoon tea break. Alternatively, provide a late morning coffee break followed by a later lunch, and then continue through to the close of the meeting. It is helpful to base the refreshment and catering stations in the same location as the trade stands so that delegates will mingle, network and visit the sponsors. If possible, arrange with the venue that the sponsors are given lunch prior to the delegates.

Volunteers

In addition to your planning team you may need to find willing volunteers (who may themselves be trusted colleagues and delegates) to assist at registration, troubleshoot on the day and generally help with the smooth running of the event. Timekeepers, runners, microphone handlers and someone to direct the delegates are all incredibly useful, allowing you the space to coordinate and oversee the event. Plan and delegate the roles beforehand so all know what is expected of them.

Publicity and booking

Finally, in relation to planning, get the event publicised. No matter how well planned, it will not succeed without delegates:

- Send out advance flyers in good time to alert and attract potential delegates.
- Follow-up with posters to include additional programme and speaker details.
- Include information on how to book a place, e.g. paper registration form, on-line registration, email.
- Provide instruction on how to make any registration payments (if delegate fees are being charged).
- Request special requirements from delegates with regard to diet and accessibility.
- Provide confirmation of booking and directions to the venue.
- Maintain a database of delegates.

If you intend running simultaneous sessions it is recommended that you ask delegates to indicate their choice of session on the booking form. This is particularly important in terms of the capacity of the breakout rooms and will minimise confusion on the day, although there will always be delegates who change their minds at the last minute.

There may be other specific issues not included here but the information provided above should set out the main ingredients in preparation for the day. The next step is to deliver the study day.

The day itself

You will have checked out the venue, presentations and facilities during the last few weeks leading up to the study day. The venue organisers will have been briefed on layout for the rooms, and your team briefed on their roles. Refreshments and catering will be booked, the trade sponsors agreed and your delegates will of course be looking forward to the day.

Be certain to arrive at the venue in good time for last minute checks or preparation and confirm with the venue hosts if any fire alarm tests are scheduled during the day. Assemble your team and check that everyone knows what they are doing, and what they should do if they become aware of any problems. As the speakers, chairs and facilitators arrive be sure to meet them, offer your thanks for their contribution and check for any unexpected problems. If you've never met them previously and will be unable to recognise them, ensure that your welcome team points them in your direction as soon as they register. For this purpose, a useful tip is to wear something noticeable such as a bright jacket so that you can easily be pointed out.

Registration

Arrange your delegate packs in batches alphabetically and keep a few spare packs for the unexpected arrival whose application form did not arrive in time. If you are charging a delegate fee, consider how you will manage any 'on-the-day' or late payments. Some events ask delegates to 'sign in' but this is not always essential, and if you have large numbers, this can cause a registration backlog, which is not a good start to the day.

Housekeeping

At the start of the event, during the opening address and welcome, there are a number of housekeeping items that you will need to inform your delegates of. This usually includes:

- Any scheduled fire alarms and action to be taken in the event of a fire alarm, plus any other health and safety information relevant to the venue.
- Location of sponsors, refreshment areas and toilets.
- Where smoking is allowed.
- Request that all delegates switch off their mobile phones or turn them to silent. If anyone has to take an essential call, respectfully ask them to leave the room to do so.

Timekeeping

In addition to introducing the speakers, your chairpersons are tasked with keeping speakers to time and managing questions from the audience. If you intend that questions should be offered after each speaker you will need to factor that into the timing. It is sometimes simpler to bring all speakers from one session back to the podium to take questions together. Whichever you decide, the chair should make this clear at the start of the session and limit questions according to available time. If the topic stimulates lengthy debate or more questions than there is time for, the speakers may be prepared to take questions from individuals at the break — but do not suggest this unless you have first confirmed with the speakers. Try to ensure that the speakers can easily see a clock to assist them with their own timekeeping.

Moving the delegates

If you include simultaneous sessions in your study day the delegates will need to move between rooms. Although potentially difficult to coordinate and more time consuming than a single auditorium, the benefits may well outweigh the disadvantages, especially with an audience from diverse backgrounds. Smaller groups are easier to manage allowing for active participation and discussion by its members. While the larger group contains a greater pool of knowledge, fewer members can participate in discussion. Furthermore, simultaneous smaller groups allow exploration of multiple topics that can be shared with the larger group in a feedback session.

To avoid confusion ensure that you have adequate signage around the venue and the programme indicates the particular room for each session. A useful tip is to apply coloured adhesive spots to name badges that will correspond to specific sessions. Helpers and facilitators can then quickly identify the correct session for the individual.

Refreshments and lunch

Allow sufficient time for delegates to eat, drink, stretch, take some air and of course to network with colleagues and the sponsors during the breaks, but not so much time that they become bored. Additionally, it is often counterproductive to provide more than a minimum of seating at lunchtime as delegates will tend to sit back and relax rather than circulate. Ensure that vegetarian food, foods that might cause a reaction (e.g. nut allergy) and special dietary requirements are clearly marked.

Closing remarks

Round off the day with a summary of the key points covered, any particular issues raised during the day and ideas for action when the delegates return to the workplace. Finally, remind delegates to complete their evaluation forms and place in a designated area before leaving and, if not included in their delegate packs, to collect their certificate of attendance.

Evaluating the day

It is essential to evaluate the day, considering all verbal and written feedback from the delegates, speakers, sponsors and your event team. Aim to assemble your planning team and volunteers for a post-meeting debrief as soon as possible after the event. Depending on your event, some key questions should include:

- What went well?
- What was less successful?
- Were there any 'disasters'?
- Were you within budget?
- Was the catering of a good standard?
- Did the venue meet all your requirements?
- Would you use the same venue again and if not, why not?
- How were the speakers rated?
- How was the administration rated?
- Were the sponsors happy?
- What are the lessons learned?
- What changes will you make next time?
- IS THERE a next time?

Finally sit back, pour yourself a cool drink of your choosing and relax — until next time that is!

Conclusions

Planning is essential for a successful study day. You will need to consider a number of practical elements, and having a team can help broaden the skill set, enhance creativity, formulate new ideas and act as a catalyst. If you take the time to plan the event strategically from the very start, communicating with all involved and ensuring that the required facilities are available and within budgetary constraints, the easier it will be to add the finer details. Most importantly, enjoy your day, and celebrate your success!

Checklist summary

✓ Assemble a planning and support team well in advance of your chosen date and use their skills to your best advantage.

✓ Link the day to a current 'hot topic' or seminal publication.

✓ Select a suitable venue that addresses all your needs.

✓ Use speakers who are engaging, informative and knowledgeable about their subject.

✓ Vary the style of sessions during the day to maximise attention and interest.

✓ Be kind to the trade sponsors — you need them as much as they need you.

✓ Reflect and learn from the experience.

✓ Celebrate your success!

References

1.   Belbin Associates. Belbin team roles, December 2014. http://www.belbin.com/rte.asp?id=8.

2.   Live Recruitment. 5 benefits of teamwork for anyone working in events, December 2014. http://www.live-recruitment.co.uk/5-benefits-of-teamwork-for-everyone-working-in-events.

3.   Johnstone AP. Attention breaks in lectures. *Education in Chemistry* 1976; 13: 49-50.

4.   Washington University, St Louis. Are you with me? Measuring student attention in the classroom, May 23rd 2013. The Teaching Center. http://teachingcenter.wustl.edu/Journal/Reviews/Pages/student-attention.aspx#.VKq0UU1yZki.

Chapter 30

Policies and guidelines — how to write them, how to keep up with them

Hannah Grainger BSc (Hons) MSc PGCE (PCET)
Cell Salvage Co-ordinator, Welsh Blood Service, Cardiff, UK
Tony Davies BSc (Hons) MSc CSci FIBMS
Patient Blood Management Practitioner, NHS Blood & Transplant and Serious Hazards of Transfusion scheme, Manchester, UK

- "A guideline must be easy to find, read and follow."

- "A guideline does not replace the need for the practitioner to think!"

- "The best guidelines are produced with input from ALL stakeholders, rather than an individual person or group."

- "Guidelines are consensus opinion of best practice, not the law."

- "Guidelines evolve — so should your practice."

Background

The blood transfusion process has never been more regulated, with rules and guidance arising variously from statutory law, national and international sources, haemovigilance schemes, professional organisations and patient groups, all with the aim of improving the quality, safety and appropriateness of blood component provision.

The European Union produced a series of directives in 2002, 2004 and 2005 [1] in an attempt to increase confidence of member states that the same standards of collection, testing, storage and distribution of blood applied across the Union.

These directives have been transposed into criminal law in the UK as the *Blood Safety and Quality Regulations (BSQR) (SI50, 2005)* [2]. These regulations set out requirements for donor selection, premises, equipment, testing and personnel in order to ensure that the highest standards of quality and safety are met and maintained.

While the BSQR provides the overarching regulatory framework for blood transfusion in the UK, there are a number of other organisations, including the National Institute for Health and Care Excellence (NICE) who provide guidance that may be evidence-based or by consensus of expert opinion, and this will be professionally mandated rather than statutory.

Key aims of policies and guidelines

Quality is a term used at many levels within transfusion, from quality control of reagents and equipment to ensure they are working correctly, through quality assurance to provide confidence that all systems influencing the production of a blood component are working as expected, quality management systems for applying good principles and practices across the transfusion process (Figure 1), to the actual regulations themselves. Guidelines and policies related to these quality systems are aimed at ensuring we can provide:

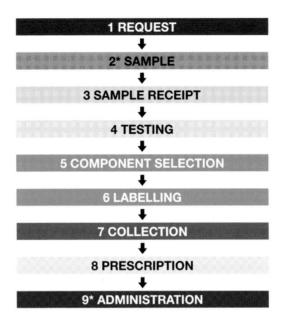

Figure 1. Graphic of critical points in the transfusion process, with the asterisked steps indicating where positive patient identification is vital — guidelines can impact on any one or more than one of these steps. *Reproduced with permission from the 2013 Annual SHOT Report, 2014. Bolton-Maggs PHB (Ed), Poles D, Watt A, Thomas D, on behalf of the Serious Hazards of Transfusion (SHOT) Steering Group.*

- A safe and pleasant experience for blood donors.
- Accurately labelled and tested blood components provided to hospitals.
- Timely, accurate and appropriate transfusion of blood components to patients.
- Minimum standards throughout, from donor to patient.

From a national point of view, there is a safety overview by organisations such as the Advisory Committee on the Safety of Blood Tissues and Organs (SaBTO), who advise the various Departments of Health (NHS England, Welsh Assembly Government, etc) on appropriate measures to take to ensure that the blood supply is as safe and secure as possible. These may include the importation (and pathogen inactivation) of plasma for clinical use for younger patients from areas of the world where variant Creutzfeldt-Jacob disease (vCJD) is of low incidence, the provision of components screened for Cytomegalovirus (CMV) and the most appropriate presentation of platelets (apheresis vs. pooled) in order to minimise the risk of vCJD.

Through the publication of national guidelines, these requirements, reviewed on a regular basis, are built into standards of collection, processing and issue in order to provide a framework to achieve accreditation and used to demonstrate assurance that an organisation is delivering a quality service.

Part of the quality system of any organisation involves consideration of what guidance is available, or needs writing, that will influence the way that organisation provides its services. This guidance can then provide the structures necessary to operate to accredited standards.

One of the most widely used guidelines in the UK is the 'Red Book'; more properly titled *Guidelines for the Blood Transfusion Services in the United Kingdom* [3]. This book (and associated on-line version) is produced by the Joint Professional Advisory Committee for the UK Blood Services (JPAC) who has oversight of definitions, requirements and procedures applied to the Blood Services in England (NHSBT), Wales (WBS), Scotland (SNBTS) and Northern Ireland (NIBTS).

Using standards from the UK regulations as a starting point, the Red Book defines in some detail donor suitability, blood collection, testing, processing, quality assurance limits and storage of every type of blood component made, ensuring that all blood components conform to a strict, and measurable, specification.

This also means that hospitals can be confident in recording in their own operating procedures, and assuring their clinicians exactly what they are giving their patients in terms of, for example, grams of haemoglobin, numbers of platelets and grams of fibrinogen. Within hospital transfusion laboratories there will be any number of guidelines seeking to provide a standardised, consistent and best practice approach to the provision of blood component support for patients.

A good guideline will be structured, easy to follow and applicable to a range of institutions from large teaching trusts to small community hospitals — the principles of good practice apply equally to all.

One of the key organisations for transfusion guidelines production in the UK is the British Committee for Standards in Haematology (BCSH) who produce and review guidance based on audit, consensus opinion and (less so, but increasingly) evidence from research.

Guidance on the specification for a laboratory information technology system (LIMS) and basic serological procedures include requirements for safe and secure blood grouping, antibody testing and compatibility testing. These provide the very basics on which to set up laboratory systems from scratch and have the added advantage that they are taken note of by manufacturers who want to sell equipment (analysers, computers, bar code readers) that will be fit for purpose.

In addition, further guidance, produced in collaboration with obstetricians and midwives as well as transfusion experts, will define how samples are taken and tested during pregnancy, and the principles of administration of anti-D immunoglobulin prophylaxis, allowing multidisciplinary procedural documentation to be produced that can be confidently followed by both the laboratory and the clinical area.

The Royal College of Obstetricians and Gynaecologists is one example of a royal society producing their own good practice guidance under the title 'Green Top', and some of these guidelines will mirror what is written by the BCSH with regard to blood transfusion in general and the frequency of testing and administration of anti-D Ig during pregnancy.

Aside from obstetrics, there is guidance available on the use of red blood cells in critical care, cell salvage, selection of blood components for specific indications, including haemoglobinopathies and neonatal transfusion, the use of plasma components and the provision of blood components in the major haemorrhage setting.

The important thing to remember is that while guidelines are very useful to structure practice and training, there is a temptation to always follow them slavishly without a good understanding of the practice that they are trying to define. It may be that a particular clinical situation requires some thinking 'outside the box' to achieve a good outcome for the patient. Haemovigilance schemes such as SHOT (Serious Hazards of Transfusion) regularly consider cases of delay and poor practice 'waiting for the perfect match' according to guidelines when a suitable alternative may be more readily available, and this is where good training and independent thinking on behalf of healthcare professionals comes to the fore.

How to write them

Regardless of the level at which guidelines and policies are being written, be it national or local, no such document is the output of a solo practitioner. A truly robust guideline is developed by a multidisciplinary group, often with differing opinions, who will challenge the guideline or policy during its development.

Very often a local policy will be based on pre-existing guidelines, turning what may be nationally agreed standards of practice into a document reflective of the practices of the individual organisation.

A good starting point in the development of a policy/guideline is to ask the following questions (Figure 2):

* Why do we need it?
* Where will it be used?
* What is the scope of the policy/guideline?
* Who is going to write it/be involved in its development?
* When is it needed?

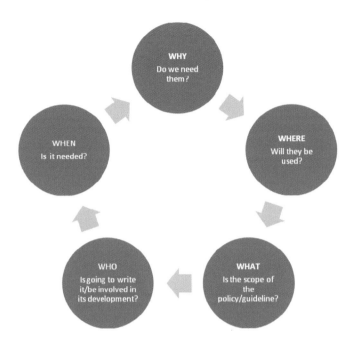

Figure 2. The five Ws of writing a policy or guideline — the important questions to ask.

Why — do we need it?

The answer is probably that there is a need to ensure minimum standards of practice adhered to, which if not met, could result in some form of detrimental outcome. The policy or guideline is an overarching document that outlines standards of practice, but it also needs to be a workable document to allow it to be implemented in all of the affected areas. For example, a statement "all sample tubes must be kept by the telephone where they are easily accessible" may work well for one department, but not for another if the telephone is at the opposite end of the department. A more generalised statement of "all sample tubes must be kept in an easily accessible area" allows affected individuals to adhere to the policy while developing a workable solution for their department.

Where — will it be used?

A policy or guideline may be local, affecting a small group of staff across several departments or the whole organisation, or could be nationally developed guidance affecting an entire industry. In either case, it must never contradict the next level of guidance that sits above it, e.g. a local policy may be written to meet the needs of just one hospital, but it must incorporate and never contradict a national guidance on the same subject.

What — is the scope of the policy/guideline?

The key to writing a good policy or guideline is making it generic enough to be useable by all those affected whilst ensuring it is specific enough that all of the key objectives of the policy can be met without open interpretation. A massive haemorrhage policy is just that — it's a policy about massive haemorrhage, it is not a rewrite of the transfusion policy! It may be that certain aspects of policies will cross over and that it is right for them to do so because of the adverse consequences that could occur if these were overlooked. However, it may equally be as simple to make reference to another document within the new policy or guideline. It is important to clearly define the scope of the policy, not only to guide its development, but to guide the end user as to what the policy does and does not cover.

Who — is going to write it/be involved in the development of the policy/guideline?

Writing by consensus is a challenge but it is also vital to ensure the policy is robust and that it forms a workable document that can be adhered to. While in general the body of the document will be written by one or two individuals, a working group is essential to scope out the contents, challenge assumptions and content, and to review and sign off each stage of the development. The working group should consist of subject matter experts, those responsible for implementing the policy, end users of the policy and in some cases even those who will be impacted on by the policy, e.g. a representative of the Jehovah's Witness community if the policy pertains to managing bloodless surgery.

When — is it needed?

We may all laugh at the joke when someone mutters "we need it yesterday", but strict deadlines are essential when there are numerous individuals involved in a project. The following deadlines may be useful (Figure 3):

- First meeting:
    - outline the scope and general content of the document;
    - allocate responsibilities for developing the document;
    - set a date for the first draft to be completed.
- First draft:
    - send out for feedback by the agreed date;
    - set a date for feedback;
    - set a date for the final draft to be completed (if there are any conflicting opinions, a face to face meeting to discuss these may be necessary).
- Final draft:
    - send out for feedback on any obvious errors or serious concerns over content by the agreed date;
    - set a date for feedback to be received;
    - set a date for sign off to be completed.
- Sign off:
    - either at a face to face meeting or via email obtain agreement by the working group that the document can be put forward for ratification by the appropriate group.

The hardest part of writing a policy is without doubt, getting started. Writing with the support of an expert group means it doesn't have to be perfect first time and a published guideline always begins with a single word.

First Meeting	• Outline the scope and general content of the document • Allocate responsibilities for developing the document • Set a date for the first draft to be completed by
First Draft	• Send out for feedback by the agreed date • Set a date for feedback • Set a date for the final draft to be completed by (if there are any conflicting opinions, a face to face meeting to discuss these may be necessary)
Final Draft	• Send out for feedback on any obvious errors or serious concerns over content by the agreed date • Set a date for feedback to be received • Set a date for sign off to be completed by
Sign Off	• Either at a face to face meeting or via email obtain agreement by the working group that the document can be put forward for ratification by the appropriate group

Figure 3. Key steps in the development of a policy or guideline — adhering to strict time lines is essential in the development of such documents to prevent them becoming out of date before they are published.

So that's it?

Writing the policy or guideline may seem like the difficult part, but in reality implementation can be much harder. Communication is vital, but hopefully, if the right people have been involved in the development, the affected areas should already know that this is coming their way. It may be that these areas will need to adapt their way of working in order to comply with the new policy, therefore advanced notice prior to the issue date is important to ensure readiness for use of the policies. It may be that standard operating procedures will need to be revised or written to take onboard the new guidance and training, and documentation of the latter is vital.

Depending on the scope of the policy and the size of the change to working practice, a period of 'bedding in' time will be necessary. A clear example of allowing time of preparedness was seen with the issue of the UK Health Service Circular *Better Blood Transfusion* (BBT) [4]. Issued in 1998, the directive gave staggered time frames varying from 6 to 18 months for achieving key objectives allowing organisations time to analyse and prepare to implement the required changes to practice.

Once policies are established in practice, it is vital that audit is used to test the effectiveness of the policy and the organisation's adherence to the policy. Results of audit(s) should be published internally and any deviations from the policy that are identified should be escalated to the appropriate group so that corrective action can be taken. Equally, it is just as important that positive results from audit are fed back to the end-users and that good practice is recognised. Local policy change that has resulted in improved practice should be published at local, national and international conferences as appropriate — successes should be celebrated.

You can be fairly certain that at some point after the policy or guideline is issued, something will change to impact upon the policy and a review will then be required. The key is to determine when that review should take place. All policies and guidelines should come with an agreed, definite review date. Where possible, the review should be completed to allow the revised policy to be published as close to the review date as possible, but it should not be done so far in advance that information may already be out of date by the time of publication. It may be that information changes well in advance of the policy review date. The question to ask is how important that information is. Is it critical to patient safety? If the answer is yes, there is no choice than to revise and reissue the policy prior to its anticipated review date. In other cases, the information may not be so important and can be added in the course of the planned review. The decision may lie with the group that developed the policy, or it may lie higher, with those that were responsible for the ratification of the policy, e.g. the hospital transfusion committee.

The effect of the policy or guideline is ongoing and its publication is only the beginning of the change.

Keeping up with the guidelines

Thanks in great part to the *Better Blood Transfusion (BBT)* initiative, the UK has developed a robust transfusion infrastructure over the past 16 years. At a national level, national and regional transfusion-related groups act not only as a source of expertise in the development of policies and guidelines but also as a mechanism through which these policies and guidelines can be fed back to the organisations affected by them. The BBT networks can also act as a central reminder when new or updated versions of guidelines are available, and point practitioners where to look for them, so they do not fall into the trap of relying on paper versions of guidelines that may well be out of date.

This ensures hospitals and blood services remain current and maintain nationally recognised minimum standards of practice. Hospitals should have transfusion/blood management committees and teams in place to act on and disseminate information locally. Regulation of both hospital blood banks and blood services by the Medicines and Healthcare products Regulatory Agency (MHRA) ensures that this national guidance is incorporated into practice to ensure standards are met throughout the UK.

Conclusions

A well-written guideline involves contributions from all stakeholders involved in the process to be described, and provides a framework of best practice based on consensus opinion from experts in the field.

However, guidelines cannot hope to cover every possible scenario that a practitioner will encounter, and thorough training and experience contribute equally to a safe and effective outcome for the patient.

Checklist summary

✓ Ensure the development of guidelines and policies are undertaken by multidisciplinary teams with expert knowledge and representation from those who will feel the impact of the policy.

✓ Ensure guidelines and policies remain up-to-date and are reviewed on a regular basis.

✓ Ensure good communication through relevant networks to raise awareness of new and revised policies and guidelines.

✓ Ensure document training and competency once policies are in use.

References

1.   EU Blood Directives 2002, 2004 and 2005.
2.   The Blood Safety and Quality Regulations (SI 50, 2005) http://www.legislation.gov.uk/uksi/2005/50/contents/made#top.
3.   Guidelines for the Blood Transfusion Services in the United Kingdom, 8th ed, 2013.
4.   UK Health Service Circular *Better Blood Transfusion* (HSC 1998/224).

Further reading

1.   Transfusion practice guidance, including:
  - patient blood management;
  - UK Cell Salvage Action Group;
  - *Handbook of Transfusion Medicine*;
  - the Red Book guidelines for UK BTS;
  - Donor Selection Guidelines;
  - Regulations and Implementation;
  - Regional and National Transfusion Committee resources;
  - Joint United Kingdom (UK) Blood Transfusion and Tissue Transplantation Services Professional Advisory Committee (JPAC) position statements.

  www.transfusionguidelines.org.

2. British Committee for Standards in Haematology: Blood transfusion guidelines. http://www.bcshguidelines.com/4_HAEMATOLOGY_GUIDELINES.html?dtype=Tra nsfusion&dpage=0&sspage=0&ipage=0#gl.

3. Serious Hazards of Transfusion (SHOT) haemovigilance scheme. www.shotuk.org.

4. National Institute for Health and Care Excellence (NICE). https://www.nice.org.uk/guidance.

5. Royal College of Obstetricians and Gynaecologists. Green Top Guidelines. http://www.rcog.org.uk/womens-health/clinical-guidance/.

6. Medicines & Healthcare products Regulatory Agency (MHRA) — Adverse blood reactions and events. http://www.mhra.gov.uk/Safetyinformation/Reportingsafety problems/Blood/index.htm.

7. SaBTO: Advisory Committee on the Safety of Blood, Tissues and Organs. Annual Report 2012 to 2013. https://www.gov.uk/government/publications/sabto-annual-report-2012-to-2013 2013.

8. British Orthopaedic Association Blue Book guidance on blood transfusion. http://www.boa.ac.uk/publications/blue-books/.

9. Blood Transfusion and the Anaesthetist. http://www.aagbi.org/sites/default/files/ bloodtransfusion06.pdf.

10. SaBTO: Advisory Committee on the Safety of Blood, Tissues and Organs. Provision of Cytomegalovirus tested blood components — position statement. http://www.dh.gov.uk/health/2012/03/sabto/.

11. JPAC: Joint UKBTS/HPA Professional Advisory Committee Position Statement on CJD, 12th November 2012. http://www.transfusionguidelines.org/document-library/position-statements/creutzfeldt-jakob-disease.

12. BSQR: Blood Safety and Quality (Amendment) (No.2) Regulations No. 2898, 2005. http://www.legislation.gov.uk/uksi/2005/2898/contents/made.

Appendix I

Steps in the hospital transfusion process

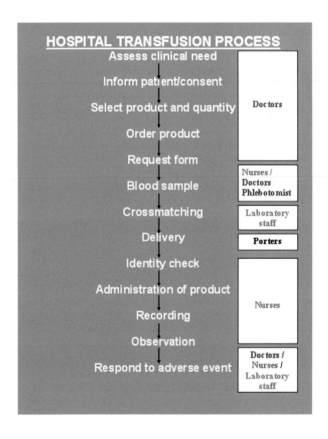

HOSPITAL TRANSFUSION PROCESS

Step	Responsible
Assess clinical need	Doctors
Inform patient/consent	
Select product and quantity	
Order product	
Request form	Nurses / Doctors Phlebotomist
Blood sample	
Crossmatching	Laboratory staff
Delivery	Porters
Identity check	Nurses
Administration of product	
Recording	
Observation	
Respond to adverse event	Doctors / Nurses / Laboratory staff

Appendix II

Safe blood administration

Positive patient identification	Positive patient identification at all stages of the transfusion process is essential. Minimum patient identifiers are:

Positive patient identification at all stages of the transfusion process is essential. Minimum patient identifiers are:

- Last name, first name, date of birth, unique identification number.
- Whenever possible ask patients to state their full name and date of birth. For patients who are unable to identify themselves (paediatric, unconscious, confused or language barrier) seek verification of identity from a parent or carer **at the bedside**. This must exactly match the information on the identity band (or equivalent).
- All paperwork relating to the patient must include, and be identical in every detail, to the minimum patient identifiers on the identity band.

Patient information and consent for transfusion

Where possible, patients (and for children, those with parental responsibility) should have the risks, benefits and alternatives to transfusion explained to them in a timely and understandable manner. Standardised patient information, such as national patient information leaflets, should be used wherever possible.

Pre-transfusion documentation

Minimum dataset in patient's clinical record:

- Reason for transfusion (clinical and laboratory data).
- Summary of information provided to patient (benefits, risks, alternatives) and patient consent.

Prescription (authorisation)

The transfusion 'prescription' must contain the minimum patient identifiers and specify:

- Components to be transfused.
- Date of transfusion.
- Volume/number of units to be transfused and the rate or duration of transfusion.
- Special requirements (e.g. irradiated, CMV negative).

Requests for transfusion

Must include:

- Minimum patient identifiers and gender.
- Diagnosis, any significant comorbidities and reason for transfusion.
- Component required, volume/number of units and special requirements.
- Time and location of transfusion.
- Name and contact number of requester.

Continued

Blood samples for pre-transfusion testing	**All patients being sampled must be positively identified.** • Collection of the blood sample from the patient into the sample tubes and sample labelling must be a continuous, uninterrupted event involving one patient and one trained and competency assessed healthcare worker. • Sample tubes must not be pre-labelled. • The request form should be signed by the person collecting the sample.
Collection and delivery of blood component to clinical area	• Before collection, ensure the patient (and staff) is ready to start transfusion and there is good venous access. • Only trained and competent staff should collect blood from the transfusion laboratory or satellite refrigerator. • Authorised documentation with minimum patient identifiers must be checked against the label on the blood component. • Minimum patient identifiers, date and time of collection and staff member ID must be recorded. • Delivery to clinical area without delay.
Administration to patient	• The final check must be conducted next to the patient by a trained and competent healthcare professional **who also administers the component**. • All patients being transfused must be positively identified. • Minimum patient identifiers on the patient's identity band must exactly match those on the blood component label. • All components must be given through a blood administration set (170-200µm integral mesh filter). • Transfusion should be completed within 4 hours of leaving controlled temperature storage.
Monitoring the patient	Patients should be under regular visual observation and, for every unit transfused, **minimum** monitoring should include: • Pre-transfusion pulse (P), blood pressure (BP), temperature (T) and respiratory rate (RR). • P, BP and T 15 minutes after start of transfusion — if significant change, check RR as well. • If there are any symptoms or signs of a possible reaction — monitor and record P, BP, T and RR and take appropriate action. • Post-transfusion P, BP and T — not more than 60 minutes after transfusion completed. • Inpatients observed over next 24 hours and oupatients advised to report late symptoms (24-hour access to clinical advice).
Completion of transfusion episode	• If further units are prescribed, **repeat the administration/identity check with each unit**. • If no further units are prescribed, remove the blood administration set and ensure all transfusion documentation is completed.

Reproduced with permission from the *Handbook of Transfusion Medicine* [1], adapted from the BCSH guideline on the administration of blood components [2].

1. UK Blood Services. *Handbook of Transfusion Medicine*, 5th ed. Norfolk D, Ed. The Stationery Office, 2013. http://www.transfusionguidelines.org/transfusion-handbook.
2. British Committee for Standards in Haematology (BCSH). Guideline on the administration of blood components, 2009. http://www.bcshguidelines.com.

Appendix III

Summary of the key recommendations of NICE NG24 on blood transfusion

Alternatives to blood transfusion for patients having surgery:

- Offer oral iron before and after surgery to patients with iron deficiency anaemia.
- Offer tranexamic acid when moderate blood loss (>500ml) is anticipated and consider intra-operative cell salvage with tranexamic acid when high-volume blood loss may occur.

Red blood cells:

- Consider a transfusion threshold of 70g/L and a target haemoglobin after transfusion of 70-90g/L. Consider transfusing single units of blood to adults who are not actively bleeding.

Platelets:

- Offer prophylactic platelet transfusions to patients with a count <10 x 10^9/L who are not bleeding, not having operations, and who have not got specified types of thrombocytopenia. Do not routinely transfuse more than a single dose of platelets.

Fresh frozen plasma transfusions:

- Do not offer these to patients who are not bleeding or who need reversal of a vitamin K antagonist.

Continued

Prothrombin complex concentrate transfusions:

- Offer these for emergency reversal of warfarin anticoagulation in patients with severe bleeding or who have a head injury with suspected intracerebral haemorrhage.

Patient information:

- Provide verbal and written information to patients and their families about the reason for transfusion, the risks, the transfusion process, the alternatives and the fact that they are no longer eligible to donate blood.

Summary of UK SaBTO consent for transfusion recommendations, 2011

Clinical recommendations:

- Valid consent for blood transfusion should be obtained and documented in the patient's clinical record by the healthcare professional.
- There should be a modified form of consent for long-term multi-transfused patients, details of which should be explicit in an organisation's consent policy.
- There should be a standardised information resource for clinicians indicating the key issues to be discussed by the healthcare professional when obtaining valid consent from a patient for a blood transfusion (available at: www.transfusionguidelines.org/transfusion-practice/consent-for-blood-transfusion-1).
- There should be a standardised source of information for patients who may receive a transfusion in the UK (leaflets provided by NHS Blood and Transplant (England) are available at: http://hospital.blood.co.uk/patient-services/patient-blood-management/patient-information-leaflets/).
- Patients who have received a blood transfusion and who were not able to give valid consent prior to the transfusion should be provided with information retrospectively.
- SaBTO good practice guidance to help identify the most effective way of providing information retrospectively when patients were unable to give prior consent is available at: www.transfusionguidelines.org/transfusion-practice/consent-for-blood-transfusion-1.

Continued

Educational recommendations:

- UK Blood Services should have an ongoing programme for educating patients and the public about blood transfusion.
- Use of the www.learnbloodtransfusion.org.uk e-learning package should be promoted by the UK Blood Services and Royal Colleges for all staff involved in the blood transfusion process.
- Consent for blood transfusion should be included in the undergraduate curriculum as part of the learning objectives outlined for the principles of consent.

Appendix V

SaBTO guidance for clinical staff to support patient consent for blood transfusion, 2011

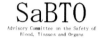

SaBTO
Advisory Committee on the Safety of
Blood, Tissues and Organs

GUIDANCE FOR CLINICAL STAFF

TO SUPPORT PATIENT CONSENT FOR BLOOD TRANSFUSION

Patient may require Blood / Blood Component Transfusion

Patients receiving a blood transfusion (red cells, platelets or plasma) whether for a medical or surgical cause should be informed of the indication for the transfusion including risks, benefits and alternatives. A record of this discussion should be documented in the patient's clinical records.

Ideally the decision to transfuse should be made with the patient or parent/carer in advance of any planned transfusion.

In the emergency setting, the information will need to be given retrospectively.

Prospective Information

Valid consent* should be obtained prior to any planned transfusion and documented in the patient's clinical record.

*Valid consent entails the provision of information on risks, benefits and alternatives available before asking the patient to give consent. This does not have to include a signature from the patient.

Retrospective Information

Patients treated in emergency setting where it was not possible to obtain valid consent pre-transfusion.

Patients who were told pre-procedure (e.g. pre-operatively) that they *might* require a transfusion then need to be informed whether they did/did not receive a transfusion.

Key issues to be discussed when obtaining valid consent

1. The following information should be discussed:
   o Type of blood / blood component
   o Indication for transfusion
   o Benefits of the transfusion
   o Risks of transfusion
   o Possible alternatives to transfusion
   o How the transfusion is administered and the importance of correct patient identification
   o Inform patient that following a blood transfusion they can no longer be a blood donor.
2. Provide written information.
3. Check if patient needs time to consider or requires further information.
4. Document the discussion in the patient's clinical records.

At discharge

1. If patient has had a transfusion, ensure that they have been informed.
2. Record information about the transfusion in the discharge summary, also stating that the patient has been informed.

Appendix VI

SaBTO consent for blood transfusion: retrospective patient information — good practice guidance, 2011

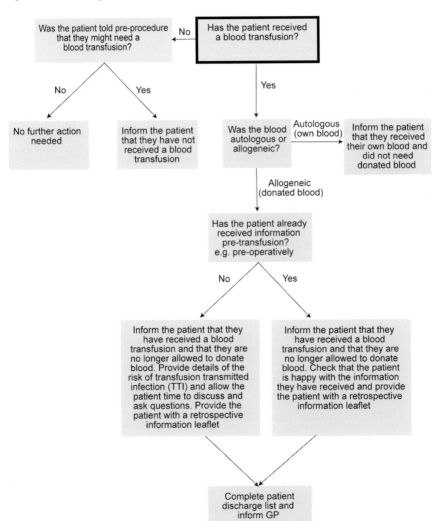

Appendix VII

Assessing a child's competence to give consent and refuse medical treatment

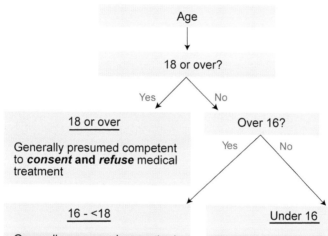

Age
↓
18 or over?

Yes → 18 or over

Generally presumed competent to *consent* and *refuse* medical treatment

No → Over 16?

Yes / No

16 - <18

Generally presumed competent to give *consent* and *refuse*

BUT:

Refusal **may be overridden** by:

• parental responsibility
• the Court

Under 16

Competent to give *consent* if 'Gillick competent'

OR (if not competent)

Obtain consent from **individual with parental responsibility**

Refusal **may be overridden** by:

• parental responsibility
• the Court

Appendix VIII

Pre-operative patient blood management algorithm

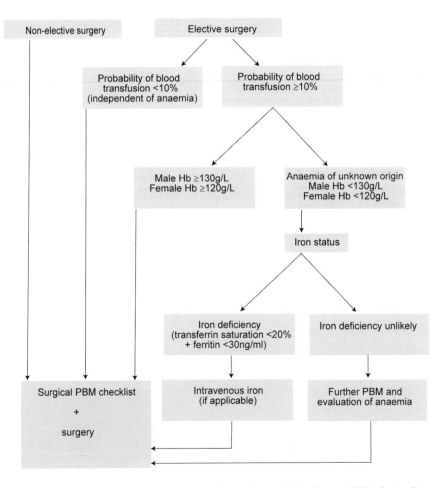

Adapted from Meybohm P, Fischer DP, Geisen C, *et al*; the German PBM Study Core Group. Safety and effectiveness of a patient blood management (PBM) program in surgical patients - the study design for a multi-centre prospective epidemiologic non-inferiority trial. *BMC Health Serv Res* 2014; 14: 576.

Flow chart outlining the management of massive haemorrhage in adults

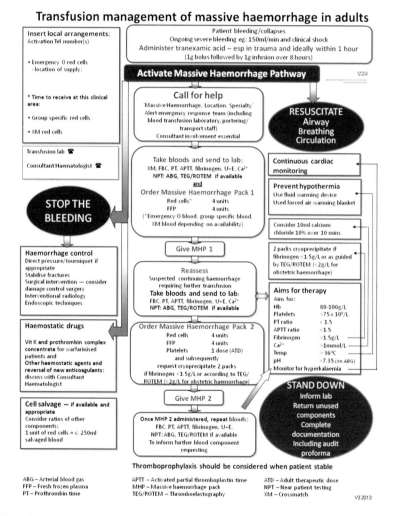

Transfusion management of massive haemorrhage in adults

Insert local arrangements:
Activation Tel number(s)

- Emergency O red cells
  - location of supply:

* Time to receive at this clinical area:

- Group specific red cells

- XM red cells

Transfusion lab ☎

Consultant Haematologist ☎

STOP THE BLEEDING

Haemorrhage control
Direct pressure/tourniquet if appropriate
Stabilise fractures
Surgical intervention — consider damage control surgery
Interventional radiology
Endoscopic techniques

Haemostatic drugs

Vit K and prothrombin complex concentrate for warfarinised patients and
Other haemostatic agents and reversal of new anticoagulants: discuss with Consultant Haematologist

Cell salvage — if available and appropriate
Consider ratios of other components:
1 unit of red cells = c. 250ml salvaged blood

Patient bleeding/collapses
Ongoing severe bleeding eg: 150ml/min and clinical shock
Administer tranexamic acid — esp in trauma and ideally within 1 hour
(1g bolus followed by 1g infusion over 8 hours)

Activate Massive Haemorrhage Pathway

Call for help
'Massive Haemorrhage, Location, Specialty'
Alert emergency response team (including blood transfusion laboratory, portering/transport staff)
Consultant involvement essential

Take bloods and send to lab:
XM, FBC, PT, APTT, fibrinogen, U+E, Ca²⁺
NPT: ABG, TEG/ROTEM if available
and
Order Massive Haemorrhage Pack 1
Red cells*   4 units
FFP   4 units
(*Emergency O blood, group specific blood, XM blood depending on availability)

Give MHP 1

Reassess
Suspected continuing haemorrhage requiring further transfusion
Take bloods and send to lab:
FBC, PT, APTT, fibrinogen, U+E, Ca²⁺
NPT: ABG, TEG/ROTEM if available

Order Massive Haemorrhage Pack 2
Red cells   4 units
FFP   4 units
Platelets   1 dose (ATD)
and subsequently
request cryoprecipitate 2 packs
if fibrinogen <1.5g/L or according to TEG/ROTEM (<2g/L for obstetric haemorrhage)

Give MHP 2

Once MHP 2 administered, repeat bloods:
FBC, PT, APTT, fibrinogen, U+E,
NPT: ABG, TEG/ROTEM if available
To inform further blood component requesting

RESUSCITATE
Airway
Breathing
Circulation

Continuous cardiac monitoring

Prevent hypothermia
Use fluid warming device
Used forced air warming blanket

Consider 10ml calcium chloride 10% over 10 mins

2 packs cryoprecipitate if fibrinogen <1.5g/L or as guided by TEG/ROTEM (<2g/L for obstetric haemorrhage)

Aims for therapy
Aim for:
Hb   80-100g/L
Platelets   >75 x 10⁹/L
PT ratio   <1.5
APTT ratio   <1.5
Fibrinogen   >1.5g/L
Ca²⁺   >1mmol/L
Temp   >36°C
pH   >7.35 (on ABG)
Monitor for hyperkalaemia

STAND DOWN
Inform lab
Return unused components
Complete documentation
Including audit proforma

Thromboprophylaxis should be considered when patient stable

ABG – Arterial blood gas
FFP – Fresh frozen plasma
PT – Prothrombin time

APTT – Activated partial thromboplastin time
MHP – Massive haemorrhage pack
TEG/ROTEM – Thromboelastography

ATD – Adult therapeutic dose
NPT – Near patient testing
XM – Crossmatch

V3 2013

Appendix X

Flow chart outlining the management of massive obstetric haemorrhage

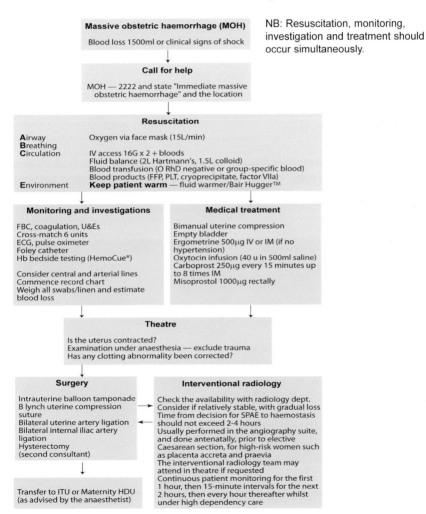

Massive obstetric haemorrhage (MOH)

Blood loss 1500ml or clinical signs of shock

NB: Resuscitation, monitoring, investigation and treatment should occur simultaneously.

Call for help

MOH — 2222 and state "Immediate massive obstetric haemorrhage" and the location

Resuscitation

Airway
Breathing
Circulation   Oxygen via face mask (15L/min)

IV access 16G x 2 + bloods
Fluid balance (2L Hartmann's, 1.5L colloid)
Blood transfusion (O RhD negative or group-specific blood)
Blood products (FFP, PLT, cryoprecipitate, factor VIIa)
Environment   **Keep patient warm** — fluid warmer/Bair Hugger™

Monitoring and investigations

FBC, coagulation, U&Es
Cross-match 6 units
ECG, pulse oximeter
Foley catheter
Hb bedside testing (HemoCue®)

Consider central and arterial lines
Commence record chart
Weigh all swabs/linen and estimate blood loss

Medical treatment

Bimanual uterine compression
Empty bladder
Ergometrine 500µg IV or IM (if no hypertension)
Oxytocin infusion (40 u in 500ml saline)
Carboprost 250µg every 15 minutes up to 8 times IM
Misoprostol 1000µg rectally

Theatre

Is the uterus contracted?
Examination under anaesthesia — exclude trauma
Has any clotting abnormality been corrected?

Surgery

Intrauterine balloon tamponade
B lynch uterine compression suture
Bilateral uterine artery ligation
Bilateral internal iliac artery ligation
Hysterectomy
(second consultant)

Transfer to ITU or Maternity HDU
(as advised by the anaesthetist)

Interventional radiology

Check the availability with radiology dept.
Consider if relatively stable, with gradual loss
Time from decision for SPAE to haemostasis should not exceed 2-4 hours
Usually performed in the angiography suite, and done antenatally, prior to elective Caesarean section, for high-risk women such as placenta accreta and praevia
The interventional radiology team may attend in theatre if requested
Continuous patient monitoring for the first 1 hour, then 15-minute intervals for the next 2 hours, then every hour thereafter whilst under high dependency care

Appendix XI

Intra-operative cell salvage machines

The following list is not exhaustive. As space is limited we could not list all manufacturers. Companies are listed in alphabetical order:

Advancis Surgical, Nottingham, UK
http://www.advancissurgical.com
Hemosep® cell salvage device (Figure 1)
© Brightwake Ltd, 2016

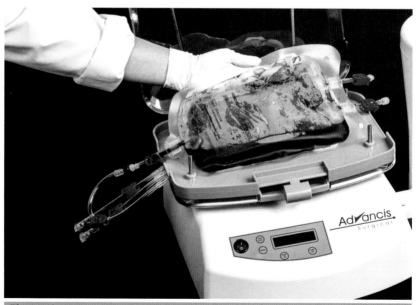

Figure 1. Hemosep® cell salvage device. *Reproduced with permission from Brightwake Ltd (trading as Advancis Surgical). © Brightwake Ltd, 2016.*

Fresenius Kabi AG, Homburg, Germany
https://www.fresenius-kabi.com
C.A.T.S.® Plus autotransfusion system (Figure 2)
© Fresenius Kabi AG, 2016

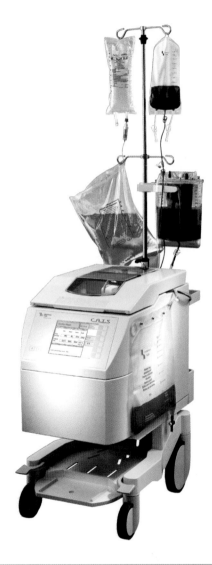

Figure 2. C.A.T.S.® Plus autotransfusion system. *Reproduced with permission from Fresenius Kabi AG. © Fresenius Kabi AG, 2016.*

Haemonetics Corporation, Braintree MA, USA

http://www.haemonetics.com

Cell Saver® Elite® autotransfusion system (Figure 3)
Cell Saver® 5+ autologous blood recovery system (Figure 4)
cardioPAT® autotransfusion system (Figure 5)
© Haemonetics Corporation, 2016

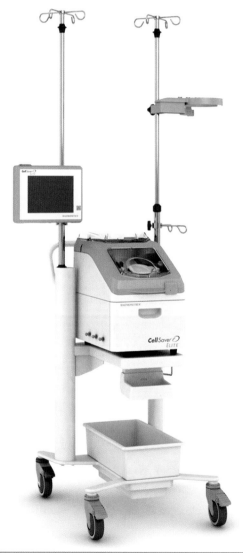

Figure 3. Cell Saver® Elite® autotransfusion system. *Reproduced with permission from Haemonetics Corporation. © Haemonetics Corporation, 2016.*

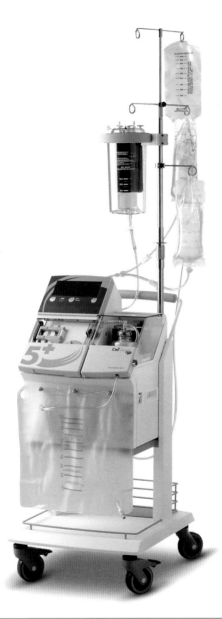

Figure 4. Cell Saver® 5+ autologous blood recovery system. *Reproduced with permission from Haemonetics Corporation. © Haemonetics Corporation, 2016.*

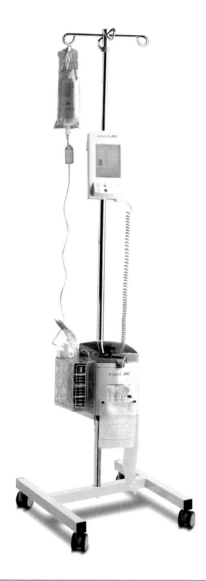

Figure 5. cardioPAT® autotransfusion system. *Reproduced with permission from Haemonetics Corporation. © Haemonetics Corporation, 2016.*

LivaNova PLC, London, UK
http://www.livanova.sorin.com
LivaNova XTRA® autotransfusion system (Figure 6)
Electa® autotransfusion system
Cobe Brat 2® cell saver
© LivaNova PLC, 2016

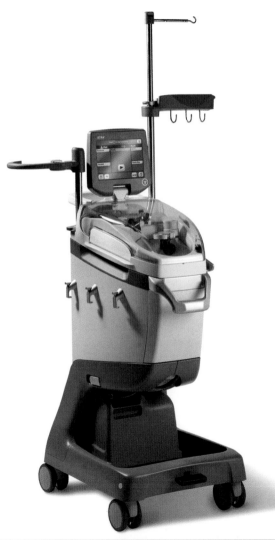

Figure 6. LivaNova XTRA™ autotransfusion system. *Reproduced with permission from LivaNova PLC. © LivaNova PLC, 2016.*

Medtronic Inc., Minneapolis, Minnesota, USA

http://www.medtronic.com
autoLog® autotransfusion system (Figure 7)
© Medtronic Inc., 2016

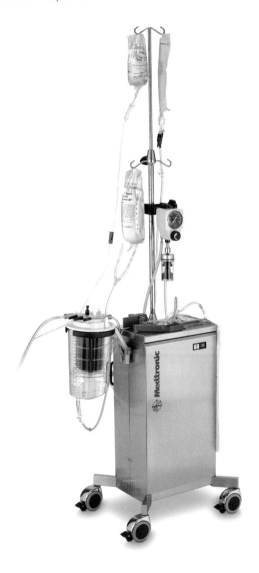

Figure 7. autoLog® autotransfusion system. *Reproduced with permission from Medtronic Inc. © Medtronic Inc., 2016.*

Terumo BCT, Inc., Lakewood, CO, USA
https://www.terumobct.com
COBE® 2991 autotransfusion system (Figure 8)
© Terumo BCT, Inc., 2016

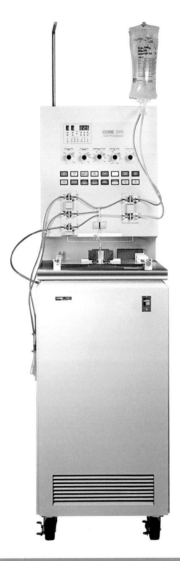

Figure 8. COBE® 2991 autotransfusion system. *Reproduced with permission from Terumo BCT, Inc. © Terumo BCT, Inc.*

Appendix XII

Useful contacts and information

American Association of Blood Banks
http://www.aabb.org

American Association of Nurse Anesthetists
http://www.aana.com

American Society of Anesthesiologists (ASA)
https://www.asahq.org

American Society of Hematology
http://www.hematology.org

Asian Society for Patient Blood Management (ASPMB)
http://www.ASPBM.net

Association of Anaesthetists of Great Britain and Ireland (AAGBI)
http://www.aagbi.org

Association of Cardiothoracic Anaesthetists
http://www.acta.org.uk

Association of Clinical Scientists
http://www.assclinsci.org

Australian National Blood Authority
http://www.blood.gov.au/ics

Australian Transfusion Safety Program
http://www.health.vic.gov.au/best

Better Blood Transfusion
www.betterblood.org.uk

Better Blood Transfusion 1 (Department of Health HSC 1998/224)
http://www.transfusionguidelines.org.uk/uk-transfusion-
committees/national-blood-transfusion-committee/better-blood-
transfusion

Better Blood Transfusion 3 (Department of Health — Health Service
Circular 2007/001)
http://www.dh.gov.uk/prod_consum_dh/groups/dh_digitalassets/docume
nts/digitalasset/dh_080803.pdf

Blood Safety and Quality Regulations (BSQR)
http://www.legislation.gov.uk/uksi/2005/50/contents/made#top

Blood Stock Management Scheme
http://www.bloodstocks.co.uk

British Blood Transfusion Society
http://www.bbts.org.uk

British Committee for Standards in Haematology Guidelines (BCSH)
http://www.bcshguidelines.com

British Medical Association
http://www.bma.org.uk

British Orthopaedic Association
http://www.boa.ac.uk

Californian Blood Bank Society
http://www.cbbsweb.org

Canadian Blood Services
https://www.blood.ca

Confidential Enquiry into Maternal and Child Health (CEMACH)
Healthcare Quality Improvement Partnership Ltd.
http://www.hqip.org.uk

European Association of Cardiothoracic Anaesthesiologists
http://www.eacta.org

European Directorate for the Quality of Medicines and Healthcare
https://www.edqm.eu/en

European Haematology Association (EHA)
http://www.ehaweb.org

European Society for Blood & Bone Marrow Transplant
https://www.ebmt.org

General Medical Council
http://www.gmc-uk.org

Give Blood
https://www.blood.co.uk

Haemophilia Society
http://www.haemophilia.org.uk

Health and Care Professionals Council (HCPC)
http://www.hpc-uk.org

Health Protection Agency - Centre for Infections
http://www.hpa.org.uk/infections

Institute of Biomedical Science
http://www.ibms.org

International Society of Blood Transfusion (ISBT)
http://www.isbtweb.org

International Society of Hematology
http://www.ishworld.org

Jehovah's Witnesses
https://www.jw.org/en

Joint United Kingdom (UK) Blood Transfusion and Tissue Transplantation Services Professional Advisory Committee
http://www.transfusionguidelines.org

Korean Research Society of Transfusion Alternatives (KRSTA)
http://www.krsta.org

Learnbloodtransfusion - interactive eLearning resource developed by the Better Blood Transfusion Continuing Education Programme
http://www.learnbloodtransfusion.org.uk

Medicines and Healthcare products Regulatory Agency (MHRA)
http://www.mhra.gov.uk

National Association of Phlebotomists
http://www.phlebotomy.org

National Blood Service
http://www.blood.co.uk

National Blood Transfusion Committee (NBTC)
http://www.transfusionguidelines.org.uk/uk-transfusion-committees/national-blood-transfusion-committee

National Comparative Audit of Blood Transfusion
http://hospital.blood.co.uk/audits/national-comparative-audit

National Institute for Biological Standards and Control
http://www.nibsc.ac.uk

National Institute for Health and Care Excellence (NICE)
http://www.nice.org.uk

National Patient Safety Agency (NPSA)
http://www.npsa.nhs.uk

Network for the Advancement of Patient Blood Management, Haemostasis and Thrombosis (NATA)
http://www.nataonline.com

NHS Blood and Transplant
http://www.nhsbt.nhs.uk

NoBlood Inc.
http://noblood.org

Northern Ireland Blood Transfusion Service
http://www.nibts.org

Nursing and Midwifery Council
http://www.nmc-uk.org

Obstetric Anaesthetists' Association (OAA)
http://www.oaa-anaes.ac.uk

Royal College of Anaesthetists
http://www.rcoa.ac.uk

Royal College of Nursing
http://www.rcn.org.uk

Royal College of Obstetricians and Gynaecologists
http://www.rcog.org.uk

Royal College of Pathologists
http://www.rcpath.org

The Royal College of Surgeons of England
http://www.rcseng.ac.uk

Safety of Blood, Tissues and Organs (SaBTO)
https://www.gov.uk/government/groups/advisory-committee-on-the-safety-of-blood-tissues-and-organs

Scottish Intercollegiate Guidelines Network (SIGN)
http://www.sign.ac.uk

Scottish National Blood Transfusion Service
http://www.scotblood.co.uk

Serious Hazards of Transfusion (SHOT)
http://www.shotuk.org

Society for the Advancement of Blood Management, Inc.
http://www.sabm.org

Society of Cardiothoracic Surgeons of Great Britain and Ireland
http://www.scts.org

Society of Clinical Perfusion Scientists of Great Britain and Ireland
http://www.sopgbi.org

Transfusion Evidence Library
http://www.transfusionevidencelibrary.com

Transfusion News
http://transfusionnews.com

Transfusion practice guidance
www.transfusionguidelines.org

UK Blood Services
https://www.blood.co.uk

UK Cell Savage Action Group
http://www.transfusionguidelines.org.uk

UK National External Quality Assessment Service (NEQAS)
http://www.ukneqas.org.uk

Welsh Blood Service
http://www.welsh-blood.org.uk

World Health Organisation
http://www.who.int/en

Index